Noninvasive Imaging of Congenital Heart Disease

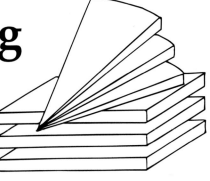

Before and After Surgical Reconstruction

by

Alvin J. Chin, MD

Director
Non-Invasive Laboratories
Children's Hospital of Philadelphia;
Associate Professor of Pediatrics
University of Pennsylvania School of Medicine
Philadelphia, Pennsylvania

with contributions by

Mark A. Fogel, MD

Assistant Professor of Pediatrics
University of Pennsylvania School of Medicine
Philadelphia, Pennsylvania

**Futura Publishing
Company, Inc.**
Armonk, NY

Library of Congress Cataloging-in-Publication Data

Chin, Alvin J.
  Noninvasive imaging of congenital heart disease: before and after
surgical reconstruction / by Alvin J. Chin: with contributions by
Mark A. Fogel.
     p.   cm.
  Includes bibliographical references and index.
  ISBN 0-87993-574-X
  1. Congenital heart disease—Imaging. 2. Congenital heart
disease—Surgery. I. Fogel, Mark A. II. Title.
  [DNLM: 1. Heart Defects, Congenital—diagnosis. 2. Diagnostic
Imaging—methods. 3. Heart Defects, Congenital—surgery. WG 220
C539n 1994]
  RC687.C48 1994
  616.1'2043—dc20   93-39613
                                                          CIP

Copyright 1994
Futura Publishing Company, Inc.

Published by
Futura Publishing Company, Inc.
135 Bedford Road
Armonk, NY 10504-0418

LC #: 93-39613
ISBN #: 0-87993-574-X

Every effort has been made to ensure that the information in this book is as up to date and as accurate as possible at the time of publication. However, due to the constant developments in medicine, neither the author, nor the editor, nor the publisher can accept any legal or any other responsibility for any errors or omissions that may occur.

Printed in the United States of America on acid-free paper.

To my wife
    Catherine Norton Marchand

    and

To my daughters
    Fiona and Meredith

Preface

The last 10 years have seen an explosion of uses for ultrasound in the identification and management of congenital heart disease. Two developments in particular have revolutionized the application of ultrasound: the popularization of the subcostal window as the starting window of choice in the newborn and the development of Doppler color flow mapping instrumentation. These advances have allowed cardiologists to noninvasively obtain *both* anatomy and physiology, the combination of which had hitherto been obtainable only by catheterization.

The purpose of the book is to outline how cardiac ultrasound can be utilized to diagnose even the most complex congenital malformations preoperatively and how both anatomy and physiology can be assessed after surgical reconstruction. Areas that are not covered in detail are systolic and diastolic ventricular function assessment, the use of transesophageal windows, and the use of ultrasound in studying cardiovascular development. These will be the subject of a future work. The chapters are organized in "segmental" fashion, drawing on the van Praagh classification scheme. Chapter 4 of Part I is a brief description of the salient features of van Praagh's nomenclature system that relate to echocardiographic imaging.

Preoperative (Part I) and postoperative (Part II) sections of the book are each concluded with chapters on magnetic resonance (MR) imaging by Mark A. Fogel. The state of MR imaging in 1993 is roughly analogous to the state of ultrasound imaging in 1983; clinical uses of MR overwhelmingly focus on display of morphology rather than hemodynamics.

The book is aimed primarily at cardiology fellows and cardiovascular technologists in training; however, cardiac surgeons, anesthesiologists, neonatologists, radiologists, and invasive cardiologists may find it useful as well. Cardiologists who treat adults with congenital heart disease may especially benefit from Part II.

Acknowledgments

The teaching of John P. Owens and John D. Murphy piqued my interest in congenital heart disease. During my cardiology fellowship, Roberta G. Williams encouraged me to utilize cardiac ultrasound as a tool to help in post-operative management. I am grateful to the late William J. Rashkind for offering me the opportunity to develop a noninvasive imaging center. William I. Norwood has been an inspiration for much of the center's clinical research.

I would like to recognize the help and support of the many physicians and technologists who have worked in the Non-Invasive Laboratories at Children's Hospital, Philadelphia since 1985. In particular, Beth Ann Aglira Andrews, BHS, RCVT, Audrey Alston Jones, CCPT, and Jane M. Vetter, RCVT, have played a crucial role in maintaining quality control, systematically teaching trainees, and participating in clinical investigations.

Burton Tabakin, Nathaniel Reichek, and Peter Lang helped me with many thoughtful discussions. The opportunity to work with superb cardiac pathologists and surgeons simultaneously during my years of formal training fostered the formulation of many subsequent applications of ultrasound. I have especially appreciated the mentorship of Aldo R. Castañeda and William F. Friedman.

Finally, the book would not have come to fruition without the editorial supervision of Steven Korn and Linda Shaw and the secretarial assistance of Kimberly Persick.

Contents

Part II: Imaging of the Postoperative Patient

Part I

Imaging of the Preoperative Patient

Chapter 1

Instrumentation

The instrumentation involved in echocardiography has evolved rapidly in the past decade to include a variety of Doppler techniques. A brief summary of the basic principles follows. The reader is referred to several other texts[1-3] for a more detailed discussion.

Ultrasound frequencies in clinical use range from 2.0 to 30.0 MHz, i.e., 2 million to 30 million cycles per second. Ultrasound beams obey the laws of reflection and refraction. As the beam travels through a homogeneous medium, there is neither reflection nor refraction. When it strikes an "object" (acoustic interface), part of the energy is reflected and part is refracted. Because many of the objects or targets are irregular in shape and reflect sound in multiple directions, only a small amount of transmitted energy actually returns to the transducer. The size of the object relative to the incident wavelength (reciprocally related to frequency) determines whether the beam is reflected from the object. A higher frequency beam (i.e., shorter wavelength) has a greater ability to resolve or distinguish objects that are close to each other; however, because so much energy is reflected by small objects (interfaces), less energy penetrates to "deeper," i.e., more distant objects. Thus, although the acoustic impedance of the medium affects penetration, the transmitted frequency also has a profound effect. Soft tissue, bone, and air (contained in lung) all "attenuate" ultrasound. Prosthetic valves produce "shadows." The electric signal generated by the reflected echo is displayed as a certain distance from the origin of the beam. How well motion of the target is visualized depends on the pulse repetition frequency.

Beam production is affected by several factors including the particular piezo-electric material, the number of crystals, and the diameter of the elements. Essentially two approaches dominated the early 1980s: use of a single large element or multiple small elements. (The former was used in mechanical scanners with oscillating transducers, the latter in electronic scanners with phased array transducers.)

To create a "sector" with an oscillating transducer, the active element is physically moved through a given arc. To create a sector with a phased array transducer, the beam is directed by changing the sequence of the firing of individual elements. In modern scanners, this is controlled by a computer.

An advantage of the single large element was a reduced problem with side lobes, extraneous beams of ultrasound generated from the edges of piezo-electric elements. Since the receiver does not know the location of the side lobes, any echoes returned from objects struck by side lobes will be displayed as if they were generated by the main beam.

The principal advantage of phased array systems[4,5] is that multiple types of ultrasound information can be acquired *simultaneously*, rather than sequentially. The addition of Doppler techniques thus made the phased array approach virtually mandatory. For example, continuous wave Doppler requires two transducers: one to transmit and one to receive. Although this is straightforward for a phased array system, it is harder to implement in a mechanical system.

As the beam propagates, it begins to diverge after a certain depth; this is why better images are produced when objects are in the near field. This distance till divergence is shorter with small diameter elements. To increase the distance before beam divergence, one can increase the acting element diameter or increase the transmitted frequency.

Attempts to alter the far field center on focusing (either by physically modifying the transducer or by electronic means). In the single large element approach, this can be achieved by interposing an acoustic lens. In the multiple small element approach, including its variant (annular phased array), the wave front can be shaped by changing the firing sequence (e.g., firing the outside elements first). If one considers the beam to be formed by areas of "constructive interference" among multiple spherical wavelets, then the shape of the beam will depend on the time of origin of each wavelet. An advantage of electronic focusing is that the focal zone can be rapidly changed. The *focal zone* is where the beam is narrowest. The three-dimensional shape in the single large element approach is cylindrical and in the multiple small element approach it is essentially a rectangular solid. Amplitude also affects *beam width,* usually drawn as the half-value limit of the beam plot.

Resolution is determined by several variables: transmitted frequency, beam width, and amplitude. Beam width is the most important determinant of lateral resolution (perpendicular to the direction of the ultrasound beam). The narrower the beam width, the better the lateral resolution. Transducer frequency is the most important determinant of axial resolution (parallel to the direction of the beam).

Although the variables mentioned so far are largely outside the operator's control, variables that can be manipulated by the operator are: depth, line density, sector angle (or arc), pulse repetition frequency, and frame rate.

Finally, in the early 1980s, Doppler echocardiography began to take on increasing importance. The Doppler effect was first described in the 1840s. If the source of a transmitted wave is stationary, then the wavelength (or its reciprocal, frequency) is constant. If the source is moving toward the receiver, the wavelength decreases (the frequency increases). The reverse occurs if the source is moving away from the receiver.

$$\text{If } f_d = f_r - f_t, \text{ then } v = f_d \cdot C_s / 2\, f_t \cos \theta$$

where v = velocity; f_d = Doppler shift frequency; f_r = received frequency; f_t = transmitted frequency; C_s = velocity of sound; θ = angle between the beam and the path of the target.

Since $\cos \theta$ only deviates significantly from 1 at $\theta > 20°$, the optimal way to obtain velocity information is by keeping the beam parallel to the moving target. (Note that this is the opposite of what is best for two-dimensional imaging.) It is fortunate that typical values of f_d lie within the audible range; thus, the operator can hear it as the exam is being performed.

The major advance in Doppler technology was the development of pulsed Doppler as a means of range definition. By gating, one can determine the velocity of a target at a specified depth. There is, however, a limit to the velocities that can be measured with pulsed Doppler. The pulse repetition frequency limits the maximal velocity which can be detected to $C_s^2/8f_tR$ where R = range, or depth. The upper limit of f_d that can be detected unambiguously is $\frac{1}{2}$ the pulse repetition frequency. Velocities that exceed this Nyquist limit

(i.e., alias) are displayed as "wrap around." To circumvent this limit, continuous wave Doppler must be utilized to characterize maximal velocity, once pulsed Doppler has identified that there is high-velocity *turbulent* flow in a given anatomical location. (Flow is laminar when the spatial velocity gradient is smooth and continuous and the streamlines are linear and aligned.[2])

In adults, there is usually only one area of disturbed flow in any patient; therefore, to complete a physiological assessment with pulsed and continuous wave Doppler is rarely tedious. In infants with congenital heart defects, however, as many as 10 areas of disturbed flow can coexist. With the advent of color flow mapping instruments, the entire heart, great arteries, and large veins could be screened rapidly for regions of physiological interest. More precise characterization could then be carried out with pulsed Doppler and finally with continuous wave Doppler. In the postoperative patient, color flow mapping is especially valuable as a means of detecting jets with unusual trajectories, e.g., at the perimeter of surgically placed patches. Indeed, full hemodynamic analysis on a routine basis in the postoperative patient would probably be impractical without color flow mapping.

The principles of Doppler color flow imaging have been reviewed in several recent publications.[3,6] Only a short summary will be given here. The entire sector arc is comprised of several hundred lines of information. Each frame is updated every $\frac{1}{30}$ second. Lines of color flow data are alternated with lines of anatomical scan data. Because of time limitations, all color flow systems are multigated. The gates are characterized by the time it takes for a pulse to hit the target and return to the receiver.

Color has been used to display direction and velocity. By convention, red indicates flow toward the transducer, and blue indicates flow away. (This is counter to the convention in astronomy.) Rather than saturation or brightness, hue (the primary sensation of color) has been selected to indicate velocity. Which velocity is displayed? At each gate (spatial location), only one color is displayed—that which represents the *mean* velocity in that gate. Thus, the examiner should remember that Doppler color flow mapping is only a screening tool and cannot be used to quantitate the gradient across turbulent flow regions. It guides the examiner to sites that must be interrogated in more detail by pulsed and continuous wave Doppler technique.

To understand how to improve estimates of mean velocity, remember that, in addition to transmitted frequency, pulse repetition frequency and "packet size" can be altered. Pulse repetition frequency is the number of pulse "trains" per second. Packet size is the number of pulse trains emitted before the system moves on to the next line. Between 3 and 16 pulse trains can be used. To increase pulse repetition frequency, one must decrease the distance to the target. The more pulse trains, the better the estimate of mean velocity.

Present color flow systems automatically readjust frame rate and line density once the operator selects sector angle and depth (distance to target). The important principle to remember is that tradeoffs are constantly being made between accurate velocity estimation, frame rate, sector angle, depth, and line density. Because of the high heart rates in pediatric patients, high frame rate is especially important; line density is probably the second most important aspect to the clinician. Given these constraints, depth and sector angle should be minimized by the operator.

Aliasing occurs just as with conventional pulsed Doppler. It can be reduced by using lower frequency transducers. The color display in a red-toward mapping schema progressively increases hue until the aliasing point is reached at which there is reversal of color. The *brightest* hues of red and blue are adjacent at the aliasing point. In pediatric patients, aliasing is a significant problem. The greatest utility of Doppler color flow mapping is as a surveillance tool that can interrogate many chambers and valves simultaneously; thus, it is necessary to minimize aliasing lest normal flow strikes the operator's eye as abnormal. Low-frequency transducers should thus be used after anatomical display (with high-frequency transducers) is completed. Distance to the target region should also be reduced by the operator whenever possible. Although aliasing is the predominant clue that "high-velocity" flow exists, color flow systems also have another feature that may alert the operator to the presence of turbulent flow. Although only mean velocity is estimated (and thus a

high peak velocity cannot be quantitated), spectral broadening is displayed by variance mapping. A third color, sometimes green, is added to a standard velocity-only red-blue map. Flow toward the transducer with turbulence results in yellow display. Flow away from the transducer with turbulence results in a cyan color.

Since alternative maps have been used with a *dark red-orange to yellow* spectrum for forward flow and *blue-purple to light blue* spectrum for backward flow, a variance display in green can only be used with the standard red-blue map.

With so many advances in instrumentation in the last decade, what improvements remain to be made? Certainly the major disadvantage of phased array systems is their bulkiness. Portable systems may yet be possible with the miniaturization of powerful microprocessors. Another improvement would be systems capable of speech recognition; these would be advantageous in the intensive care unit or operating unit where patients and beds are tethered to a variety of support equipment making simultaneous manual manipulation of the transducer and the machine controls awkward.

Future software improvements may permit three-dimensional displays of morphology and flow mapping. Several limitations have retarded progress so far. First, the frame rates have necessitated huge storage capacity, at prohibitive cost. Second, automatic border detection is more difficult than in either computed tomography or magnetic resonance scanning. Third, reconstruction algorithms have traditionally employed parallel slice acquisition, which is impractical from surface windows in the infant. The new Omni-plane probe should allow rotational imaging protocols.

References

1. Feigenbaum H. *Echocardiography*, 4th edition, Lea & Febiger, Philadelphia, 1986.
2. Taylor KJW, Burns PN, Wells PNT (eds). *Clinical Applications of Doppler Ultrasound*. Raven Press, New York, 1988.
3. Kisslo J, Adams DB, Belkin RN. *Doppler Color Flow Imaging*. Churchill Livingstone, New York, 1988.
4. von Ramm OT, Thurstone FL. Cardiac imaging using a phased array ultrasound system. I. System design. *Circulation* 1976; 53:258–262.
5. Kisslo J, von Ramm OT, Thurstone FL. Cardiac imaging using a phased array ultrasound system. II. Clinical technique and application. *Circulation* 1976; 53:262–267.
6. Mitchell DG. Color Doppler imaging. *Radiology* 1990; 177:1–10.

Chapter 2

Methodology

A. Qualitative Morphology

The goal of ultrasonographic imaging is to provide high-resolution imaging of the heart, great vessels, and major thoracic branches of the great vessels. Thus, a methodology should be chosen that is applicable *generally*, not selectively. A methodology should not require any assumptions about the patient (e.g., that normally aligned great arteries are present, or that levocardia exists, etc.).

As understanding of cardiac pathology grew in the 1970s, more and more diagnostic sophistication was demanded of echocardiographers. Although initial examinations in pediatric cardiac ultrasound were conducted on unsedated subjects, by the early 1980s it was obvious that the median length of examination time needed to provide morphological accuracy similar to axial angiography was 45 to 60 minutes. Thus, the routine administration of premedication for outpatients became standard practice in many laboratories. Other benefits of sedation soon emerged.

First, skeletal muscle tone (e.g., in the abdomen) diminishes, making it easier for any examiner, especially the novice, to manipulate the transducer in many windows without upsetting the infant. Second, having uninterrupted sedative effect allows the examiner to proceed through a scanning protocol *sequentially* on a consistent basis; one need not start in the subcostal window, stop when the infant cries, have to move on to the precordial window, and return to the subcostal window only when the crying has abated. Finally, when Doppler echocardiography emerged as an important physiological measurement technique, sedation was mandatory to achieve and maintain steady-state conditions.

The basic principle in any morphology recognition scheme (e.g., aerial reconnaissance, undersea canyon exploration, or cardiac imaging) is to move progressively from wide field of view to smaller fields of view. By far the widest field of view in the infant is afforded by the subcostal window. Historically, first attempts at pediatric cardiac ultrasonic imaging used precordial windows, presumably borrowing from initial developments in the adult setting. Although the use of the subcostal window in infants and in children had been proposed by several investigators, Bierman[1] was the first to point out the major advantage in *starting* from the subcostal window. The first sweeps developed were the frontal (coronal) and sagittal.

Bierman advocated initiating the examination with a display of the abdominal great vessels (aorta, azygos, inferior vena cava). The classic format has been that used by computed tomography (and magnetic resonance imaging) with ventral structures displayed at the top. The "transverse" view of the body at a level just superior to the renal poles, with the spine cross-section in the middle, is the starting point for the exam (Figure 1). To ascertain whether the transducer is oriented correctly, angle the transducer to one of the patient's sides and watch to see if the display on the monitor moves in the appropriate direction. Thus, if the transducer is aimed toward the patient's right hemiabdomen, the display should move so that the spine occupies the leftward aspect of the sector (i.e., leftward is used to mean the patient's left) and the structures to the right of the spine should occupy the center of the sector. If the display moves so that the spine occupies the rightward aspect of the sector, the transducer is 180° "reversed." Either the transducer or the display should then be flipped 180° before proceeding. It is unreliable to use the presence or absence of the liver (or other organs) to determine whether the transducer is correctly oriented; the liver may in fact be on the right side of the spine, on the left side of the spine, or relatively symmetrical (e.g., in heterotaxy syndrome).

Once proper orientation has been achieved, the transducer is angulated cranially until the heart is reached. The display on the monitor is then reoriented so that superior is at the top and inferior is at the bottom. The "frontal" (coronal) sweep is thus a series of images from inferior and posterior (Figures 2–6) to superior and anterior; only at the most anterior reaches of the sweep does it provide *true* coronal pictures of the mediastinum. The position of the cardiac apex is obvious on the frontal sweep and affects how much the examiner will emphasize the left oblique or right oblique sweep (see Chapter 3, section B).

The left oblique sweep is performed by rotating the transducer 30° to 45° clockwise from the previous position.[2] The trajectory of the sweep is from the patient's right hip to left shoulder (Figures 7–9). This is the cornerstone of imaging for the *levocardia* patient. The portion of the sweep that displays the ventricles is analogous to Bargeron's angiographic long axial oblique view (Figures 10–14). There is the left obliquity together with the approximately 30° of cranial angulation.

The sagittal sweep is performed by further clockwise rotation until the transducer is 90° different from its initial position. The trajectory of the sweep is from one side to the other (Figures 15–21). (The most convenient starting site in levocardia is the right side since in situs solitus, the superior vena cava and the inferior vena cava are almost directly vertically oriented and thus can be displayed simultaneously.)

The right oblique sweep[3,4] is performed by rotating the transducer 30°–45° counterclockwise from its frontal starting position (Figure 22). The trajectory is from the patient's left hip to right shoulder. In *dextrocardia* patients, this becomes a very helpful sweep for displaying the ventricles and sometimes for displaying the atria (see Chapter 3).

An argument could be made to then proceed to the window with the next widest field of view—the suprasternal window; however, I have found that the best pictures necessitate extending the patient's neck, which requires placing a roll or pillow under the shoulders. To manipulate the infant to this extent is to risk waking him up; thus, I have usually left suprasternal imaging to the end. (In the near future when deeper sedation is instituted, it may be possible to proceed as follows: subcostal to suprasternal to parasternal to apical.)

The next part of the exam, therefore, involves the parasternal window.[5] [Note that the recognition of proper orientation for the "parasternal long axis" view (Figure 23) *depends* on the presence of normally aligned great arteries, i.e., the aorta arises from the left ventricle. Thus, it is difficult to conceive of how the parasternal long axis cut could ever be utilized as a universal starting point, since many congenital malformations do *not* have normally aligned great arteries.] From the view in which aortic root and left ventricular body are simultaneously displayed, angulation medially yields the "right ventricular inflow" view. The "parasternal short axis" sweep is typically begun by obtaining a circular display of the left ventricle and then sweeping toward the right shoulder, i.e., toward the base of the heart (Figure 24).

The apical window[6] is utilized primarily for the four-chamber view (Figure 25). Tilting cranially yields the "five-chamber" view, which is actually the four chambers of the heart plus the aortic root (Figures 26 and 27).

The "suprasternal" window[7] is actually an area that includes not only the suprasternal notch but also the "high parasternal" regions on either side of the sternum (Figure 28). (Again, care should be taken to ensure that the transducer is correctly oriented by beginning with a frontal cut and angling to one side to see whether the display on the monitor moves in the appropriate direction.) The sector is displayed so that superior is at the top and inferior at the bottom. The frontal sweep is typically begun from the view of the superior vena cava (Figures 29–32); the transducer is angled anteriorly and then posteriorly. The left oblique cut is performed by rotating the transducer 30°–45° counterclockwise from the starting position and placing the transducer footprint in the high right parasternal region and aiming at the left hip (Figure 33). The sagittal cut is performed by rotating the transducer 90° from its initial frontal position. The footprint is usually best situated in the suprasternal notch or in the high left parasternal region.

B. Quantitative Morphology

In 1992, use of quantitative information about morphology in the management of congenital heart disease still lags behind the use of qualitative descriptions. In the next 10 years, the gap should close.

Although normal values for most chambers and vessels are available, what would be more helpful is "normal" values for chambers and vessels in *each* congenital lesion. Moreover, since a "program of surgical therapy" is now available for each lesion, the determination of normal values for chambers and pathways *after* a surgical palliation would enable the cardiologist to screen for pathway obstruction and ventricular dysfunction. For example, the pulmonary venous pathway following Fontan[8] or Senning[9] procedures has been studied in detail. Finally, the characterization of what minimum size of mitral valve, left ventricle, and outflow tract can sustain the systemic circulation should help cardiac surgeons decide whether to aim for a two-ventricle repair.

In the fetus, it should be possible to predict whether a ventricle will be hypoplastic if serial measurements can be made during gestation. Normal values for the fetus are shown in Figures 34–47.

C. Physiology

Normal values for velocities in the fetus are shown in Figures 48–61.

1. Stenotic Lesions

Stenotic lesions can be divided into *discrete* and *long-segment*[10] and also into *fixed* and *dynamic*. Virtually all discrete stenoses (Figures 62 and 63) are also fixed. Long-segment stenoses can be either fixed (e.g., aortic arch hypoplasia) or dynamic (e.g., subpulmonary stenosis in tetralogy of Fallot).

The quantitative characterization of a discrete *arterial* stenosis is most conveniently performed by measuring the velocity proximal and distal to the stenosis and employing the simplified Bernoulli formula: $P = 4 (V_2^2 - V_1^2)$, where V_2 = the velocity distal to the stenosis and V_1 = the velocity proximal to the stenosis. The most reliable way to measure V_1 is to use pulsed Doppler, rather than using the continuous wave trace of V_2 (see Figure 64) since the best angle for V_2 may not be the best angle for V_1.

The derivation of this formula is discussed by Holen.[11] Although many investigators[12] have advocated using $P = V_2^2$, in pediatric patients it is better to get into the habit of not neglecting V_1. For example, with large ventricular septal defect and valvar pulmonic stenosis, the velocity proximal to the pulmonary cusps can be over 2 m/sec. If the velocity distal to the cusps is measured to be 3.0 m/sec, then by neglecting the proximal velocity, the operator would be significantly overestimating stenosis severity.

The estimation of discrete *atrioventricular valve* stenosis is more difficult. The pressure half-time method[13] has not proved very clinically useful in infants for at least two reasons. First, the vast majority of infants with mitral stenosis (MS) have a coexistent atrial septal defect (ASD) so that the hemodynamic consequence of MS is *not* a high left atrial pressure but rather a large left-to-right shunt. Second, the heart rate is sufficiently fast that the E-F downslope is quite short, increasing the possibility of error.

Several methods have been tried to circumvent the problems with pressure half-time. The estimation of mean gradient may offer some insight in cases with intact atrial septum. In cases with significant ASD, mea-surement of annulus diameter may be a more reliable predictor of severity of stenosis although measurement of annulus diameter can be applied *only* to cases of mitral hypoplasia since in other types of mitral stenosis the obstruction is caused not by too small an annulus but by interchordal spaces that are too cramped. Analogous issues arise in the quantitation of tricuspid stenosis.

With venous stenosis,[14] a combination of anatomical display and color flow mapping, followed by pulsed Doppler interrogation,[15] is probably the best approach (Figures 65–68).

Interrogating a tricuspid regurgitation jet (Figures 69 and 70) is a good "cross-check" for evaluating right ventricular outflow tract obstruction.[16]

2. Regurgitant Lesions

Arterial valve regurgitation and atrioventricular valve regurgitation will be discussed separately. For arterial valve regurgitation, the color Doppler parameters proposed by Perry et al.[17] have been widely accepted as clinically useful in the noninvasive semiquantitative assessment of native aortic valve regurgitation. The jet width/outflow width ratio appears to correlate well with angiographic severity. Pulmonary valve regurgitation (high-pressure type) can theoretically be assessed using similar color Doppler parameters; however, the Doppler evaluation of low-pressure pulmonary regurgitation has not yet been studied quantitatively, but one rough guide to severe pulmonary regurgitation would be the detection of diastolic reversal in the branch pulmonary arteries.

Prosthetic aortic valve regurgitation is usually paravalvar since the vast majority of artificial valves implanted in infants and children are mechanical. Criteria for judging severity have not yet been proposed.

In chronic regurgitation, the assessment of ventricular performance is the predominant factor in clinical management. Thus, precise regurgitant volume estimates are of limited value.

Atrioventricular valve regurgitation (Figure 71) has proved more problematic to quantify than arterial valve regurgitation. Although we initially found reasonably good agreement between jet area/left atrial area ratio (Figure 72) and the angiographic grading of native mitral valve regurgitation, we have recently changed our "cut-off" values from 0.20 and 0.40, as suggested by Helmcke[18] for adults, to 0.30 and 0.50 as the best partitions in the pediatric age group between mild and moderate and between moderate and severe degrees of regurgitation, respectively. (This should not be too surprising since adult cardiologists have recently noted a need for different criteria in transesophageal imaging[19] as compared with transthoracic imaging because of the shorter distance to target.) We also discovered that the regurgitant jet area indexed to body surface area correlated well with angiographic severity when cut-off values of 4 cm²/m² and 10 cm²/m² were employed.[20]

Regurgitant jet area as displayed by Doppler color flow mapping is affected by several factors,[21–24] including compliance and size of receiving chamber, color gain setting, carrier frequency, pulse repetition frequency, wall impingement, and driving pressure. Since gain controls are not standardized within the ultrasound industry, the cut-off values mentioned above thus can only be assumed true for a single instrument. Without prospective trials and analogous study of other commercially available instruments, it is difficult to know whether widespread acceptance of color Doppler parameters will occur.

Other methods not involving regurgitant jet area are under study. In adults, regurgitant jet width[25] may be better than regurgitant jet area. Regurgitant flow rate and volume have been calculated by measuring momentum[26] and combining it with peak orifice velocity and distal centerline velocity. The proximal isovelocity surface area method[27–30] looks promising in adults; however, in-vivo validation has yet to be reported in the pediatric population. This method assumes that flow is symmetrically disposed around an axis normal to the regurgitant orifice so that all velocities will be equal at the same radial distance from the orifice. By the continuity principle, $Q = 2\pi r^2 V_r$ where V_r is the velocity at the radial distance r from the orifice. The first aliasing limit is displayed on all current Doppler color flow mapping instruments, so it represents a convenient site to obtain r and V_r. Simpson[31] has recently suggested using the point of second alias to better ensure a hemispherical "velocity shell."

In chronic regurgitation, serial assessment of ventricular performance is more important clinically than measurement of regurgitant volume.

3. Left-to-Right Shunts

One of the largest contributions of Doppler color flow mapping appears to be its use in (a) estimating size of ventricular septal defects, (b) visualizing systemic-to-pulmonary artery shunts (Figures 73 and 74), and (c) ruling out the presence of any significant shunting (Figure 75). Although absolute defect size or defect

size indexed to body surface area would probably correlate well with hemodynamic importance, it is often not easy to precisely determine the edges of VSDs preoperatively because of attached or overlying tricuspid valve tissue. Measuring color Doppler jet width, however, appears to be quite feasible. Pulmonary/systemic flow ratio can be estimated, although this information is not usually crucial prior to surgical repair in the infant <1 year of age.

Postoperatively, the presence of patch material has made recognition of peripatch VSDs by two-dimensional imaging alone unreliable, whereas color Doppler jet width can be conveniently measured 1 week after surgery and correlates well with the need for reoperation in the first 12 postoperative months.[32]

The ruling out of residual ASDs, residual systemic-to-pulmonary artery shunts (Figure 76), as well as hemodynamically important ventricular-level shunts is relatively fast. Pulmonary/systemic flow ratio can be estimated; however, in cases where its magnitude affects surgical decision-making, cardiac catheterization is still needed.

4. Right-to-Left Shunts

Doppler color flow mapping has been a major aid in the detection of ductal (Figure 77) and ventricular-level right-to-left shunts and may also help in identifying atrial-level right-to-left shunts (Figure 9). One limitation of the technique in the latter situation is the low velocity typically seen. This may be lower than the threshold velocity to appear on the color display. Thus, choosing an angle of incidence becomes important in order to maximize the chances that low-velocity flow will be visible.

D. Altered Electrical Activation

Although this has been reported most frequently in fetal imaging studies (Figures 78 and 79), this has also been applied to postnatal imaging, especially in patients after Fontan and Mustard surgery. The most common arrhythmic sequela of intra-atrial surgery is atrial flutter. If it is impossible to rule out from a surface ECG, two-dimensional echocardiographic imaging can display the regional high-frequency atrial contractions, and the degree of atrioventricular block can be quantitated.

References

1. Bierman FZ, Williams RG. Subxiphoid two-dimensional imaging of the interatrial septum in infants and neonates with congenital heart disease. *Circulation* 1979; 60:80–90.

2. Chin AJ, Yeager SB, Sanders SP, Williams RG, Bierman FZ, Burger BM, Norwood WI, et al. Accuracy of prospective 2-dimensional evaluation of the left ventricular outflow tract in complete transposition of the great arteries. *Am J Cardiol* 1985; 55:759–764.

3. Isaaz K, Cloez JL, Danchin N, Marcon F, Worms AM, Pernot C. Assessment of right ventricular outflow tract in children by two-dimensional echocardiography using a new subcostal view. *Am J Cardiol* 1985; 56:539–545.

4. Marino B, Ballerini L, Marcelletti C, Piva R, Pasquini L, Zacche C, Giannico S, et al. Right oblique subxiphoid view for two-dimensional echocardiographic visualization of the right ventricle in congenital heart disease. *Am J Cardiol* 1984; 54:1064–1068.

5. Feigenbaum H. *Echocardiography,* 4th edition. Lea & Febiger, Philadelphia, 1986.

6. Silverman NH, Schiller NB. Apex echocardiography: a two- dimensional technique for evaluating congenital heart disease. *Circulation* 1978; 57:503–511.

7. Snider AR, Silverman NH. Suprasternal notch echocardiography: a two-dimensional technique for evaluating congenital heart disease. *Circulation* 1981; 63:165–173.

8. Fogel M, Chin AJ. Imaging of pulmonary venous pathway obstruction in patients after the modified Fontan procedure. *J Am Coll Cardiol* 1992; 20:181–190.

9. Chin AJ, Sanders SP, Williams RG, Lang P, Norwood WI, Castaneda AR. Two-dimensional echocardiographic assessment of caval and pulmonary venous pathways after the Senning operation. *Am J Cardiol* 1983; 52:118–126.

10. Yoganathan AP, Valdes-Cruz LM, Schmidt-Dohna J, Jimoh A, Berry C, Tomura T, Sahn DJ. Continuous-wave Doppler velocities and gradients across fixed tunnel obstructions: studies in vitro and in vivo. *Circulation* 1987; 76:657–666.

11. Holen J, Aaslid R, Landmark K, Simonsen A. Determination of pressure gradient in mitral stenosis with a non-invasive ultrasound Doppler technique. *Acta Med Scand* 1976; 199:455–460.

12. Yoganathan AP, Cape EG, Sung H-W, Williams FP, Jimoh A. Review of hydrodynamic principles for the cardiologist: applications to the study of blood flow and jets by imaging techniques. *J Am Coll Cardiol* 1988; 12:1344–1353.

13. Hatle L, Angelsen B. *Doppler Ultrasound in Cardiology.* Lea & Febiger, Philadelphia, 1982.

14. Reynolds T, Appleton CP. Doppler flow velocity patterns of the superior vena cava, inferior vena cava, hepatic vein, coronary sinus, and atrial septal defect. *J Am Soc Echo* 1991; 4:503–512.

15. Ding ZP, Oh JK, Klein AL, Tajik AJ. Effect of sample volume and location on Doppler-derived transmitral inflow velocity values. *J Am Soc Echo* 1991; 4:451–456.

16. Chang AC, Vetter JM, Gill SE, Franklin WH, Murphy JD, Chin AJ. Accuracy of prospective two-dimensional/Doppler echocardiography in assessment of reparative surgery. *J Am Coll Cardiol* 1990; 16:903–912.

17. Perry GL, Helmcke F, Nanda NC, Byard C, Soto B. Evaluation of aortic insufficiency by Doppler color flow mapping. *J Am Coll Cardiol* 1987; 9:952–9.

18. Helmcke F, Nanda NC, Hsiung MC, Soto B, Adey CK, Goyal RG, Gatewood RP. Color Doppler assessment of mitral regurgitation with orthogonal planes. *Circulation* 1987; 75:175–183.

19. Smith MD, Harrison MR, Pinton R, Kandil H, Kwan OL, DeMaria AN. Regurgitant jet size by transesophageal compared with transthoracic Doppler color flow mapping. Circulation 1991; 83:79–86.

20. Wu Y-T, Chang AC, Chin AJ. Semiquantitative assessment of mitral regurgitation by Doppler color flow imaging in patients aged <20 years. *Am J Cardiol* 1993; 71:727–732.

21. Krabill KA, Sung H-W, Tamura T, Chung KJ, Yoganathan AP, Sahn DJ. Factors influencing the structure and shape of stenotic and regurgitant jets: an in-vitro investigation using Doppler color flow mapping and optical flow visualization. *J Am Coll Cardiol* 1989; 13:1672–1681.

22. Aragam JR, Flachskampf FA, Weyman AE, Thomas JD. Variation in the color Doppler area of a regurgitant jet with changes in the absolute chamber pressure: an in vitro study. *J Am Soc Echo* 1992; 5:421–426.

23. Stevenson JG. Two-dimensional color Doppler estimation of the severity of atrioventricular valve regurgitation: important effects of instrument gain setting, pulse repetition frequency, and carrier frequency. *J Am Soc Echo* 1989; 2:1–10.

24. Chen C, Thomas JD, Anconina J, Harrigan P, Mueller L, Picard MH, Levine RA, et al. Impact of impinging wall jet on color Doppler quantitation of mitral regurgitation. *Circulation* 1991; 84:714–720.

25. Tribouilloy C, Shen WF, Quere J-P, Rey J-L, Choquet D, Dufosse H, Lesbre J-P. Assessment of severity of mitral regurgitation by measuring regurgitant jet width at its origin with transesophageal Doppler color flow imaging. *Circulation* 1992; 85:1248–1253.

26. Thomas JD, Liu C-M, Flachskampf FA, O'Shea JP, Davidoff R, Weyman AE. Quantification of jet flow by momentum analysis: an in vitro color Doppler flow study. *Circulation* 1990; 81:247–259.

27. Bargiggia GS, Tronconi L, Sahn DJ, Recusani F, Raisaro A, DeServi S, Valdes-Cruz LM, et al. A new method for quantitation of mitral regurgitation based on color flow Doppler imaging of flow convergence proximal to regurgitant orifice. *Circulation* 1991; 84:1481–1489.

28. Rodriquez L, Anconina J, Flachskampf FA, Weyman AE, Levine RA, Thomas JD. Impact of finite orifice size on proximal flow convergence: implications for Doppler quantification of valvular regurgitation. *Circ Res* 1992; 70:923–930.

29. Baumgartner J, Schima H, Kuhn P. Value and limitations of proximal jet dimensions for the quantitation of valvular regurgitation: an in vitro study using Doppler flow imaging. *J Am Soc Echo* 1991; 4:57–66.

30. Utsunomiya T, Ogawa T, Doshi R, Patel D, Quan M, Henry WL, Gardin JM. Doppler color flow "proximal isovelocity surface area" method for estimating volume flow rate: effects of orifice shape and machine factors. *J Am Coll Cardiol* 1991; 17:1103–1111.

31. Simpson IA. Quantitative color Doppler flow mapping (editorial). *Circulation* 1993; 87:1762–1764.

32. Rychik J, Norwood WI, Chin AJ. Doppler color flow mapping assessment of residual ventricular septal defect after reparative surgery. *Circulation* 1991; 84(Suppl II):III153–III161.

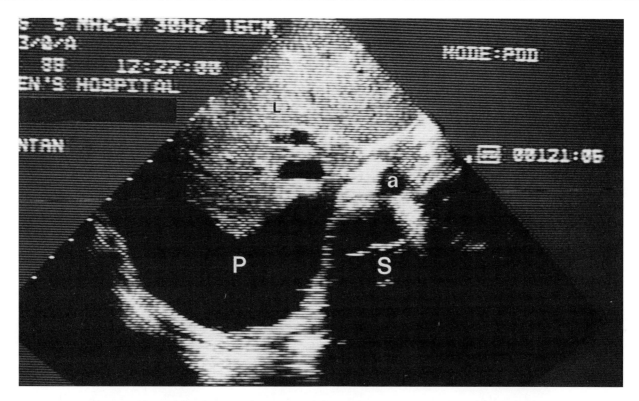

Figure 1: Transverse abdominal view. a = abdominal aorta; L = liver; P = right pleural effusion; S = vertebral column.

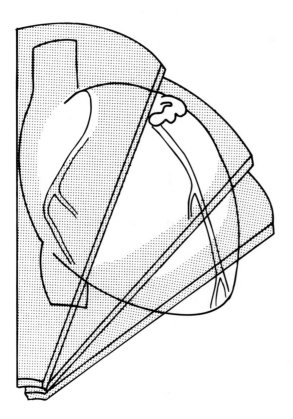

Figure 2: Subcostal frontal sweep. Note that only at the most anterior aspects of this sweep are *true* coronal views achieved.

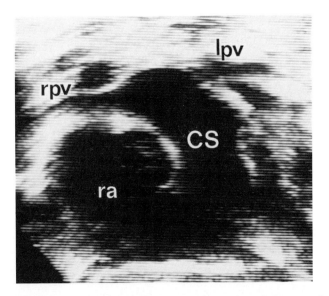

Figure 3: Subcostal frontal sweep. At the most inferior portions of this sweep, the coronary sinus (CS) can be displayed. This infant had total anomalous pulmonary venous connection to the coronary sinus. lpv = left pulmonary vein; ra = right atrium; rpv = right pulmonary vein.

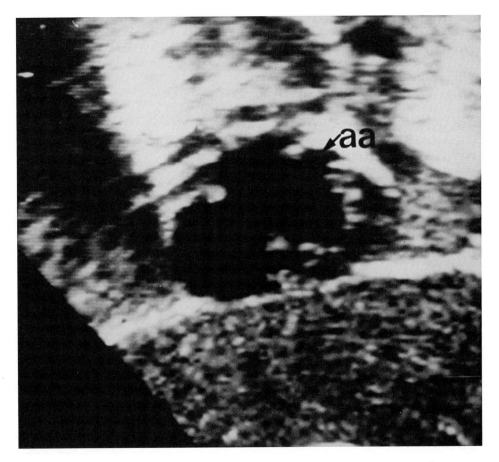

Figure 4: Subcostal frontal sweep. At a slightly higher plane (than in Figure 3), other structures can be seen. The orifice of the left atrial appendage (aa) can be visualized.

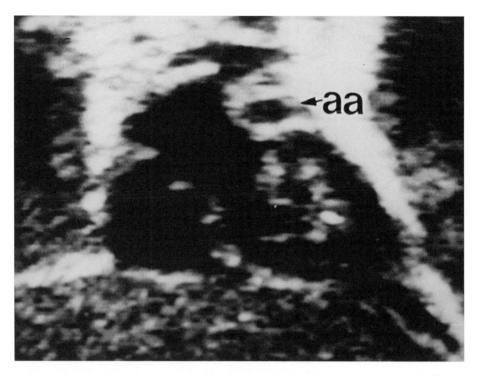

Figure 5: Subcostal frontal sweep. At a still higher plane, the tip of the left atrial appendage (aa) can be seen. The right pulmonary artery origin is coming into view.

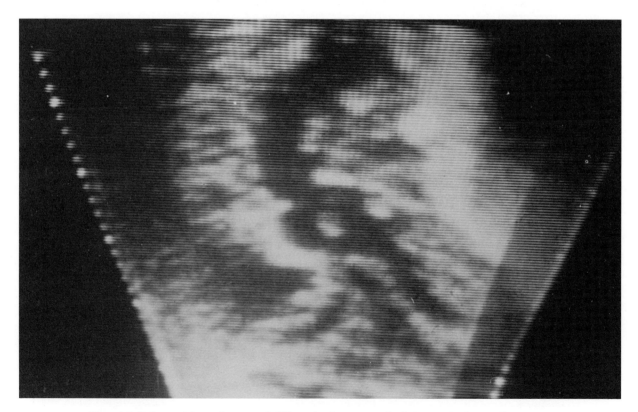

Figure 6: Subcostal frontal sweep. Still later in the sweep, the left ventricular outflow tract comes into view. This patient has undergone arterial switch repair.

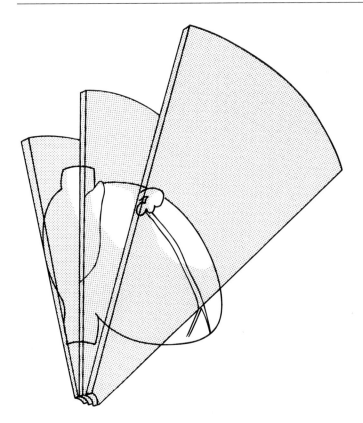

Figure 7: Subcostal left oblique sweep. The trajectory of the sweep is from the patient's right hip toward his left shoulder. A mirror-image of this trajectory produces the right oblique sweep.

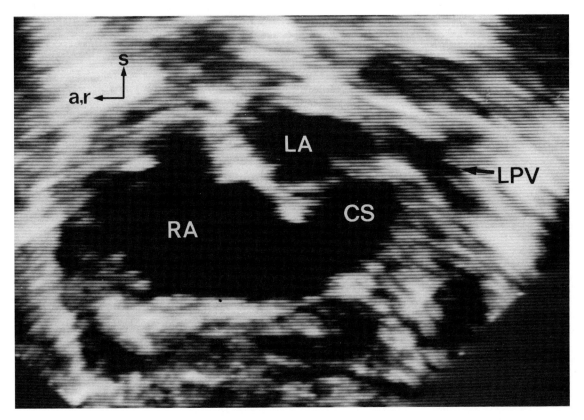

Figure 8: At an early point in the sweep, the right superior vena cava is displayed, along with the coronary sinus (CS). LA = left atrium; LPV = left pulmonary vein; RA = right atrium.

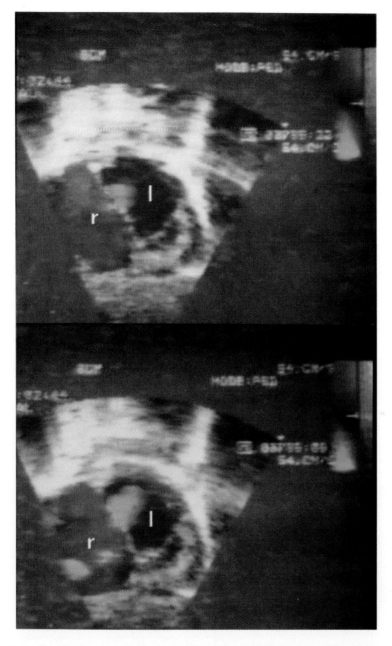

Figure 9: At a slightly later point in the sweep, the coronary sinus is no longer seen; the superior portion of the atrial septum is visualized. This patient has a right-to-left (r to l) shunt at the atrial level.

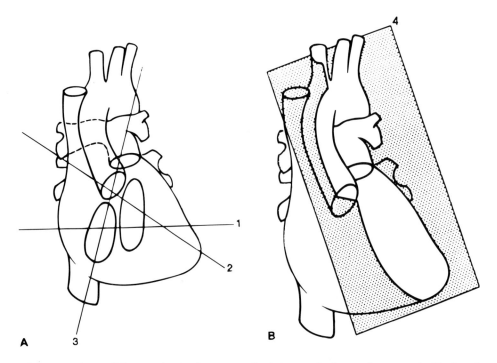

Figure 10: At a still later point in the sweep, the left ventricular outflow tract is displayed in a manner analogous to Bargeron's long axial oblique angiographic view.

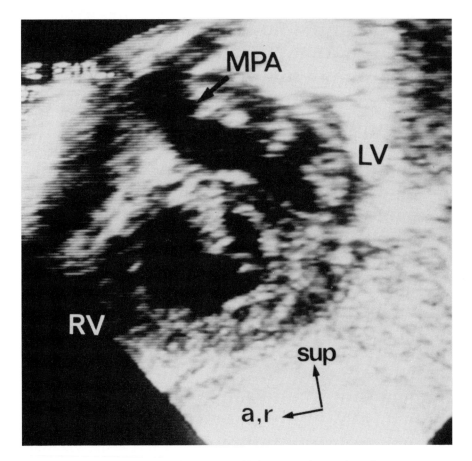

Figure 11: Subcostal long axial oblique view of left ventricular (LV) outflow tract in transposition of the great arteries. MPA = main pulmonary artery; RV = right ventricle.

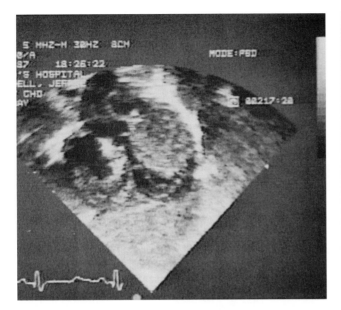

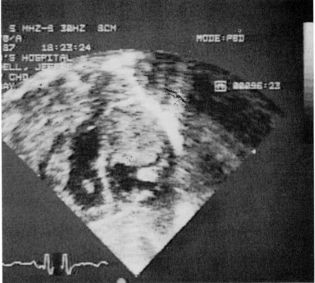

Figure 12: Subcostal long axial oblique view of left ventricular tumor impinging on outflow tract.

Figure 13: Plane slightly leftward of that in Figure 12, showing right ventricular outflow tract.

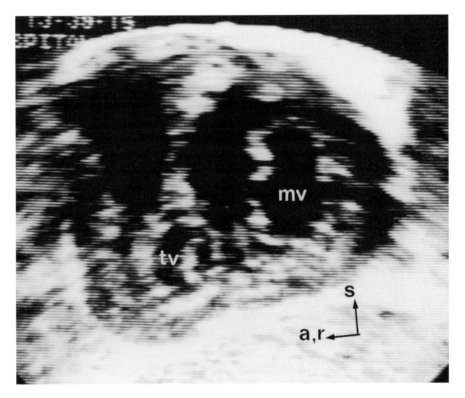

Figure 14: Subcostal long axial oblique view of a patient with mild hypoplasia of the tricuspid valve (tv) and right ventricular inflow. The gain has been decreased so that the left septal surface is just barely seen. mv = mitral valve.

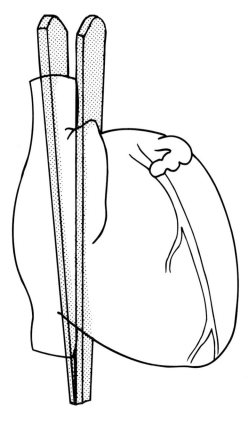

Figure 15: The subcostal sagittal sweep. As shown, the easiest way to begin is to display the superior vena cava and inferior vena cava simultaneously.

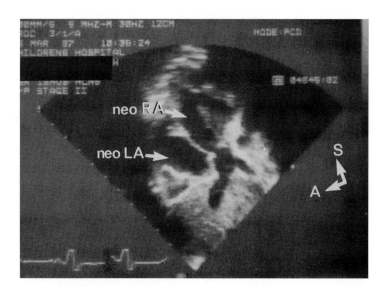

Figure 16: Subcostal sagittal view of patient who has undergone Fontan procedure. neoLA = neo-left atrium; neoRA = neo-right atrium.

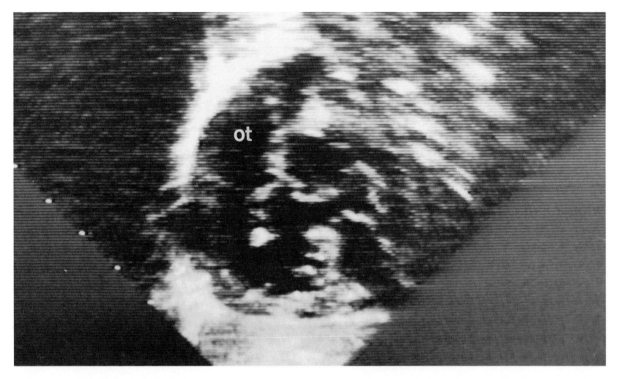

Figure 17: A later point in the sagittal sweep. The atria in this case of common atrioventricular canal are no longer visible. The right ventricular outflow tract (ot) is seen.

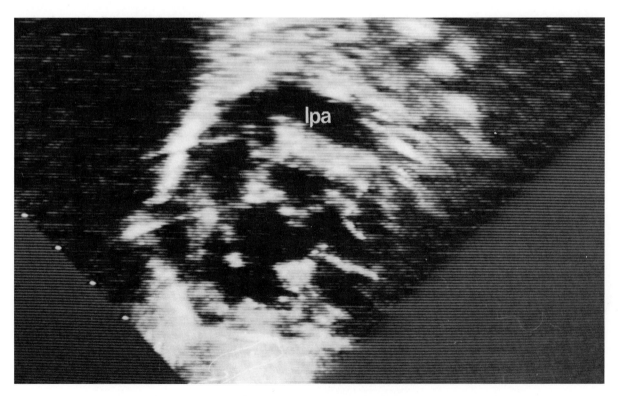

Figure 18: Slightly leftward of the plane in Figure 17. The left pulmonary artery (lpa) appears as a continuation of the main pulmonary artery.

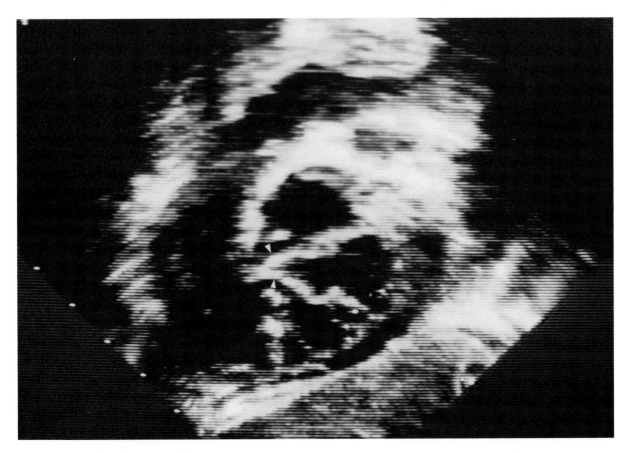

Figure 19: Subcostal sagittal view of common atrioventricular canal patient whose septal commissure (arrowheads) was not sutured.

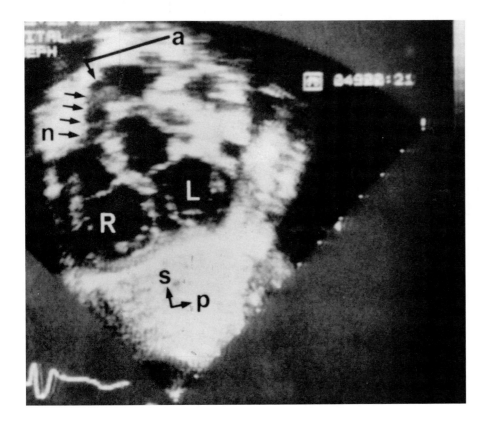

Figure 20: Subcostal sagittal view of neo-pulmonary artery stenosis after arterial switch.

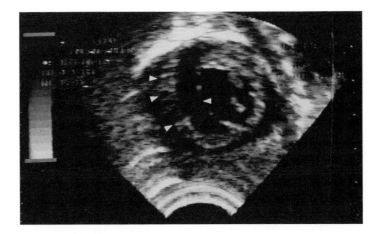

Figure 21: A view that is even more leftward than the plane in Figure 18. The left septal surface (single arrow) is smoother than the right septal surface (three arrows). This patient has D-looped ventricles.

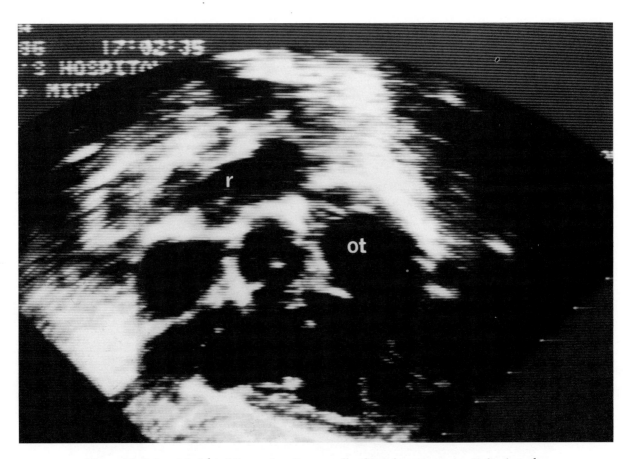

Figure 22: Subcostal right oblique view. In normally aligned great arteries, it displays the right ventricular outflow tract (ot) and the right (r) pulmonary artery–main pulmonary artery junction. This patient had undergone pulmonary artery banding.

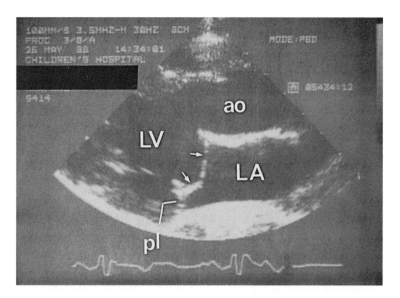

Figure 23: Parasternal long axis view. The anterior mitral leaflet (unlabeled arrows) prolapses in this patient with Marfan's syndrome. ao = aortic root; LA = left atrium; LV = left ventricle; pl = posterior leaflet of the mitral valve.

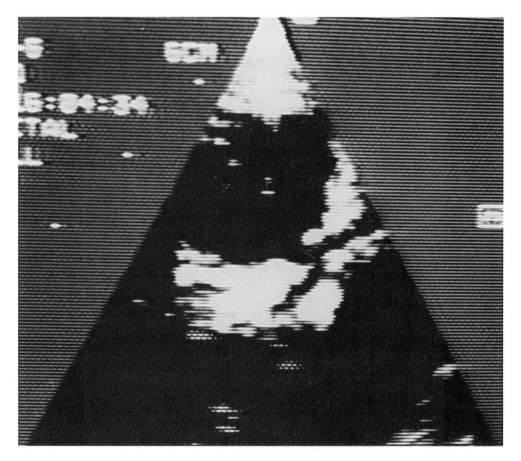

Figure 24: Parasternal short axis view of the pulmonary root. This patient had anomalous origin of the left coronary artery from the pulmonary artery.

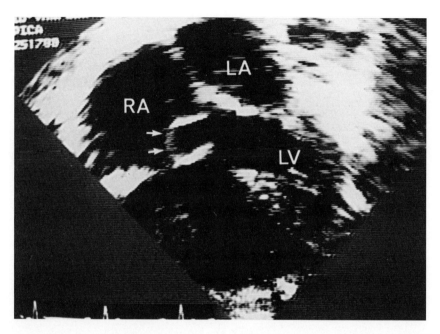

Figure 25: Apical four-chamber view of a sinus of Valsalva aneurysm (arrows) protruding into the right atrium (RA). LA = left atrium; LV = left ventricle.

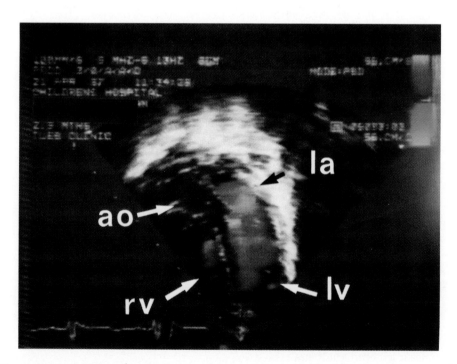

Figure 26: Apical "five-chamber" view, showing left ventricular (lv) inflow. ao = aorta; la = left atrium; rv = right ventricle.

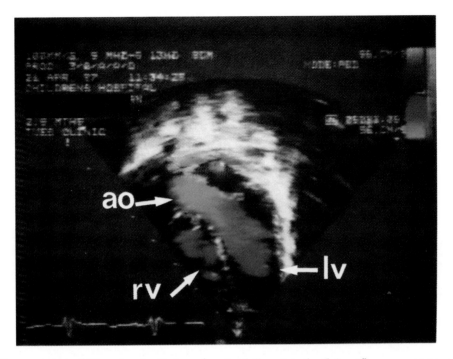

Figure 27: Apical "five-chamber" view, showing left ventricular (lv) outflow. ao = aorta; rv = right ventricle.

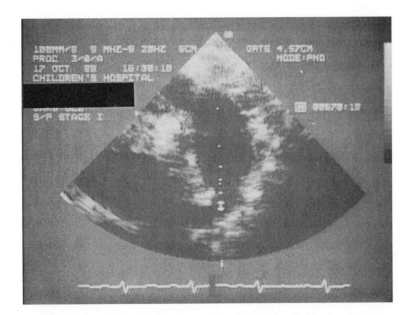

Figure 28: High parasternal sagittal view of distal arch following Norwood procedure for hypoplastic left heart syndrome.

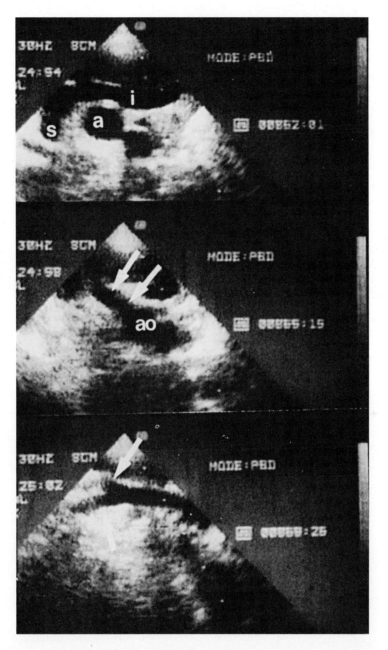

Figure 29: Suprasternal frontal sweep. **Top:** The innominate vein's (i) usual position above the ascending aorta (a) is shown. s = right superior vena cava. **Middle:** A plane slightly posterior to that in top panel. The innominate artery (arrows) courses to the patient's right. **Bottom:** The transducer is angled toward the right shoulder. The innominate artery is seen to bifurcate into the common carotid artery (arrow) and the subclavian artery.

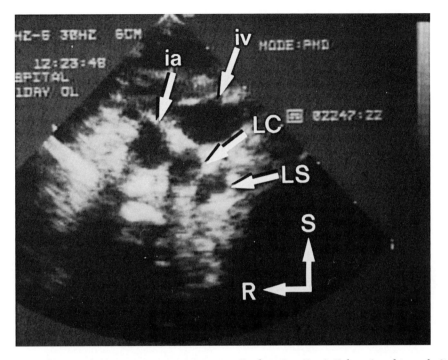

Figure 30: Suprasternal frontal sweep. Occasionally the takeoffs of all three brachiocephalic vessels can be seen simultaneously. ia = innominate artery; iv = innominate vein; LC = left common carotid artery; LS = left subclavian artery.

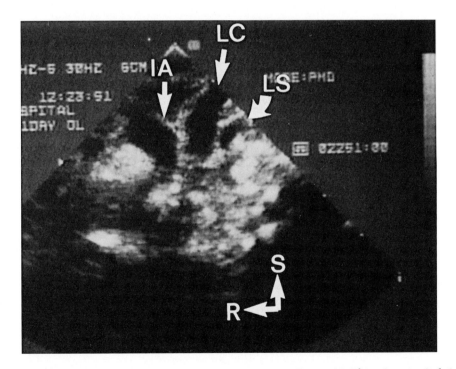

Figure 31: Suprasternal frontal sweep, same patient as in Figure 30. This plane is slightly posterior to Figure 30. This patient has a left aortic arch. IA = innominate artery; LC = left common carotid artery; LS = left subclavian artery.

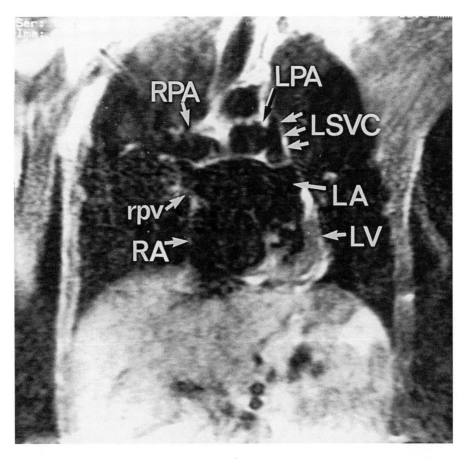

Figure 32: Frontal magnetic resonance scan showing left superior vena cava (LSVC). RPA = right pulmonary artery; LPA = left pulmonary artery; rpv = right pulmonary vein; LA = left atrium; LV = left ventricle; RA = right atrium.

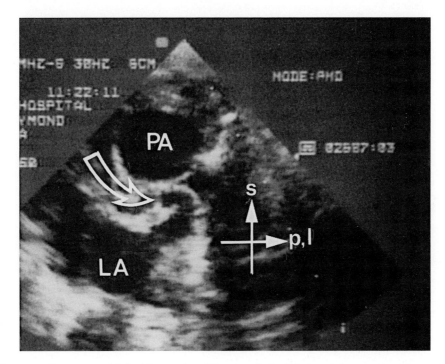

Figure 33: Suprasternal left oblique view. The morphologic left atrial appendage (arrow) is well seen. PA = pulmonary artery; LA = left atrium.

Cardiac area

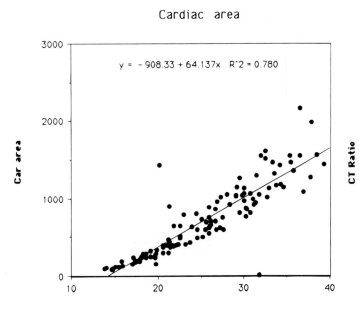

Figure 34: Normal values for cardiac "area" on fetal echocardiographic exam. The abscissa is gestational age (GA) in weeks. The ordinate is mm². [This figure and succeeding ones (through Figure 61) are used with permission of Dr. Zhi-yun Tian.]

CT Ratio

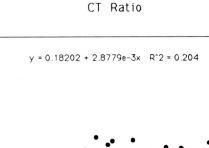

Figure 35: Normal values for "cardiothoracic (CT) ratio."

Dimension of SVC

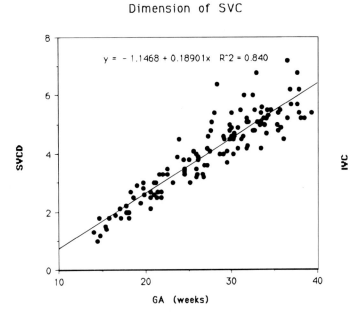

Figure 36: Normal values for superior vena cava (SVC), in mm.

Dimension of IVC

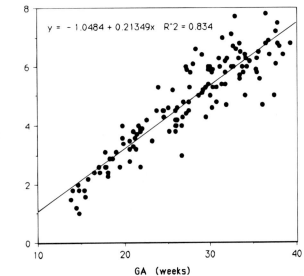

Figure 37: Normal values for inferior vena cava (IVC), in mm.

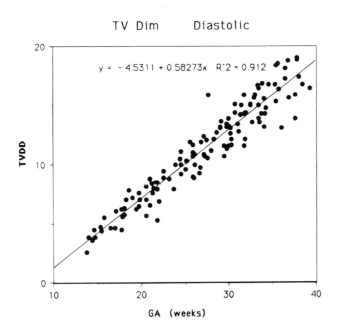

Figure 38: Normal values for tricuspid valve (TV) annulus dimension (Dim) in diastole, in mm.

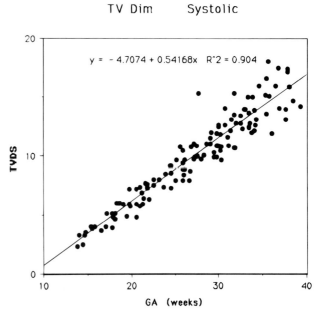

Figure 39: Normal values for tricuspid valve (TV) annulus dimension (Dim) in systole, in mm.

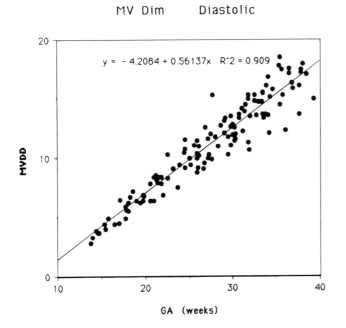

Figure 40: Normal values for mitral valve (MV) annulus dimension (Dim) in diastole, in mm.

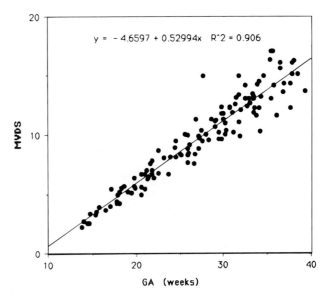

Figure 41: Normal values for mitral valve (MV) annulus dimension (Dim) in systole, in mm.

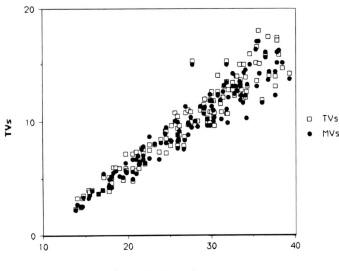

Figure 42: Normal values for mitral valve in systole (MVs) and tricuspid valve in systole (TVs). Note how closely the two correspond throughout the second two trimesters. Near term, the tricuspid valve is slightly larger.

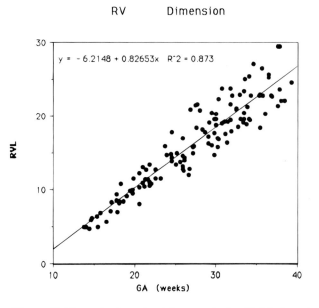

Figure 43: Normal values for right ventricular (RV) inflow dimension, in mm.

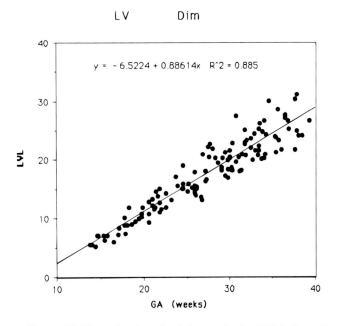

Figure 44: Normal values for left ventricular (LV) inflow dimension, in mm. The LV is slightly larger than the RV.

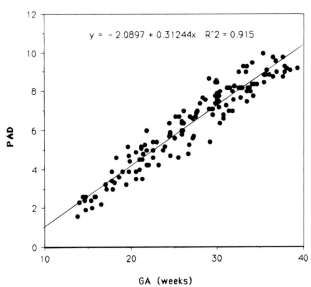

Figure 45: Normal values for pulmonary root (PA) dimension, in mm.

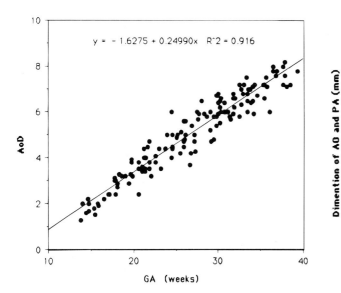

Figure 46: Normal values for aortic root dimension (AoD), in mm.

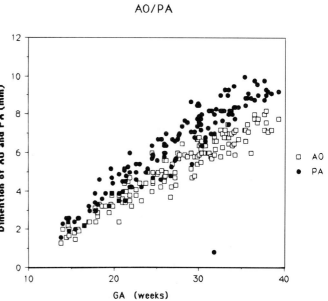

Figure 47: Normal values for aortic (AO) and pulmonary (PA) roots. The aortic root is smaller than the pulmonary root throughout the second two trimesters.

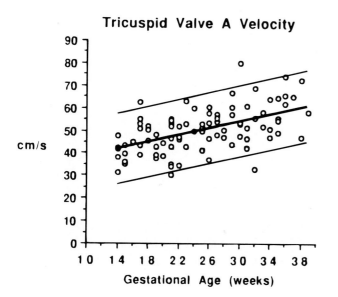

Figure 48: Normal values for a wave velocity in tricuspid valve.

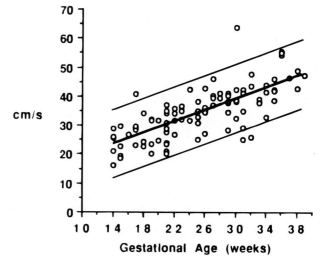

Figure 49: Normal values for e wave velocity in tricuspid valve.

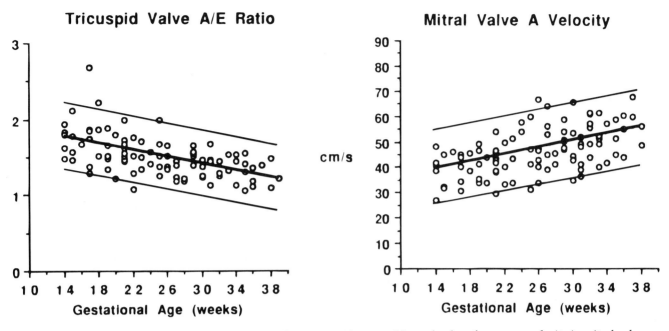

Figure 50: Normal values for a/e ratio in tricuspid valve.

Figure 51: Normal values for a wave velocity in mitral valve.

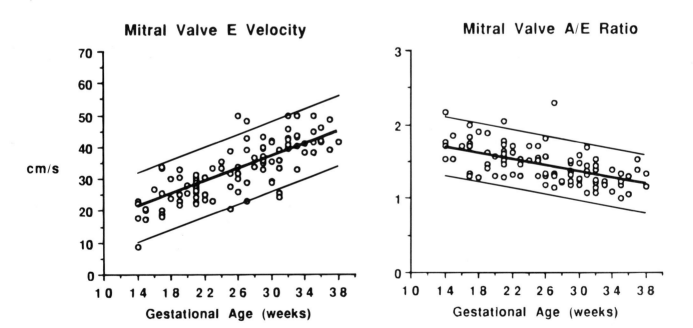

Figure 52: Normal values for e wave velocity in mitral valve.

Figure 53: Normal values for a/e ratio in mitral valve.

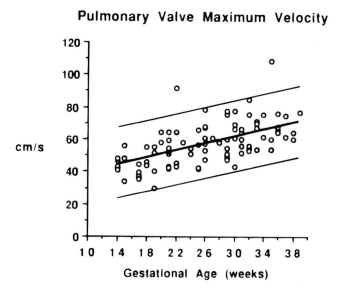

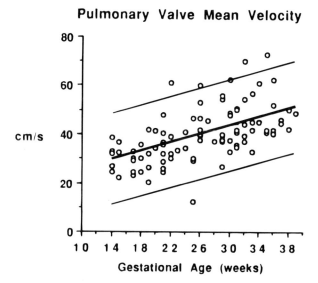

Figure 54: Normal values for peak velocity in the pulmonary root.

Figure 55: Normal values for mean velocity in the pulmonary root.

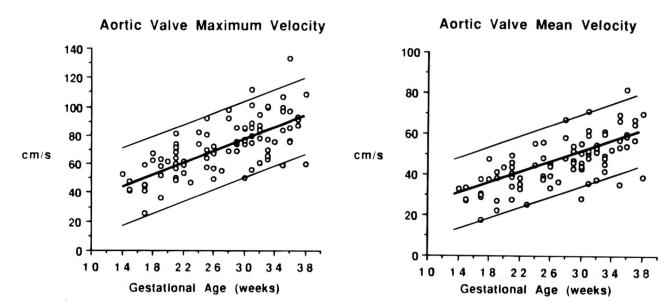

Figure 56: Normal values for peak velocity in the aortic root.

Figure 57: Normal values for mean velocity in the aortic root.

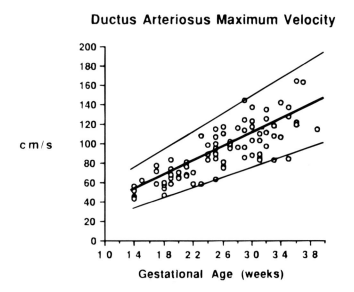

Figure 58: Normal values for peak velocity in the ductus arteriosus.

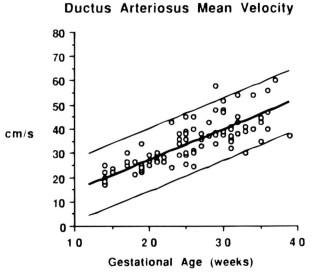

Figure 59: Normal values for mean velocity in the ductus arteriosus.

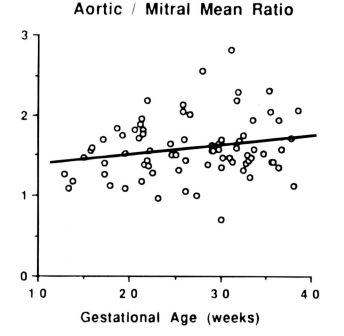

Figure 60: Normal values for ratio of aortic mean velocity to mitral mean velocity.

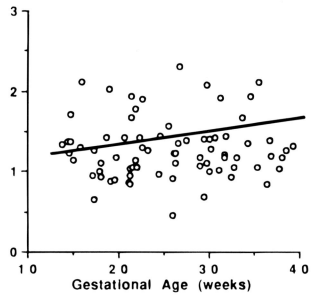

Figure 61: Normal values for ratio of pulmonary mean velocity to tricuspid mean velocity.

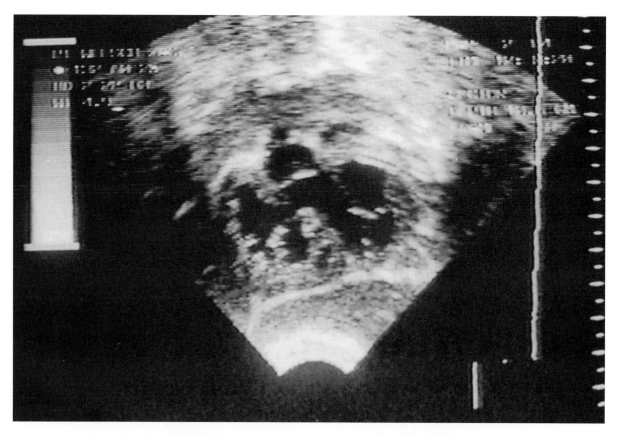

Figure 62: Subcostal long axial oblique view of transposition of the great arteries with large ventricular septal defect after pulmonary artery banding.

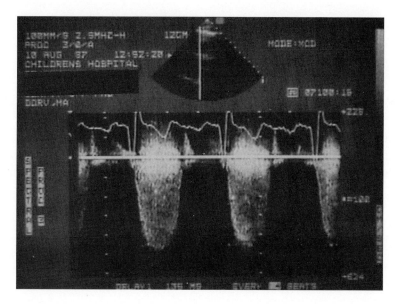

Figure 63: Continuous wave Doppler assessment of velocity distal to the band (4.7 m/s).

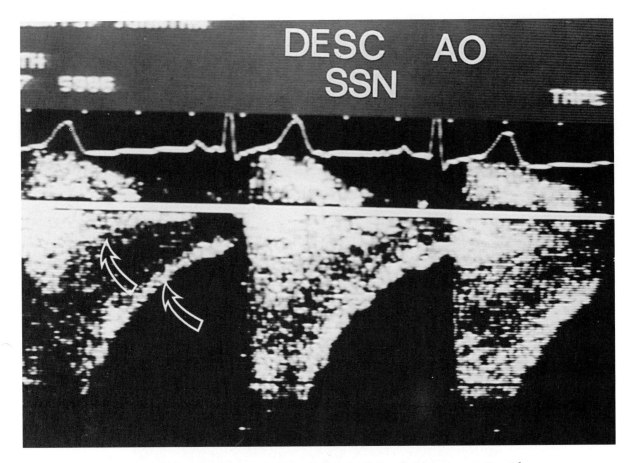

Figure 64: Continuous wave Doppler assessment of velocity distal to a coarctation. The arrows show the two dominant jets—the one proximal to the constriction and the one distal to the constriction.

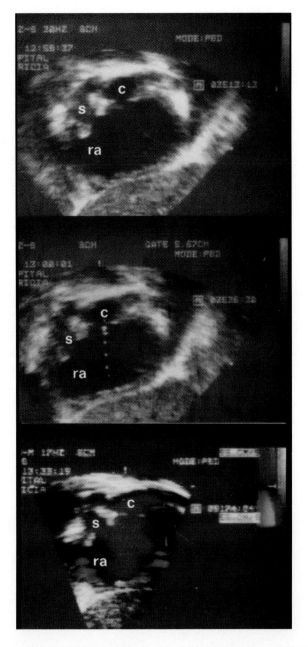

Figure 65: Top panel: Subcostal left oblique view of a heterotaxy patient following repair of total anomalous pulmonary venous connection. The pulmonary venous confluence (c) has been anastomosed to the left side of a common atrium. s = right superior vena cava; ra = right atrium. **Middle panel:** Pulsed Doppler sample volume has just been moved from the confluence to the atrium. **Bottom panel:** Color flow mapping does not show much change in mean velocity.

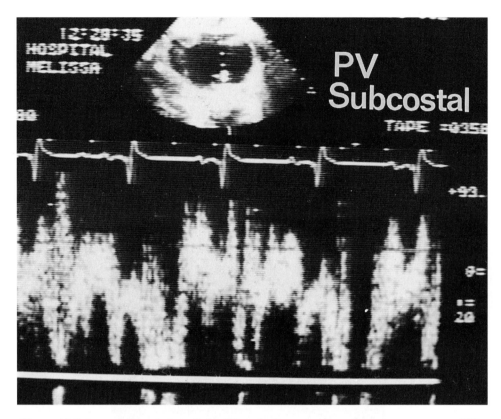

Figure 66: Subcostal frontal view. Pulsed Doppler interrogation of pulmonary venous (PV) flow in a patient similar to Figure 65 shows low-velocity, laminar flow.

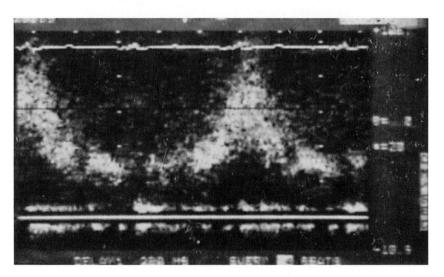

Figure 67: Pulsed Doppler interrogation of pulmonary venous confluence in a patient with severe obstruction. Note the low-velocity, continuous, laminar flow.

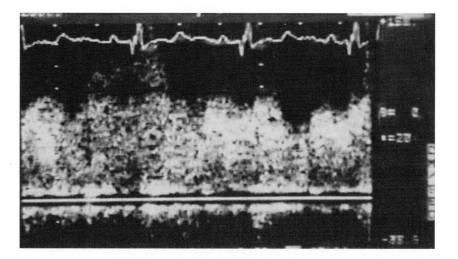

Figure 68: Pulsed Doppler interrogation of atrium adjacent to narrowed anastomosis, same patient as in Figure 67. Note the high-velocity, continuous, turbulent flow.

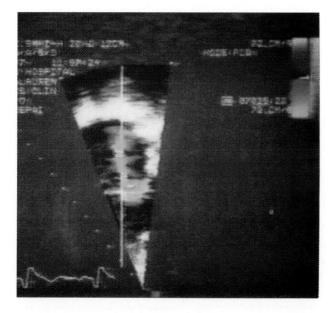

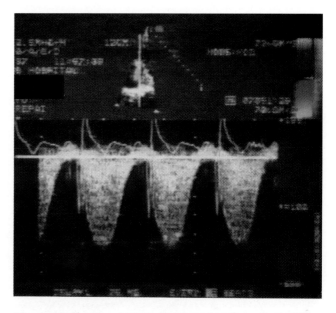

Figure 69: Alignment of continuous wave cursor with tricuspid regurgitant jet in a patient who has undergone repair of tetralogy of Fallot, apical view.

Figure 70: The tricuspid regurgitant jet in the patient of Figure 69 is 4.8 m/s.

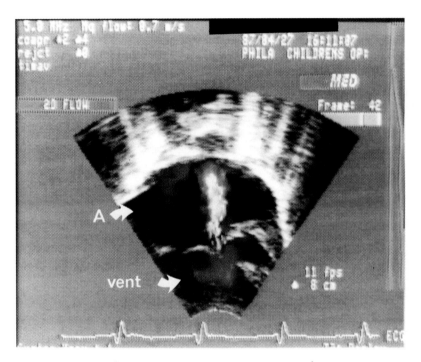

Figure 71: Regurgitant of the common atrioventricular valve in a heterotaxy patient, apical view.

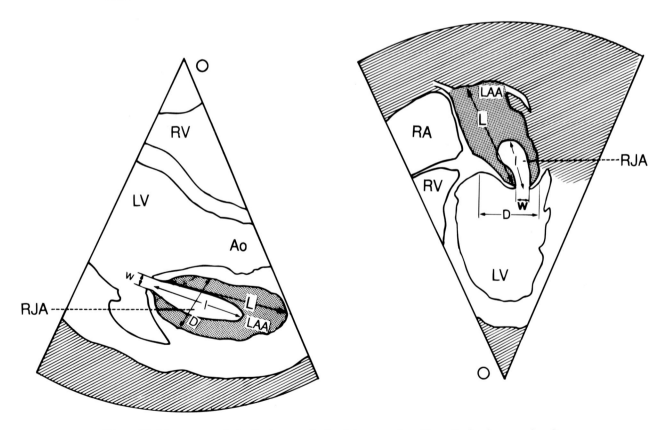

Figure 72: Measurement of mitral regurgitation jet parameters. D = mitral valve annulus dimension; l = length of jet; L = depth of left atrium; LAA (shaded area) = left atrial area; RJA = regurgitant jet area; w = jet width at the level of leaflets. Used with permission of American Journal of Cardiology.

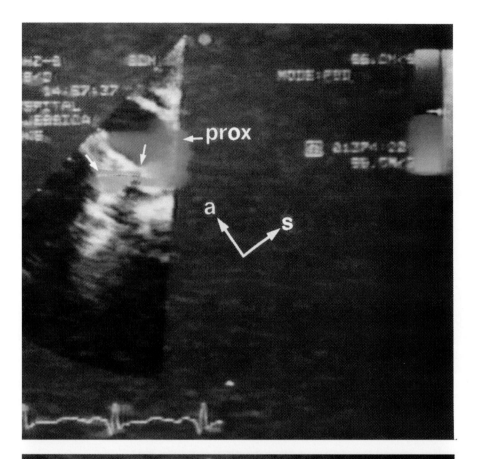

Figure 73: Doppler color flow mapping (high parasternal sagittal view) of central shunt in a patient who has undergone the Norwood procedure. The shunt takes off from the underside of the arch gusset. In systole, flow enters the shunt (unlabeled arrows) from the proximal (prox) arch.

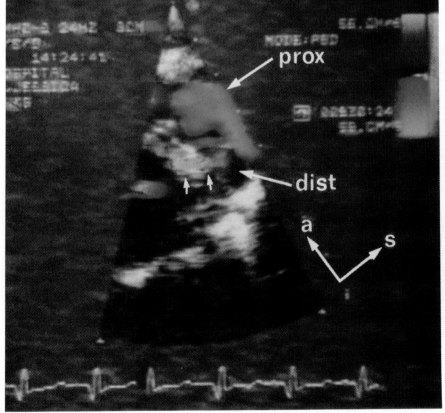

Figure 74: Same patient as in Figure 70. In diastole, flow enters the shunt (unlabeled arrows) from the distal (dist) arch.

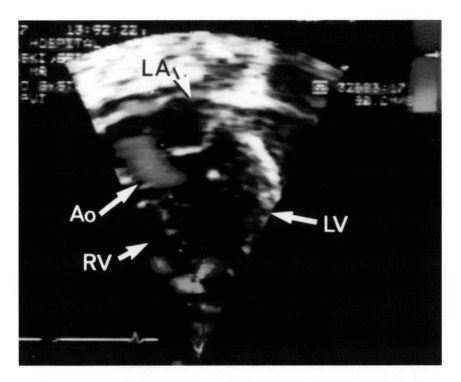

Figure 75: Apical "five-chamber view" showing residual apical muscular ventricular septal defect. LA = left atrium; Ao = aorta; RV = right ventricle; LV = left ventricle.

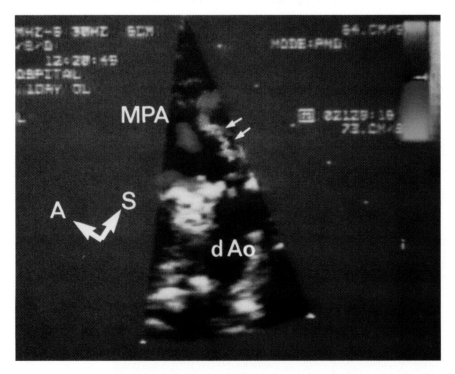

Figure 76: High parasternal view showing residual ductus arteriosus (arrows). MPA = main pulmonary artery; dAo = descending aorta.

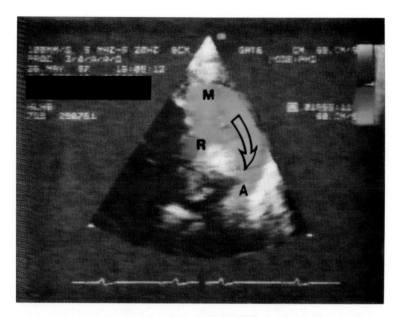

Figure 77: High parasternal view of right-to-left ductal flow (arrow). A = descending aorta; M = main pulmonary artery; R = right pulmonary artery takeoff.

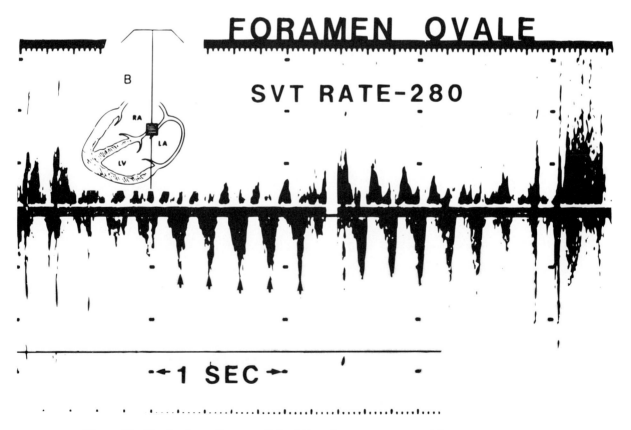

Figure 78: Fetal echocardiogram. Pulsed Doppler interrogation of flow across foramen ovale, showing supraventricular tachycardia (SVT).

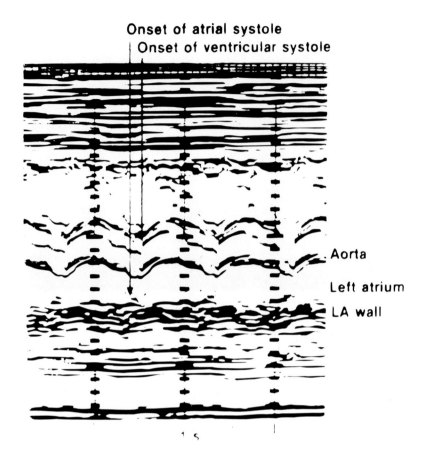

Figure 79: Fetal echocardiogram. Two-dimensional image-directed M-mode showing atrial contractions. Ventricular contractions are inferred from aortic valve openings.

Chapter 3

Malposition of the Heart

In this book, position of the heart will be arbitrarily defined by the trajectory of the ventricular apices. Levocardia is when the ventricles point to the patient's left. Mesocardia is when the ventricles point due anteriorly (Figure 1). Dextrocardia exists if the ventricles point to the patient's right (Figure 2).

A. Levocardia

When levocardia is discovered on the frontal sweep, the atrial configuration is such that one atrium is posterior and leftward while the other is anterior and rightward. Exceptions to this rule are exceedingly rare; the only example this author has seen was a case of levocardia in a situs inversus patient (Figure 3). Since situs inversus totalis is relatively uncommon and levocardia in that setting extremely rare, it may be quite some time before we find out if this exception is reproducible.

Thus, the relative uniformity of atrial and ventricular spatial configurations make the scanning protocol discussed in Chapter 2, section A consistently feasible.

B. Dextrocardia

Although many authors[1-5] have studied dextrocardia, detailed descriptions of imaging techniques have been lacking.

When dextrocardia (ventricular apex pointing to the right) is discovered on the initial subcostal frontal sweep, a slightly more complicated scanning protocol

is used in our laboratory. In levocardia, the atrial (or, more precisely, the *venous aspect* of the atria) are consistently positioned so that one is posterior and leftward while the other is anterior and rightward; however, in dextrocardia, the atria can be arranged in three ways. In one arrangement (type A), one atrium is posterior and rightward while the other is anterior and leftward (Figure 2). The atria can also be arranged side by side (type B). Finally, one atrium can be posterior and leftward while the other is anterior and rightward (type C), just as in the case of levocardia!* Thus, the frontal sweep should elucidate which one of the three configurations is present. Choice of subsequent subcostal sweeps to optimally display atrial anatomy is dependent on the type of configuration identified.

If one atrium is posterior and rightward while the other is anterior and leftward (type A), then the transducer should be rotated counterclockwise to produce a right oblique orientation and the trajectory of the sweep should be from left hip to right shoulder. Sagittal sweep from the patient's left to the patient's right should also yield helpful information.

If the atria are side by side (type B), we have found that oblique scans do not add significant data but that a sagittal sweep does help.

Finally, if one atrium is anterior and rightward and the other is posterior and leftward (type C), we use the same sweeps as are employed in levocardia.

The atrial configuration similarly affects the choice of suprasternal planes.

The ventricular and great artery anatomy is displayed best by the subcostal (or suprasternal) right oblique sweep and the sagittal sweep.

In our laboratory, we examined 19 consecutive dextrocardia patients using the scanning protocol just

---

* In an examination of 16 postmortem specimens with dextrocardia from the Cardiac Registry of the Children's Hospital of Philadelphia, it appeared that *any* atrial situs (and any ventricular loop!) could be seen with each atrial configuration. Type A (4 patients): {S,D,S} 2, {A,L,L} 2, type B (4 patients): {S,D,D,} 1, {S,L,L} 1, {I,L,I} 1, {I,L,L} 1; type C (8 patients): {A,L,L} 3, {S,D,S} 2, {A,D,S} 1, {S,L,L} 1, {I,L,I} 1.

outlined. Twelve subsequently had surgical or postmortem observations that could be utilized as a reference standard. The comparison between two-dimensional echocardiographic findings and surgery (or autopsy) is shown in Table I.

Out of a possible 60 anatomical diagnoses (appendage morphology, systemic and pulmonary vein connection sites), only two errors were made.

In many dextrocardia patients, the great arteries also point in a different trajectory. For example, in normally aligned great arteries in levocardia, the right pulmonary artery points to the right lateral aspect of the thoracic cage while the left pulmonary artery points posteriorly. In "dextrocardia with normally aligned great arteries," the right pulmonary artery usually points posteriorly and the left pulmonary points to the left lateral aspect of the thoracic cage. In fact, the pulmonary sinuses of Valsalva may be due anterior (or even anterior and *rightward*) to the aortic sinuses of Valsalva, and yet the great arterial situs would still be designated as solitus (normal) (see Chapter 4, section B, 3).

Table I

Comparison of Two-Dimensional Echocardiographic Findings and Surgery (or Autopsy) in Patients with Dextrocardia

Patients	Cardiac Segments (Atrial, Loop, G.A.)	Atrial Append	RSVC	LSVC	IVC or Azygos	Pulmonary Veins	Errors Found at Surgery or Autopsy
BW	A,L,L	I	CS	L-sided atrium	L-sided Az	R-sided atrium	None–Autopsy
MC	A,L,L	I	R-sided atrium	L-sided atrium	R-sided atrium	to LSVC	RSVC not present–Autopsy
W	A,L,L	R Isom	R-sided atrium	L-sided atrium	R-sided atrium	R-sided atrium	Pulm veins actually infracardiac–Autopsy
DL	S,L,D	S	R-sided atrium	CS	R-sided atrium	L-sided atrium	None–Autopsy
MF	A,D,S	I	R-sided atrium	L-sided atrium	R-sided atrium	L-sided atrium	None–Autopsy
WI	S,D,D	S(LJAA)	R-sided atrium	CS	R-sided atrium	L-sided atrium	None–Autopsy
SS	S,L,X	S(LJAA)	R-sided atrium	CS	R-sided atrium	L-sided atrium	None–Surgery
MK	S,L,L	S	R-sided atrium	None	R-sided atrium	L-sided atrium	None–Surgery
GR	S,D,D	S(LJAA)	R-sided atrium	None	R-sided atrium	L-sided atrium	None–Surgery
AZ	I,L,L	L Isom	None	L-sided atrium	L-sided Az	R-sided atrium	None–Surgery
KP	S,L,L	S	R-sided atrium	None	R-sided atrium	L-sided atrium	None–Autopsy
JM	S,L,L	S	R-sided atrium	CS	R-sided atrium	L-sided atrium	None–Surgery

{A,L,L} = atrial situs ambiguous, L-ventricular loop, L-related great arteries; Append = appendages; Az = azygos; CS = coronary sinus; I = inversus; IVC = inferior vena cava; L = left; Isom = atrial appendage isomerism; LJAA = left-sided juxtaposition of the atrial appendages; LSVC = left superior vena cava; pulm = pulmonary; R = right; RSVC = right superior vena cava; S = solitus; GA = great arteries.

C. Mesocardia

Patients with mesocardia (ventricular apex pointing ventrally) are best scanned with frontal (Figure 1) and sagittal sweeps. These two sweeps yield the same information in mesocardia as do left oblique and right oblique sweeps in levocardia.

The two most common mesocardia situations are cases with underdevelopment of the right lung and those with situs solitus of the atria associated with L-ventricular loop.

D. Thoracopagus Twins

Thoracoabdominally conjoined twins[6–11] represent one of the few conditions in which cardiac imaging is easier in utero than postnatally (Figure 4). This is due to window limitation imposed by the conjunction region and the associated omphalocele.

Cardiac conjunction can occur at several levels: at both ventricular (Figures 5 and 6) and atrial (Figure 7) levels, at only the atrial level, and occasionally at the venous level only. In addition to intra-twin septal defects, inter-twin communications must be characterized.

The most difficult portion of the cardiac mass to image are the systemic and pulmonary venous connections (Figure 8).

The atrial appendages can be difficult to identify because of their unusual spatial location. The atrial septum is frequently in an unusual orientation. The identification of atrioventricular connections and ventricular "situs" is usually straightforward.

The great arteries may have unusual proximal courses; however, the aortic arch and distal pulmonary arteries have more familiar configurations (Figure 9).

Cardiac catheterization and angiography are sometimes necessary. Postnatal magnetic resonance imaging may also help.

In August 1993, the first successful salvage of one twin in a thoracopagus set was achieved by Dr. William Norwood and Dr. James O'Neill at The Children's Hospital of Philadelphia. The cardiac mass was *not* divided; rather, the great arteries of the other twin were transected. The aortic root of the latter was connected with the ascending aorta of the salvaged twin with a non-valved conduit. The plan was designed not to "normalize" the anatomy but to normalize the physiology. Preoperative imaging should be undertaken with this goal in mind.

References

1. Rao PS. Dextrocardia: systemic approach to differential diagnosis. *Am Heart J* 1981; 102:389–403.

2. Rice MJ, Seward JB, Hagler DJ, Edwards WD, Julsrud PR, Tajik AJ. Left juxtaposed atrial appendages: diagnostic two-dimensional echocardiographic features. *J Am Coll Cardiol* 1983; 1:1330–1336.

3. Huhta JC, Hagler DJ, Seward JB, Tajik AJ, Julsrud PR, Ritter DG. Two-dimensional echocardiographic assessment of dextrocardia: a segmental approach. *Am J Cardiol* 1982; 50:1351–1360.

4. Lev M, Liberthson RR, Eckner FAO, Arcilla RA. Pathologic anatomy of dextrocardia and its clinical implications. *Circulation* 1968; 37:979–999.

5. Squarcia U, Ritter DG, Kincaid DW. Dextrocardia: angiocardiographic study and classification. *Am J Cardiol* 1973; 32:965–977.

6. Seo JW, Shin SS, Chi JG. Cardiovascular system in conjoined twins: an analysis of 14 Korean cases. *Teratology* 1985; 32:151–161.

7. Sabherwal U, Tandon R, Chopra P. Cardiovascular anomalies in conjoined thoracopagus twins. *Jap Heart J* 1979; 20:897–905.

8. Mathewson JW, Waldman JD, George L, Kirkpatrick SE, Turner SW, Pappelbaum SJ. Shared coronary arteries and coronary venous drainage in thoracopagus twins. *J Am Coll Cardiol* 1984; 3:1019–1025.

9. Sanders SP, Chin AJ, Parness IA, Benacerraf B, Greene MF, Epstein MF, Colan SD, et al. Prenatal diagnosis of congenital heart defects in thoracoabdominally conjoined twins. *N Engl J Med* 1985; 313:370–374.

10. Marin-Padilla M, Chin AJ, Marin-Padilla TM. Cardiovascular abnormalities in thoracopagus twins. *Teratology* 1981; 23:101–113.

11. Gerlis LM, Seo JW, Ho SY, Chi JG. Morphology of the cardiovascular system in conjoined twins: spatial and sequential segmental arrangements in 36 cases. *Teratology* 1993; 47:91–108.

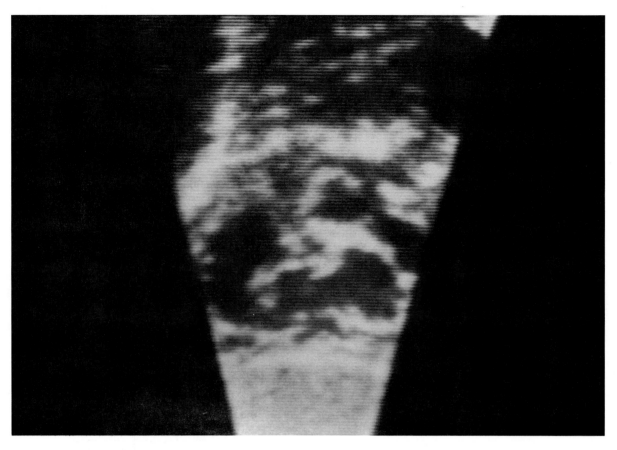

Figure 1: Subcostal frontal view of mesocardia. Note the atrioventricular valves opening directly at the observer.

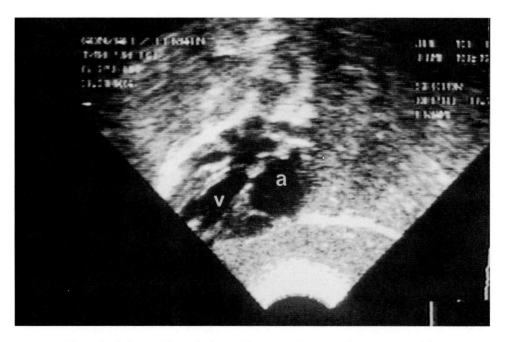

Figure 2: Subcostal frontal view of dextrocardia. a = atrium; v = ventricle.

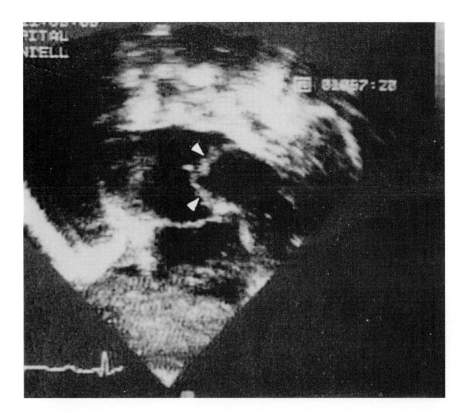

Figure 3: Subcostal frontal view of a rare patient with levocardia in whom one atrium is posterior and rightward and in the other is anterior and leftward. Note the orientation of the posterior part of the atrial septum.

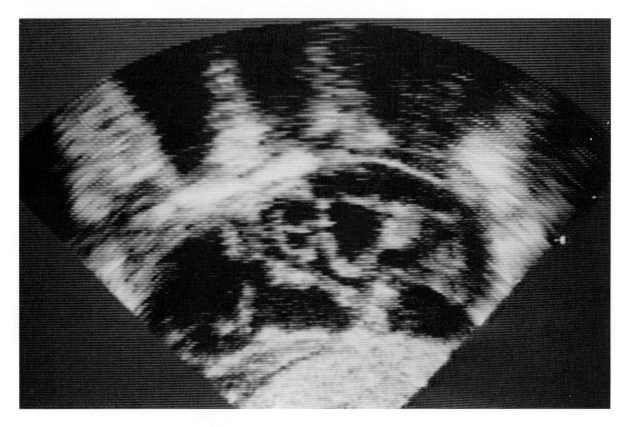

Figure 4: Subhepatic frontal view, thoracopagus twins. Note the ventricular-level conjunction.

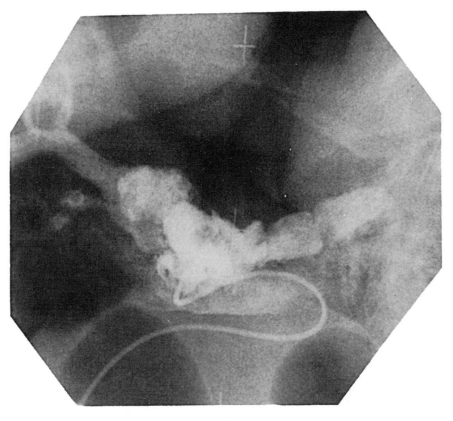

Figure 5: "Frontal" angiogram showing ventricular conjunction.

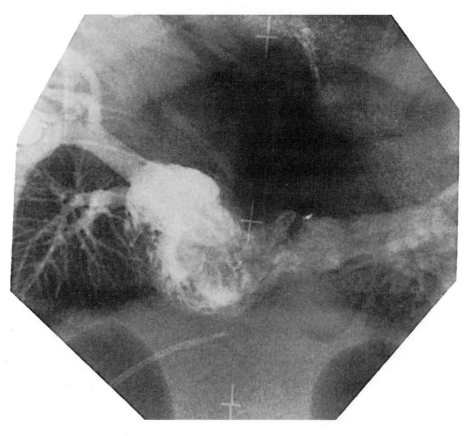

Figure 6: The conjoined ventricle is a morphological left ventricle.

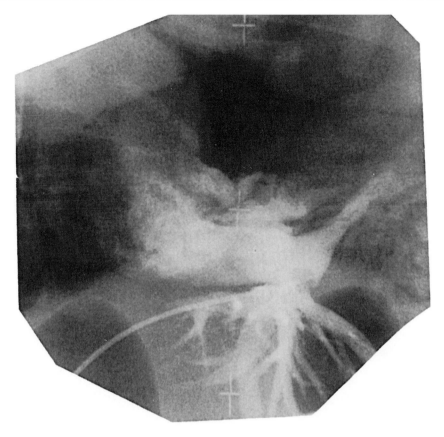

Figure 7: Atrial-level conjunction is present as well.

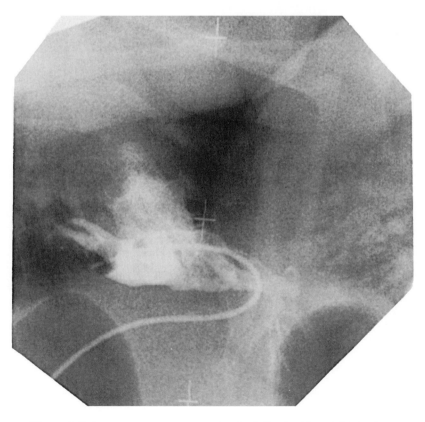

Figure 8: Pulmonary-venous connection is defined with atrial injection.

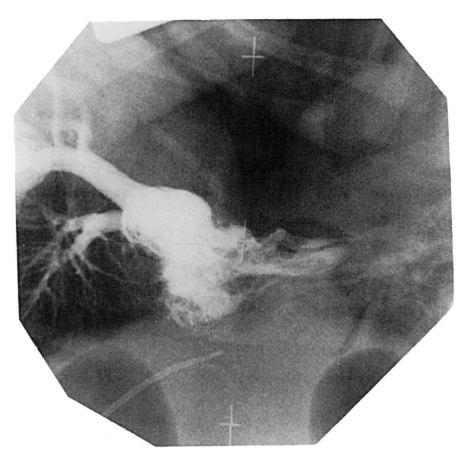

Figure 9: The aortic arch is seen. This twin had pulmonary stenosis.

Chapter 4

Segmental Diagnosis of the Heart

A. Background

While the etiology of most congenital heart malformations has not been discovered, the need for some system of nomenclature is widely accepted. The issue that has caused decades of controversy is which system to adopt. Two widely promoted systems are those of Van Praagh (modified by Weinberg) and Anderson. Because it is beyond the scope of this text to review the advantages and disadvantages of each, the reader is referred to discussions of these systems.[1,2]

Both systems will probably have to be reanalyzed and reorganized when a more complete understanding of *in utero* cardiac development is achieved. For example, it may turn out that a chamber may be best identified by certain *molecular* signatures! The current description of the sequence in human cardiac development has been reported by Streeter[3] and O'Rahilly.[4] The sequence of cardiac development in the chick has been described, and that in the mouse has also been investigated. The genomes of the chick and mouse are partly known, and the Human Genome Project has as its goal the complete sequencing of the genome of *Homo sapiens*. Recently, investigations have begun in other species as well.

The modified Van Praagh nomenclature system will be utilized in this text. Underpinning both this system and that of Anderson is the basic principle of Lev[5] termed *the morphological method*—a chamber is assigned a name based on particular gross anatomical features, *not* on spatial position. (The embryologic terms that are used in this text, e.g., septum secundum, sinus venosus defect, septal band, etc., are not meant to imply that the derivation of that structure is fully understood. Often the usage of a term becomes widespread despite the paucity of data justifying it.)

B. Cardiac Segments

There are three main segments: atrial situs, ventricular loop, and great arterial situs. There are two main alignments: atrioventricular and ventriculo-arterial.

1. Atrial Situs

An atrium is defined as a chamber that is immediately proximal to a ventricle. Most atria actually consist of two parts: a smooth portion and a trabeculated portion. The trabeculated portion is the appendage. The smooth portion consists of the systemic, coronary, and pulmonary veins. From observations of human embryo collections, it appears that the precursor for the appendages is the *primitive atrium* section of the straight heart tube and that for the smooth portion of the right and left atria are *sinus venosus* and *common pulmonary vein*, respectively.

The morphological right atrium is defined as that which has a morphological right atrial appendage; if an inferior vena cava is uninterrupted, i.e., passes through the liver, then the atrium that receives it is virtually always the right atrium. A morphological right atrial appendage has a broad base (Figure 1), rather than an os. It has a pyramidal configuration.

The morphological left atrium is defined as that which has a morphological left atrial appendage (Figure 2). In those with a well-formed septum primum attaching to the superior limbic band (septum secundum), the atrium on the side of the attachment points is the morphological left atrium.

Even when the appendages are *juxtaposed* instead of each lying to its own side of the arterial portion of the heart, each appendage still maintains its distinctive anatomical trademarks.

Atrial situs is designated either S (solitus), I (inversus), or A (ambiguous). Although the most rigorous definition involves the concept of *chirality,* or handedness, discussed below, sidedness of atrial virtually always corresponds to handedness.

2. Ventricular Loop

The fact that the heart tube does in fact loop has allowed the designation of ventricular "situs" to be built on "handedness" of the ventricle, not spatial position. Unlike atria, the sidedness of a ventricle often does not correlate well with handedness; thus, the more rigorous definition serves us better.

A morphological right ventricle is the one that is more coarsely trabeculated. The largest trabecula is one that runs from the apex toward the arterial outflow and bifurcates at its arterial end (Figure 3). It is termed *septal band* in the Van Praagh nomenclature system (and *septomarginal trabecula* in the Anderson nomenclature system) and can be seen by day 60 of fetal development.

A D-loop right ventricle is one in which the inflow (Figure 4), outflow, and septal surface conform to the axes of perpendicularly outstretched thumb, index finger, and middle finger of a right hand. Thus, the morphological right ventricle can be identified as a D-loop even when it is directly superior to, rather than to the side of, the morphological left ventricle.

An L-loop right ventricle is one in which the inflow, outflow, and septal surface conform to the axes of perpendicularly outstretched thumb, index finger, and middle finger of a left hand (Figures 5 and 6).

A morphological left ventricle is the less coarsely trabeculated one (Figure 7). The septal surface is smooth at its arterial end, a phenomenon already visible by the fifth month of fetal development.

3. Great Arterial Situs

The most reliable indicators of *which great vessel is which* are as follows:

a. the aorta is the vessel from which the first brachiocephalic artery arises

b. the aorta is the vessel from which the coronary arteries arise

c. the main pulmonary artery is the vessel that bifurcates into two branch pulmonary arteries.

Great arterial situs is the aspect of Van Praagh's nomenclature system that is the most difficult to use. The definitions of the four designations are as follows. S (solitus) signifies that there is a clockwise twist of the main pulmonary artery around the aorta (Figures 8 and 9) and requires that the ventriculo-arterial alignment be normal. I (inversus) refers to a counterclockwise twist of the main pulmonary artery around the aorta. D refers to any situation in which the aorta is to the right of the pulmonary artery and the ventriculo-arterial alignment is *not* normal. L refers to any situation in which the aorta is to the left of the pulmonary artery and the ventriculo-arterial alignment is not inversus.

The principal difficulty in applying these designations is their dependence on the particular ventriculo-arterial alignment. For example, many double-outlet right ventricle cases have a clockwise twist of the main pulmonary artery around the aorta but because the ventriculo-arterial alignment is not normal, the great arterial situs is termed D rather than S.

4. Atrioventricular Alignments

There are *two* components to these alignments: *atria-to-atrioventricular valve connections* and *atrioventricular valve-to-ventricle connections*. Within the former, there are four basic categories: normal, common atrioventricular canal, atrioventricular valve atresia (right or left), and the rare double-outlet atrium. Within atrioventricular valve-to-ventricle connections, there are three basic categories: normal, common-inlet, or double-inlet.

5. Ventriculo-arterial Alignments

There are six ventriculo-arterial alignments: normal, inversus, double-outlet right ventricle, double-outlet left ventricle, transposition of the great arteries, and anatomically corrected malposition. *Normal* is defined as aorta above the left ventricle (LV) and pulmonary artery above the right ventricle (RV) but with continuity between the aorta and an atrioventricular (AV) valve lying within the LV. *Inversus* is the mirror-image of normal. *Double-outlet right ventricle (DORV) and double-outlet left ventricle (DOLV)* are each divided into three cases: bilateral infundibulum, unilateral infundibulum, and absent infundibulum. For bilateral infundibulum, each great artery has to be >50% above the RV to be a DORV. Likewise, each great artery has to be >50% above the LV to be a DOLV. For unilateral infundibulum, the great artery with infundibulum has to be >50% above the RV and the great artery without infundibulum has to have continuity with the AV valve lying within the RV to be considered a DORV. The analogous situation applies to DOLV. For absent infundibulum, each great artery must be in continuity with the AV valve lying in the RV to be a DORV. The analogous criteria apply to DOLV. *Transposition of the great arteries* applies when the aorta is more than 50% above the RV and the pulmonary artery is more than 50% above the LV. Finally, in *anatomically corrected malposition*, the aorta is above the LV and the pulmonary artery is above the RV, but there is no continuity between aorta and the AV valve lying within the LV.

As would be expected, cases in which there is atresia of the main pulmonary artery are termed: "tetralogy of Fallot with pulmonary atresia" if there is aortic-mitral continuity, "right ventricular aorta with pulmonary atresia" if the aorta is aligned above the RV and there is not aortic-mitral continuity, and "left ventricular aorta with pulmonary atresia" if the aorta is aligned above the LV and there is not aortic-mitral continuity.

Cases of atresia of the ascending aorta are exceedingly rare, but criteria analogous to those for main pulmonary artery atresia should be used.

C. Heterotaxy

1. General Considerations

Heterotaxy can be defined as incomplete lateralization of the organs. Although there are few animal models, one that has been worked on extensively is the *iv/iv* mouse. The *iv/iv* mouse[6] exhibits random lateralization of the organs. Approximately 50% have D-looped ventricles and 50% have L-looped ventricles.

Recently, Brueckner[7] has mapped the *iv* gene to chromosome 12 in the mouse. A recently discovered gene *inv* has been mapped to mouse chromosome 4. Homozygosity for the *inv* gene is sufficient to produce 100% reversal of embryonic rotation and of stomach orientation but is not sufficient to always specify polarity of the heart and spleen.[8]

2. Spleen

Most but not all patients have abnormal splenic development.[9] The most frequently observed defects are: asplenia,[10–13] polysplenia,[14,15] and accessory spleens. The most reliable imaging techniques are magnetic resonance imaging and ultrasound.

3. Bronchi/Lungs[16–18]

The right and left bronchi are arranged in eparterial and hyparterial fashion, respectively, in a normally lateralized individual. Eparterial means situated above the pulmonary artery; hyparterial means situated below the pulmonary artery. The lungs are tri-lobed on the right and bi-lobed on the left. In heterotaxy syndrome, the bronchi can be "solitus," "inversus," bilaterally eparterial, or bilaterally hyparterial. The lungs can be solitus, inversus, bilaterally tri-lobed, or bilaterally bi-lobed.

4. Stomach

The stomach can be right-sided, left-sided, or midline.

5. Liver

The liver is typically symmetrical, but it can be solitus or inversus.

References

1. Weinberg PM. Systemic approach to diagnosis and coding of pediatric cardiac disease. *Pediatr Cardiol* 1986; 7:35–48.
2. Miller GAH, Anderson RH, Rigby ML. *The Diagnosis of Congenital Heart Disease*. Castle House, Tunbridge Wells, 1985.
3. Streeter GL. Developmental horizons in human embryos: description of age groups XIX, XX, XXI, XXII, and XXIII. *Contrib Emb* 1951; 34:165–196.
4. O'Rahilly R. The timing and sequence of events in human cardiogenesis. *Acta Anat* 1971; 79:70–75.
5. Lev M. The pathologic diagnosis of positional variations in cardiac chambers in congenital heart disease. *Lab Invest* 1954; 3:71–82.

6. Seo JW, Brown NA, Ho SY, Anderson RH. Abnormal laterality and congenital cardiac anomalies: relations of visceral and cardiac morphologies in the iv/iv mouse. *Circulation* 1992; 86:642–650.

7. McGrath J, Horwich AL, Brueckner M. Duplication/deficiency mapping of situs inversus viscerum (iv), a gene that determines left-right asymmetry in the mouse. *Genomics* 1992; 14:643–648.

8. Yokoyama T, Copeland NG, Jenkins NA, Montgomery CA, Elder FFB, Overbeek PA. Reversal of left-right asymmetry: a situs inversus mutation. *Science* 1993; 260:679–682.

9. Layman TE, Levine MA, Amplatz K, Edwards JE. "Asplenic syndrome" in association with rudimentary spleen. *Am J Cardiol* 1967; 20:136–140.

10. Campbell M, Deuchar DC. Absent inferior vena cava, symmetrical liver, splenic agenesis, and situs inversus, and their embryology. *Br Heart J* 1967; 29:268–275.

11. Anderson C, Devine WA, Anderson RH, Debich DE, Zuberbuhler JR. Abnormalities of the spleen in relation to congenital heart malformations of the heart: a survey of necropsy findings in children. *Br Heart J* 1990; 63:122–128.

12. VanMierop LHS, Wiglesworth FW. Isomerism of the cardiac atria in the asplenia syndrome. *Lab Invest* 1962; 11:1303–1315.

13. Freedom RM. Aortic valve and arch anomalies in the congenital asplenia syndrome: case report, literature review and re-examination of the embryology of the congenital asplenia syndrome. *Johns Hopkins Med J* 1974; 135:124–135.

14. Peoples WM, Moller JH, Edwards JE. Polysplenia: a review of 146 cases. *Pediatr Cardiol* 1983; 4:129–137.

15. Garcia OL, Mehta AV, Pickoff AS, Tamer DF, Ferrer PL, Wolff GS, Gelband H. Left isomerism and complete atrioventricular block: a report of six cases. *Am J Cardiol* 1981; 48:1103–1107.

16. Partridge JB, Scott O, Deverall PB, Macartney FJ. Visualization and measurement of the main bronchi by tomography as an objective indicator of thoracic situs in congenital heart disease. *Circulation* 1975; 51:188–196.

17. Caruso G, Becker AE. How to determine atrial situs? *Br Heart J* 1979; 41:559–567.

18. Devine WA, Debich DE, Taylor SR. Symmetrical bronchial pattern with normal atrial morphology. *Int J Cardiol* 1988; 20:395–398.

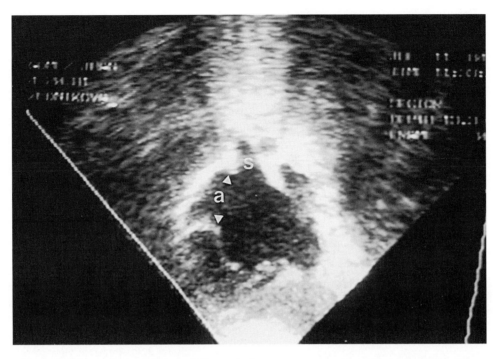

Figure 1: Subcostal sagittal view. Adjacent to the superior vena cava (s) is a broad-based appendage (a). The pyramidal shape is characteristic of a morphological right atrial appendage.

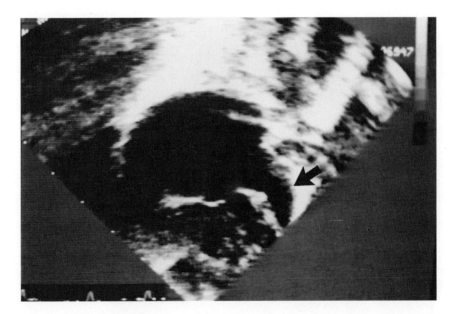

Figure 2: Apical view. Adjacent to the atrioventricular groove is a finger-like appendage (arrow). This configuration is characteristic of a morphological left atrial appendage.

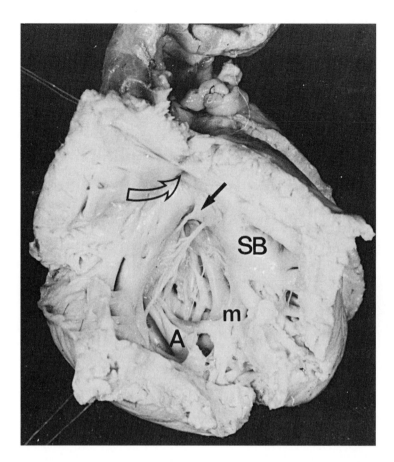

Figure 3: Postmortem view of right ventricle. The closed arrow points to the medial papillary muscle insertion at the bifurcation of the septal band (SB). The open arrow points to the arterial outflow. A = anterior papillary muscle; m = moderator band.

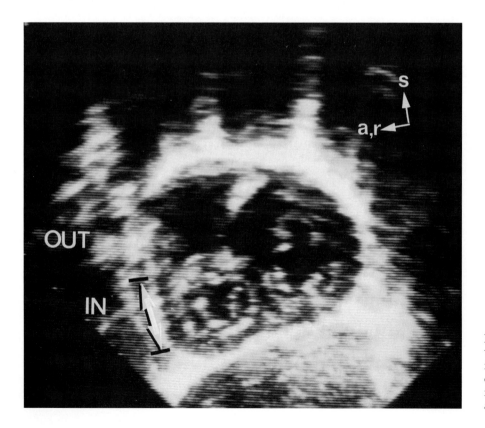

Figure 4: Subcostal left oblique view. The moderator band, as it runs from the free wall to the septum, divides the right ventricle into inflow (IN) and outflow (OUT). This is a D-loop right ventricle.

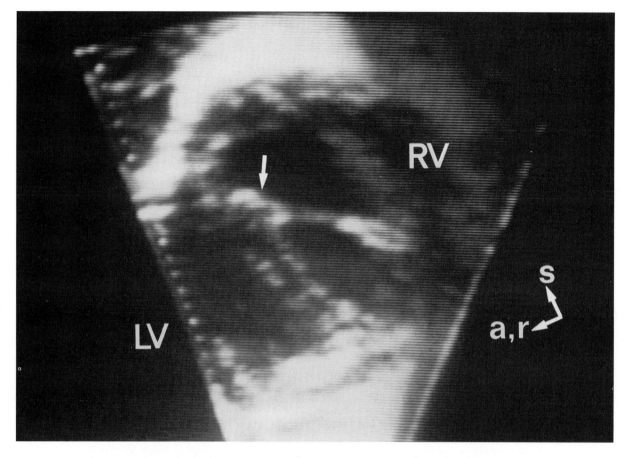

Figure 5: Subcostal left oblique view of right ventricle in L-loop. The medial papillary muscle (arrow) can be seen. LV = left ventricle; RV = right ventricle.

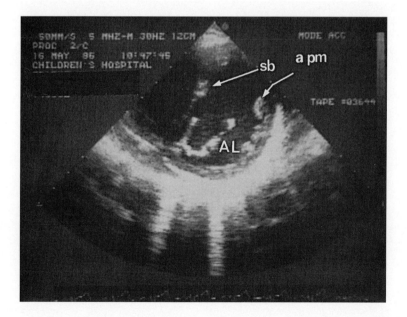

Figure 6: Parasternal short axis view. The anterior papillary muscle (apm) and septal band (sb) are characteristic of a right ventricle. This is L-loop. AL = anterior tricuspid leaflet.

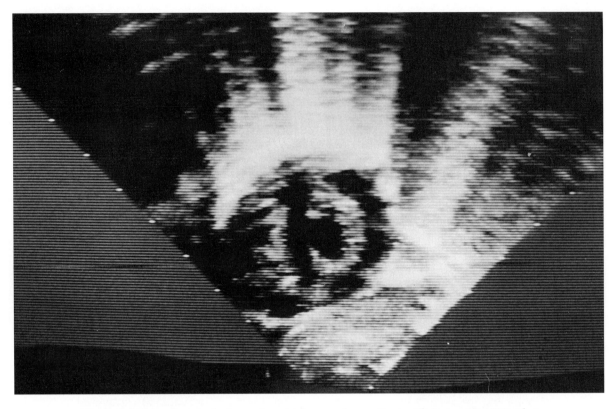

Figure 7: Leftward part of subcostal sagittal sweep in a patient with levocardia. Note that the posterior ventricle's septal surface is much smoother than the anterior ventricle's septal surface. Thus, the posterior ventricle is the left ventricle; the anterior ventricle is the right ventricle.

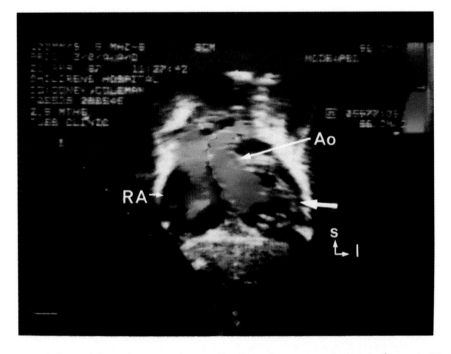

Figure 8: Subcostal frontal sweep of normally aligned great arteries. Note the aorta (Ao) starts posterior, inferior, and to the left. Its trajectory takes it anterior and rightward. RA = right atrium.

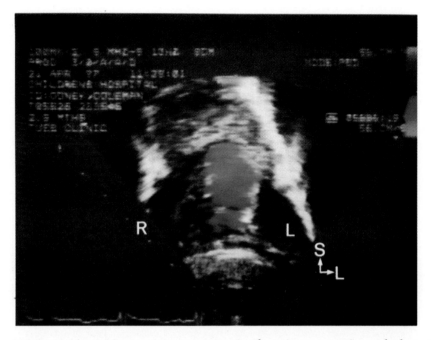

Figure 9: Subcostal frontal sweep continues anteriorly. The pulmonary outflow, which starts in an anterior and rightward location, progresses so that it lies posterior and to the left of the aorta. This clockwise twist of the main pulmonary artery around the aorta defines solitus great arteries.

Chapter 5

Atria

A. Appendage Morphology

A noninvasive technique for determining appendage morphology would be valuable for determination of atrial situs. Two-dimensional echocardiography (2-D echo) has been used to *infer* atrial appendage morphology based on (a) the position of the abdominal aorta and the inferior vena cava relative to the vertebral column and (b) the pattern of hepatic venous connection.[1] However, we have noted a significant number of cases in which this inferential method of determining atrial situs by 2-D echo led to conclusions regarding atrial appendage morphology which proved erroneous at postmortem examination; thus, we believe that the *appendages themselves* should be imaged.

Although it is difficult to consistently display atrial appendages using only frontal and sagittal subcostal views,[2] we examined 300 consecutive patients under 2 years of age using additional subcostal axial views[3] to assess how often the distinctive shape of each appendage and its junction with the rest of the atrial chamber could be recognized.

We began by displaying the abdominal great vessels in a transverse projection at a level just cephalad to the superior renal poles. (Although Huhta[1] has reported that this is approximately at the T_{10} level, we did not attempt to test that hypothesis.) The transducer was angled progressively more cranially to track the inferior vena cava and hepatic veins until they connected to the heart. We deliberately chose this view to follow the course of the inferior vena cava rather than using a parasagittal view; subtle details such as the inferior vena cava *crossing the midline* immediately prior to entering an atrium cannot be reliably assessed by using

parasagittal views of the abdomen. Likewise, deciding the descending aorta's position vis-a-vis the middle of the spine is much easier using transverse scans. For example, a typical right aortic arch descends on the right in the upper thorax but crosses to the left just above the diaphragm; this crossing is hard to appreciate using parasagittal views. The pattern of hepatic venous connection was traced using both transverse and parasagittal views. In cases with an azygos vein, this was tracked until the entrance site was identified. Data on the abdominal great vessels and the hepatic veins were first used to infer atrial appendage morphology, according to the algorithm proposed by Huhta (Figure 1).[1]

The examination was continued by imaging the atrial appendages directly. Although the morphological left atrial appendage (LAA) can sometimes be displayed in a subcostal four-chamber cut (Figure 2, top), the use of a "long axial oblique" view[3] allows the examiner to better distinguish the appendage from the left pulmonary veins (Figure 2, bottom). The morphological right atrial appendage (RAA) is often seen in a subcostal parasagittal view; however, the axial oblique cut usually displays the crista terminalis better (Figure 3).

An atrial appendage was judged to be morphologically *right* if it displayed a blunt shape and had a broad junction with the rest of the atrial chamber. If a distinct ridge (crista terminalis) could be visualized at the superior aspect of the junction, this also signified a morphologically RAA. Another way of diagnosing a broad junction was if the posterior extent of the junction of the appendage with the rest of the atrium was far from the atrioventricular groove.

An appendage was judged to be morphologically

left if it displayed a narrow junction with the rest of the atrial chamber[4] and if the junction, or os, had the same or smaller width as the proximal portion of the appendage (Figure 2). If the posterior extent of the junction of the appendage to the rest of the atrium was near the atrioventricular groove, this also signified a morphologic LAA (Figure 2). The overall shape of an LAA was not used as a diagnostic criterion, since it is quite variable and can be "Z-shaped."[5]

If both appendages were judged to be morphological RAAs, the designation right (atrial) isomerism was applied.[6] Left (atrial) isomerism was diagnosed if both appendages were judged to be morphological LAAs.

In the 291 cases with visceral (hepatic) situs solitus or inversus, we examined how frequently atrial appendage morphology could be displayed by 2-D echo. In the nine cases with visceral heterotaxy (symmetrical liver with or without abnormal gastric situs), we compared 2-D echo determination of atrial appendage morphology to that predicted by the inferential method.

In the 291 cases without visceral heterotaxy, a morphological RAA could be imaged successfully in *all* patients; it was right-sided in 285, left-sided in three, and juxtaposed to the left in three patients. The long axial oblique view emerged as an easier way of verifying the diagnosis of complete left-sided juxtaposition of the atrial appendages than the previously proposed method of identifying septum secundum orientation.[2,7] In the three patients with this lesion, the right atrium had a concave or straight (instead of convex) right anterior border in this view. The posterior extent of the junction of the superior appendage with the rest of the atrium was far from the atrioventricular groove in all three of these cases, so that even though the appendages were arranged in a superior-inferior orientation, the chirality[8] of the appendages was clearly solitus.

A morphological LAA was imaged successfully in 279 patients (96%); it was left-sided in 276, and right-sided in three patients.

Of the nine cases with visceral heterotaxy, five had a solitus arrangement of atrial appendages on 2-D echo, two had an inversus arrangement, and two had right (atrial) isomerism (Figure 4). Of note, in four of these nine cases, the inferential method predicted an atrial situs *different* from the diagnosed by direct 2-D echo visualization of appendage morphology (Table I).

Both of the cases with inversus appendage arrangement of 2-D echo and one of the five cases with solitus appendages would have been deemed right isomerism on the basis of abdominal aorta and inferior vena cava positions together with the pattern of hepatic venous connection (see Table I, Figures 5 and 6). All three of these cases demonstrated aortocaval juxtaposition to the right of the spine and did not manifest total anomalous hepatic venous connection.

Another of the five cases with solitus atrial appendages by 2-D echo would have been classified as inversus by the inferential method. In this case, the abdominal aorta was to the right of the spine while the inferior vena cava was to the left (Figure 7).

Autopsy or angiography examinations, available in three of the four cases in which there was discordance between the two methods of determining atrial appendages situs (direct and inferential), agreed with the direct method.

If we are to apply the morphological method[9] of diagnosis and naming of the cardiac chambers, appendage morphology should be assessed to determine atrial situs. As Van Praagh[10] has stated, cardiac chambers should not be diagnosed and named in terms of the vessels of entry. Thus, the inferior vena cava (IVC) entrance site[11] should not be used since this vessel can, in a few instances, enter a chamber that all other features suggest is a morphological left atrium.[8] Another reason why the use of the IVC entrance site is difficult for the echocardiographer is that in many cases of "absence of the suprarenal portion of the inferior vena cava,"[12] even the "hepatic" segment of the IVC[8] can be impossible to identify. The hepatic drainage may be by more than one orifice; this would make it impossible to say which orifice is the "hepatic" segment of the IVC.

Other indirect indicators of atrial situs should also be discarded. Caruso and Becker[13] reported three cases in which the situs of the tracheobronchial tree[14,15] did not correctly predict the appendage situs. These authors suggest that since isomerism of the tracheobronchial tree is not invariably associated with atrial appendage isomerism, the morphology of the appendages themselves should be identified to determine atrial situs. Abdominal visceral situs is also not always predictive of thoracic situs.[16] Splenic status is not predictive of atrial appendage isomerism.[13,17] Finally, truly indeterminate appendage morphology appears to be very rare in the same way that truly indeterminate ventricular morphology is rare.[18]

In explaining the differences between our results and those of Huhta,[1] we note that it is difficult to precisely ascertain the "T_{10} level" recommended for transverse scanning of the abdominal aorta and the inferior vena cava. (Even a one-vertebra error[19] can lead to an opposite conclusion about sidedness of the inferior vena cava.) Using a transverse cut somewhat more cephalad might eliminate the confusion about sidedness of the inferior vena cava; however, it would create problems about sidedness of the lower descending

Table I

Echocardiographic Data in Four Cases of Heterotaxy: Comparison of Two Methods of Designating Atrial Situs

						Echocardiographic Data			Designation of Atrial Situs		
Abd Ao	*IVC*	*HVC*	*Drainage of Venae Cavae*	*Drainage of Pulmonary Veins*	*Appendages*	*Inferential*	*Direct*	*Autopsy/ Angio*
R	R	NL	RSVC→right-sided atrium RIVC→right-sided atrium	Left-sided	Solitus	Right isomerism	Solitus	Solitus (Angio)
R	R	PAHVC	RIVC→right-sided atrium LSVC→left-sided atrium RIVC→right-sided atrium	LPV→LSVC RPV→?	Inversus	Right isomerism	Inversus	Inversus (Autopsy)
R	R	NL	LSVC→left-sided atrium RIVC→left-sided atrium	Right-sided atrium	Inversus	Right isomerism	Inversus	NA
R	L	NL	RSVC→right-sided atrium LSVC→left-sided atrium LIVC→left-sided atrium	Right-sided atrium	Solitus	Inversus	Solitus	Solitus (Angio)

L = left; LIVC = left-sided inferior vena cava; LPV = left pulmonary veins; LSVC = left-sided superior vena cava; NA = not available; NL = normal; PAHVC = partial anomalous hepatic venous connection; RIVC = right-sided inferior vena cava; RPV = right pulmonary veins; RSVC = right superior vena cava.

aorta. In patients with solitus atria, right aortic arch, and right upper descending aorta, the aorta crosses the midline at a level higher than that of the superior renal poles and would therefore appear on the right side of the spine if a transverse abdominal cut higher than ours were employed.[20]

A limitation of the study was the relatively small number of heterotaxy patients, which was possibly explained by our requirement that the liver be symmetric; this may be too stringent an entrance criterion since occasional patients with left atrial isomerism may have a normal appearing liver.

Although we had virtually complete success in displaying appendage morphology in the patient population under 2 years of age, subcostal sweeps are difficult to perform on many older children and adults, making direct visualization of the atrial appendages problematic in these latter groups. Axial oblique-equivalent spin echo magnetic resonance imaging and transesophageal echocardiography may help.

Further investigation of other anatomical features of the atria may establish additional indicators of atrial appendage morphology. The taenia sagittalis may be a reliable indicator of a morphological RAA; however, so far we have been unable to consistently detect this structure by 2-D echo imaging. It is possible that suprasternal notch imaging using 7.5 MHz transducers may display the pectinate muscle architecture sufficiently to establish atrial situs.

As improvements in the surgical management of heterotaxy occur, accurately establishing the atrial situs of every patient is becoming more important.[21–23] Finally, the association of left atrial appendage isomerism (Figure 8) with conduction abnormalities also makes accurate appendage indentification valuable to the clinician.

B. Juxtaposition of the Atrial Appendages

Left-sided juxtaposition of the atrial appendages (LJAA)[24-30] occurs when the right atrial appendage, instead of lying to the right and anterior of the great arterial trunks, is situated posterior and to the left of them. The right atrial appendage in LJAA is invariably positioned between the area of the great arterial trunks and the left atrial appendage (Figure 9). LJAA is typically associated with several ventriculoarterial alignments (double-outlet right ventricle, transposition of the great arteries, and anatomically corrected malposition). It frequently coexists with hypoplasia of the tricuspid valve and right ventricular inflow as well as with the {S,D,L} segmental combination. Atrial septal defect creation and intra-atrial baffle procedures may be more challenging in LJAA.

Although an early report noted the difficulty of displaying the appendages themselves,[2] subsequent work has dispelled this myth. Largely through the utilization of more views [i.e., adding the left oblique sweep (Figures 10–13) and the right oblique cut to the frontal and sagittal sweeps developed earlier], both the morphological right atrial appendage and the morphological left atrial appendage can be identified consistently in the infant from the subcostal window. In the frontal sweep, if both great arteries lie at the right edge of the heart border, the examiner should expect to find the appendages juxtaposed at the left heart border.

In most infants, the two juxtaposed appendages can also be displayed from the suprasternal window. Larger children present more difficulty to the examiner; parasternal short axis views can usually display the fact that a portion of the right atrium extends far to the left of its usual site.

The problem with Chin's original suggestion[2] of identifying the posterior orientation of the septum secundum (Figure 14) is that in some cases of LJAA the septum secundum is very small. The unusually curved appearance reported by Rice et al. is in fact not pathognomonic of LJAA but is actually typical of features in certain atrial configurations found in dextrocardia (see Chapter 3, section B). Another reason that atrial septal morphology should not be counted on to make the diagnosis is that most LJAA patients have a very large atrial septal defect because of malalignment of the sep-

tum secundum vis-à-vis the septum primum (see Chapter 8, section B).

Right-sided juxtaposition of the atrial appendages occurs when the left atrial appendage, instead of lying to the left and anterior of the great arteries, is situated posterior and to the right of them.

C. Cor Triatriatum Dexter

Cor triatriatum dexter[31-34] occurs when the eustachian valve (Figure 15), or right venous valve of the inferior vena cava,[35] is unusually large. Normally, the valve involutes. Sometimes the tissue fenestrates, and a veil-like network, or rete Chiari, persists. If the valve persists without fenestration, it can obstruct right ventricular filling.

Subcostal left oblique (Figure 16) and sagittal views are most helpful.

D. Cor Triatriatum Sinister

Cor triatriatum sinister[36-38] (sinistrum) occurs when a left atrial "membrane" divides the left atrium into a portion receiving the pulmonary veins and a portion giving rise to the left atrial appendage. (If the left atrial appendage is superior to the membrane, the entity is best called supramitral ring.)

Although it often occurs in isolation, it can coexist with other intracardiac lesions. It is most challenging to identify in malformations with severe subpulmonary stenosis; the diminished pulmonary blood flow in such patients usually masks the physiological significance of the left atrial membrane.

The membrane can be identified in any of several views from the subcostal window (Figures 17 and 18). Color Doppler imaging is probably best done from apical and parasternal windows.

The most challenging part of cor triatriatum is to visualize the distal (low-pressure) chamber. The proximal (high-pressure) chamber is often so bulbous that it virtually obliterates the low-pressure chamber.

E. Isolated Atrial Inversion

So-called isolated atrial inversion {I,D,S} (or {S,L,I}) is quite rare,[39] except in heterotaxy.

References

1. Huhta JC, Smallhorn JF, Macartney FJ. Two-dimensional echocardiographic diagnosis of situs. *Br Heart J* 1982; 48:97–108.

2. Chin AJ, Bierman FZ, Williams RG, Sanders SP, Lang P. Two-dimensional echocardiographic appearance of complete left-sided juxtaposition of the atrial appendages. *Am J Cardiol* 1983; 52:346–348.

3. Chin AJ, Yeager SB, Sanders SP, Williams RG, Bierman FZ, Burger BM, Norwood WI, et al: Accuracy of prospective two-dimensional echocardiographic evaluation of left ventricular outflow tract in complete transposition of the great arteries. *Am J Cardiol* 1985; 55:759–764.

4. Sharma S, Devine W, Anderson RH, Zuberbuhler JR. Identification and analysis of left atrial isomerism. *Am J Cardiol* 1987; 60:1157–1160.

5. Van Mierop LHS. Morphological characteristics of the atria and their variations, including characteristics in the splenic syndrome. In: Godman MJ (ed). *Paediatric Cardiology 4*. Churchill Livingstone, Edinburgh, 144–152, 1981.

6. Van Mierop LHS, Wiglesworth FW. Isomerism of the cardiac atria in the asplenia syndrome. *Lab Invest* 1962; 11:1303–1315.

7. Rice MJ, Seward JB, Hagler JD, Edwards WD, Julsrud PR, Tajik AJ. Left juxtaposed atrial appendages: diagnostic two-dimensional echocardiographic features. *J Am Coll Cardiol* 1983; 1:1330–1336.

8. Van Praagh R, Weinberg PM, Matsuoka R, Van Praagh S. Malpositions of the heart. In: Adams FH, Emmanouilides GC (eds). *Moss's Heart Disease in Infants, Children, and Adolescents.*. Williams and Wilkins, Baltimore, 1983, pp 422–458.

9. Lev M. Pathological diagnosis of positional variations in cardiac chambers in congenital heart disease. *Lab Invest* 1954; 3:71–82.

10. Van Praagh R, David I, Van Praagh S. What is a ventricle? The single ventricle trap. *Pediatr Cardiol* 1982; 2:79–84.

11. Sanders SP. Echocardiography and related techniques in the diagnosis of congenital heart defects. *Echocardiography* 1984; 1:185–217.

12. Freedom RM, Ellison RC. Coronary sinus rhythm in the polysplenia syndrome. *Chest* 1973; 63:952–958.

13. Caruso G, Becker AE. How to determine atrial situs? *Br Heart J* 1979; 41:559–567.

14. Landing BH, Lawrence T-Y K, Payne VC, Wells TR. Bronchial anatomy in syndromes with abnormal visceral situs, abnormal spleen and congenital heart disease. *Am J Cardiol* 1971; 28:456–462.

15. Partridge JB, Scott O, Deverall PB, Macartney FJ. Visualization and measurement of the main bronchi by tomography as an objective indicator of thoracic situs in congenital heart disease. *Circulation* 1975; 51:188–196.

16. Chacko KA, Krishnaswami S, Sukumar IP, Cherian G. Isolated levocardia; two cases with abdominal situs inversus, thoracic situs solitus, and normal circulation. *Am Heart J* 1983; 106:155–159.

17. Freedom RM. Aortic valve and arch anomalies in the congenital asplenia syndrome. *Johns Hopkins Med J* 1974; 135:124–135.

18. Van Praagh R, Plett JA, Van Praagh S. Single ventricle: pathology, embryology, terminology, and classification. *Herz* 1979; 4:113–150.

19. Sapire DW, Ho SY, Anderson RH, Rigby ML. Diagnosis and significance of atrial isomerism. *Am J Cardiol* 1986; 58:342–346.

20. Baron MG. Right aortic arch. *Circulation* 1971; 44:1137–1145.

21. Van Mierop LHS. Diagnostic code for congenital heart disease. *Pediatr Cardiol* 1984; 5:331–362.

22. Weinberg PM. Systematic approach to diagnosis and coding of pediatric cardiac disease. *Pediatr Cardiol* 1986; 7:35–48.

23. Van Mierop LHS. Diagnostic code for congenital heart disease, supplement. *Pediatr Cardiol* 1986; 7:31–34.

24. Rosenquist GC, Stark J, Taylor JFN. Anatomical relationships in transposition of the great arteries. Juxtaposition of the atrial appendages. *Ann Thorac Surg* 1974; 18:456–461.

25. Wood AE, Freedom RM, Williams WG, Trusler GA. The Mustard procedure in transposition of the great arteries associated with juxtaposition of the atrial appendages with and without dextrocardia. *J Thorac Cardiovasc Surg* 1983; 85:451–456.

26. Melhuish BPP, Van Praagh R. Juxtaposition of the atrial appendages. A sign of severe cyanotic congenital heart disease. *Br Heart J* 1968; 30:269–284.

27. Mendelsohn G, Hutchins GM. Juxtaposition of the atrial appendages. Reinterpretation as an accessory appendage or atrial deverticulum. *Arch Pathol Lab Med* 1977; 101:409–492.

28. Allwork SP, Urban AE, Anderson RH. Left juxtaposition of the auricles with l-position of the aorta. Report of 6 cases. *Br Heart J* 1977; 39:299–308.

29. Wagner HR, Alday LE, Vlad P. Juxtaposition of the atrial appendages: report of six necropsied cases. *Circulation* 1970; 42:157–163.

30. Freedom RM, Harrington DP. Anatomically corrected malposition of the great arteries. *Br Heart J* 1974; 36:207–215.

31. Burton DA, Chin A, Weinberg PM, Pigott JD. Identification of cor triatriatum dexter by two-dimensional echocardiography. *Am J Cardiol* 1987; 60:409–410.

32. Alboliras ET, Edwards WD, Driscoll DJ, Seward JB. Cor triatriatum dexter by two-dimensional echocardiographic diagnosis. *J Am Coll Cardiol* 1987; 9:334–337.

33. Hansing CE, Young WP, Rowe GG. Cor triatriatum dexter. *Am J Cardiol* 1972; 30:559–564.

34. Thomka I, Bendig L, Szente A, Arvay A. Cor triatriatum dextrum simulating right ventricular myxoma and pulmonary stenosis. *Thorac Cardiovasc Surg* 1983; 31:114–116.

35. Limacher MC, Gutgesell HP, Vick GW, Cohen MH, Huhta JC. Echocardiographic anatomy of the Eustachian valve. *Am J Cardiol* 1986; 57:363–365.

36. Ostman-Smith I, Silverman NH, Oldershaw P, Lincoln C, Shinebourne EA. Cor triatriatum sinistrum: diagnostic features on cross sectional echocardiography. *Br Heart J* 1984; 51:211–219.

37. Schluter M, Langenstein BA, Thier W, Schmiegel WH, Krebber HJ, Kalmar P, Hanrath P. Transesophageal two-dimensional echocardiography in the diagnosis of cor triatriatum in the adult. *J Am Coll Cardiol* 1983; 2:1011–1015.

38. Jacobstein MD, Hirschfeld SS. Concealed left atrial membrane: pitfalls in the diagnosis of cor triatriatum and supravalvar mitral stenosing ring. *Am J Cardiol* 1982; 49:780–786.

39. Clarkson PM, Brandt PWT, Barratt-Boyes BG, Neutze JM. Isolated atrial inversion. *Am J Cardiol* 1972; 29:877–881.

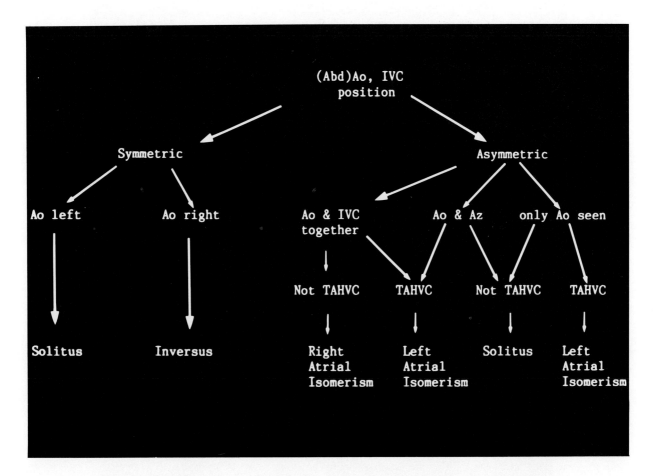

Figure 1: Algorithm proposed by Huhta[1] for designating atrial situs based on: (a) position of the abdominal aorta and inferior vena cava relative to the vertebral column and (b) the pattern of hepatic venous connection. Total anomalous hepatic venous connection was defined as "separate hepatic venous connection directly to an atrium via one or more veins." Abd = abdominal; Ao = aorta; Az = azygos vein; IVC = inferior vena cava; TAHVC = total anomalous hepatic venous connection.

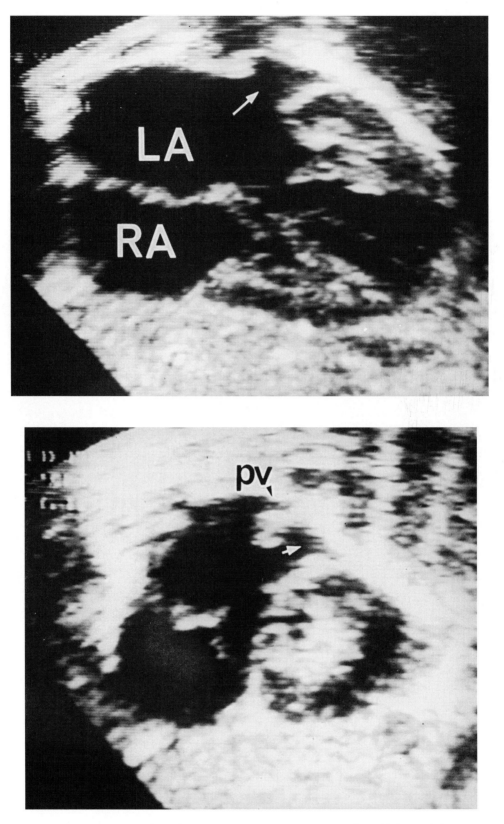

Figure 2: Top: Subcostal four-chamber view. Arrow points to orifice of left atrial (LA) appendage. RA = right atrium. **Bottom:** Long axial oblique view. Both the left superior pulmonary vein (pv) and the left atrial appendage orifice (arrow) can be displayed simultaneously.

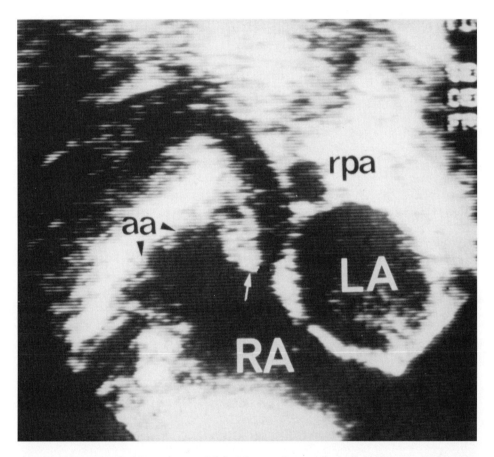

Figure 3: Long axial oblique view of the right atrial appendage (aa). The crista terminalis shown by the white arrow. rpa = right pulmonary artery; LA = left atrium; RA = right atrium.

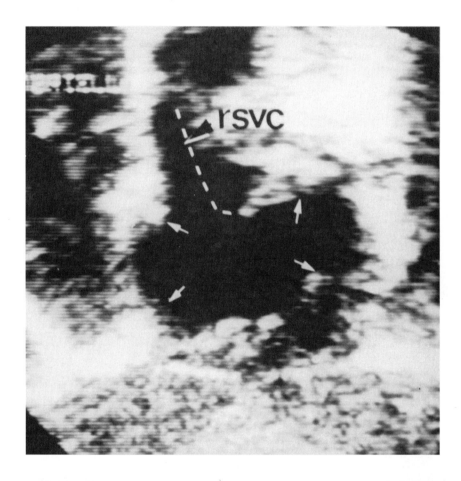

Figure 4: Top: Right atrial appendage isomerism (long axial oblique view). The junction (white arrows) of both atrial appendages with common atrium are broad. rsvc = right superior vena cava. **Bottom:** Abdominal great vessels in transverse view (same patient as above). The inferior vena cava (ivc) and the aorta (ao) are both to the right of midline. The dashed line bisects the vertebral column. r = right; l = left.

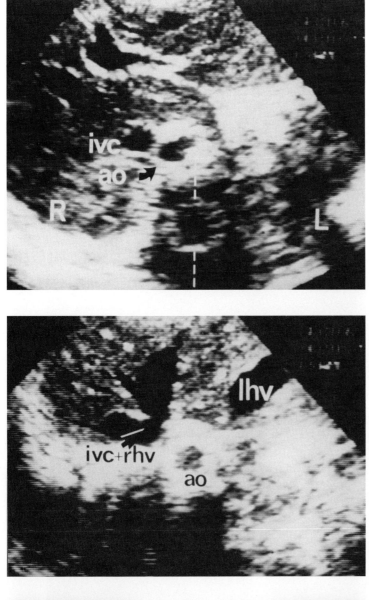

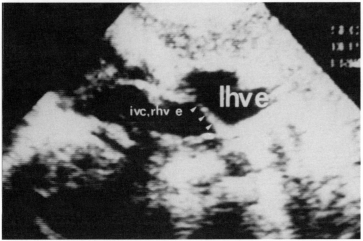

Figure 5: Inversus atrial appendages. **Top:** Transverse view of the abdomen. The inferior vena cava (ivc) and abdominal aorta (ao) both lie to the right of the midline. The dashed line shows the middle of the spine. R = right; L = left. **Middle:** Cranial angulation of transducer from above plane brings the hepatic venous system into view. The right hepatic veins (rhv) joint the ivc, while the left hepatic veins (lhv) do not. **Bottom:** Further cranial angulation displays entrance sites (e) of the ivc and right hepatic veins (rhv) on the one hand and left hepatic veins (lhv) on the other. The arrowheads show the most inferior portion of the atrial septum in this patient with heterotaxy.

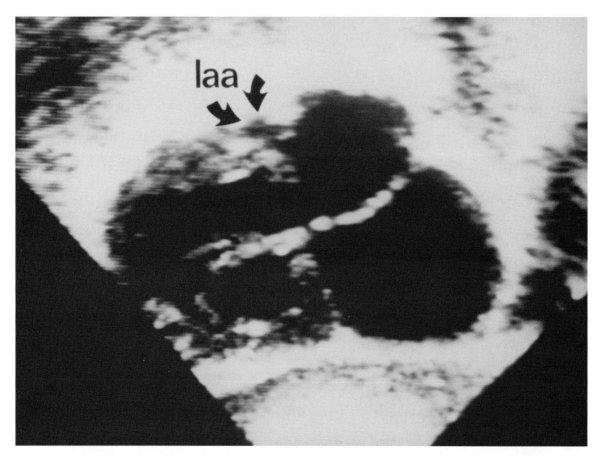

Figure 6: Subcostal four-chamber cut, same patient as in Figure 5. In this patient with dextrocardia, the right-sided appendage is seen to be a morphological left atrial appendage (laa).

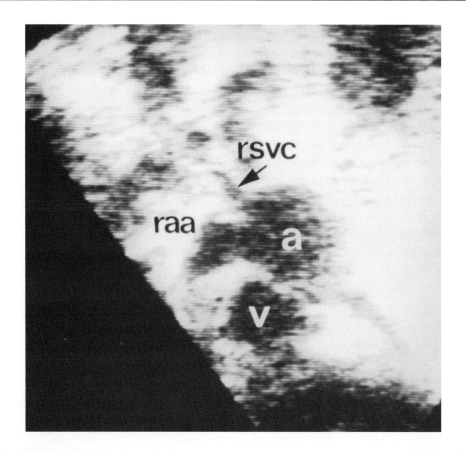

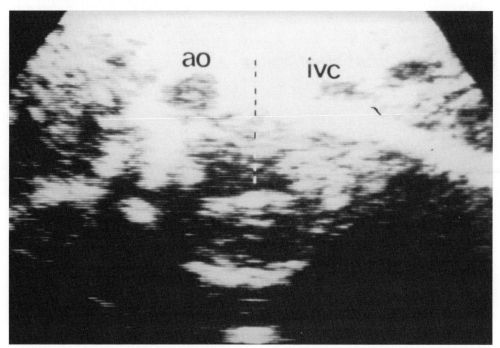

Figure 7: Top: In this patient, with solitus atrial appendages, the broad junction of the morphological right atrial appendage (raa) is displayed in this parasagittal view. a = atrium; v = ventricle; rsvc = right superior vena cava. **Bottom:** Abdominal transverse view of the same patient as above. Since the aorta is to the right of midline (dashed line) and the inferior vena cava (ivc) is to the left, the inferential method[1] (see Figure 1) would have predicted inversus atrial appendages.

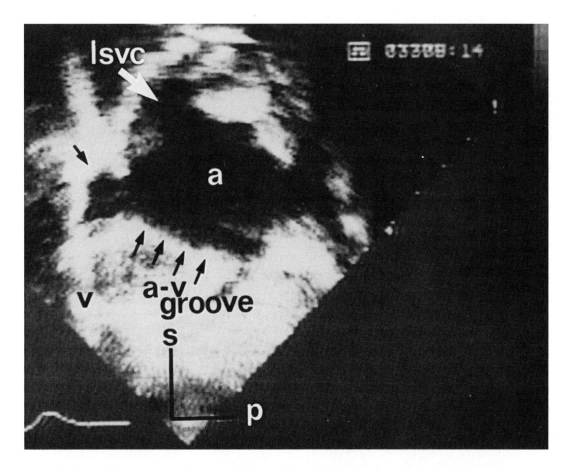

Figure 8: Subcostal sagittal view of left atrial isomerism. Note how there is no ridge adjacent to the left superior vena cava (lsvc) orifice but rather a long smooth drop until the os of the left atrial appendage (unlabeled black arrow) is seen near the left atrioventricular (a-v) groove.

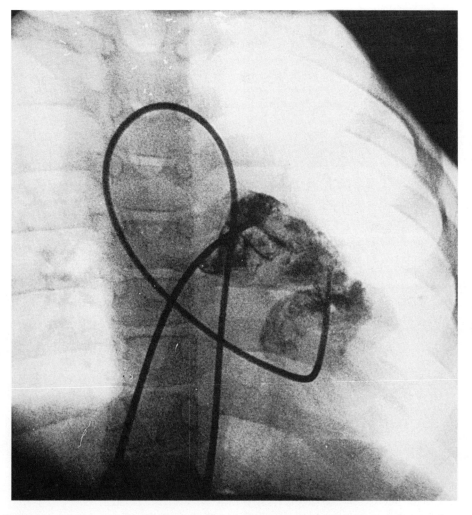

Figure 9: Anteroposterior angiogram showing left-sided juxtaposition of the atrial appendages.

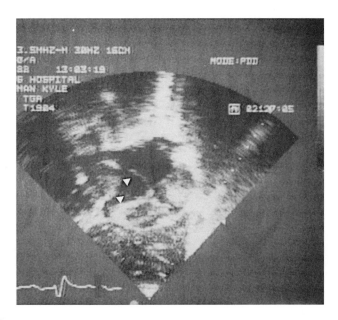

Figure 10: Subcostal left oblique view (rightward and inferior part of the sweep). Note the concave right atrial border.

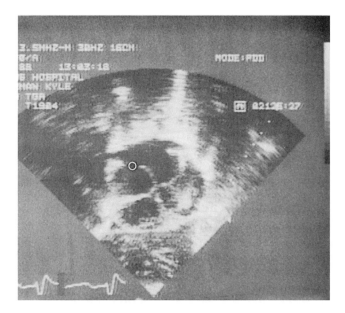

Figure 11: Subcostal left oblique view, slightly left of and superior to the plane shown in Figure 10. The malalignment-type ASD (open circle) is now visible.

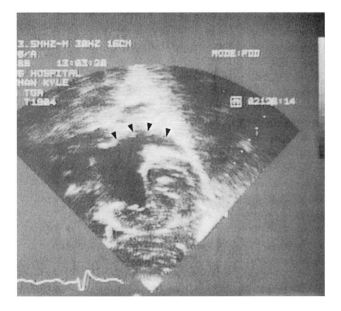

Figure 12: Subcostal left oblique view, slightly left of and superior to the plane shown in Figure 11. The ASD is no longer visible. The outline of the appendage (arrowheads) is emerging. The great arteries have not been traversed yet; thus, this appendage is posterior to the great arteries.

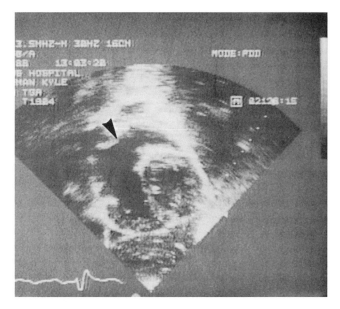

Figure 13: Subcostal left oblique view, slightly left of and superior to the plane shown in Figure 12. The base of the appendage is broad (arrow), characteristic of a right atrial appendage.

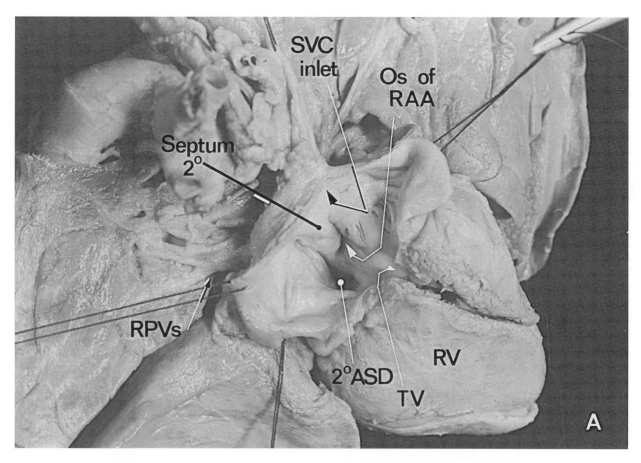

Figure 14: Postmortem view of the right atrium, showing the malalignment-type septal defect (ASD). Because the os of the right atrial appendage (RAA) is so posterior, the septum secundum (Septum 2°) is abnormally oriented. RPVs = right pulmonary veins; RV = right ventricle; SVC = superior vena cava; TV = tricuspid valve.

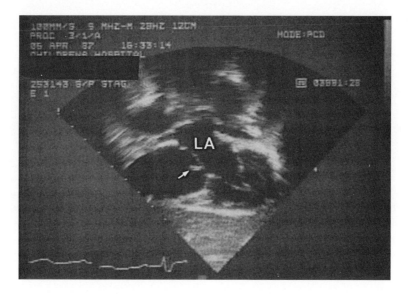

Figure 15: Subcostal frontal view of the typical eustachian valve. LA = left atrium.

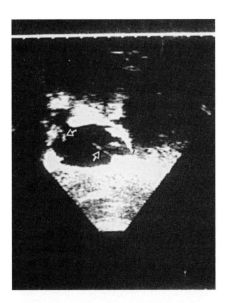

Figure 16: Subcostal left oblique view of an unusually large right venous valve (arrows) with a superior component as well.

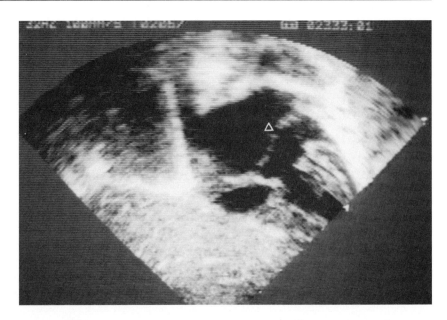

Figure 17: Subcostal frontal view of cor triatriatum. The defect (arrowhead) in the membrane is about 3 mm.

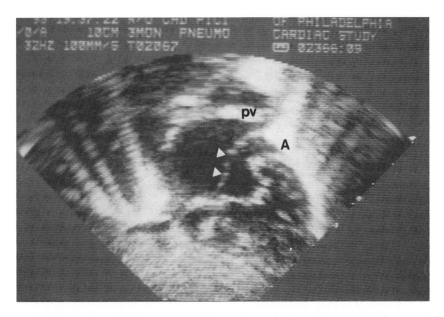

Figure 18: Subcostal right oblique view of the patient shown in Figure 17. The membrane divides the left atrium into a portion receiving the pulmonary veins (pv) and a portion giving rise to the left atrial appendage (A).

Chapter 6

Systemic Veins

A. Left Superior Vena Cava to Coronary Sinus

This anomaly can be recognized consistently only from the suprasternal window. (Thus, in older children, it may be impossible to rule out.) The frontal (Figure 1) and left oblique (Figure 2) views are the most helpful. It can be inferred from the subcostal sweep (Figures 3–5) when the coronary sinus appears dilated and there exists a circular structure (left superior cava) near the left atrioventricular groove.

B. Left Superior Vena Cava to Left Atrium

The suprasternal frontal view again establishes the presence of a left superior vena cava; however, a dilated coronary sinus cannot be visualized, and the left superior cava drains into the roof of the left atrium. Before ligation is contemplated, it is helpful to know about the presence of any bridging vein (Figures 6 and 7).

C. Absent Right Superior Vena Cava

This anomaly appears to be quite rare[1,2] (in the absence of heterotaxy). The upper body drains via a left superior vena cava.

D. Innominate Vein Under Arch

The usual position for the innominate vein (bridging vein) is cephalad to the arch. In rare cases, its course is actually inferior to the arch.[3–6]

In the suprasternal frontal view, it is identified as immediately posterior to the ascending aorta.

In the sagittal view, it appears immediately under the arch, *cephalad* to the branch pulmonary arteries.

E. Right Superior Vena Cava to Left Atrium

This rare anomaly[7–9] can be diagnosed by careful subcostal sweeps [especially left oblique and sagittal (Figure 8)]. The right upper pulmonary vein may have a common entrance (Figure 9).

F. Left Hepatic Vein to Coronary Sinus

Although heterotaxy patients frequently demonstrate anomalous hepatic venous connections, occasionally patients with completed lateralization can have such malformations. There can be anomalous hepatic vein to right atrium (independent of the inferior vena cava orifice), anomalous hepatic vein to left atrium (an extremely rare entity), or anomalous drainage of the left hepatic vein to the coronary sinus.[10,11]

The subcostal frontal sweep should allow the identification of this malformation. A long axial oblique equivalent is the best for confirming that the hepatic vein connects to the coronary sinus itself rather than to the right atrium.

G. Unroofed Coronary Sinus

A defect in the wall dividing the left atrium from the coronary sinus may occur in isolation or together with a left superior vena cava.[12–14] When it occurs in association with intracardiac anomalies, such as tetralogy of Fallot or tricuspid atresia,[15] there can be significant residual right-to-left shunting through the defect in the early postoperative period if it is not recognized at the time of repair. Resolving the thin wall is sometimes possible in the neonate who can be scanned from multiple windows (Figures 10 and 11) with 5.0 and 7.5 MHz transducers. The long axial oblique equivalent[16] is the best view (Figure 12 and Figure 6 in Chapter 8). Color Doppler displays the left-to-right shunt from the left atrium, passing through the mouth of the coronary sinus, into the right atrium. In those with right heart obstructive lesions, the recognition of this anomaly may be difficult even with color Doppler echocardiography because there is a coexistent patent foramen ovale; the mouth of the coronary sinus may not be very large and the coronary sinus septal defect (CSSD) may not be identified until the foramen ovale is closed surgically. This diagnostic problem has led some surgeons to repair tricuspid atresia with a systemic venous baffle diverting inferior vena cava blood to a superiorly located atriopulmonary anastomosis; this technique leaves the orifice of the coronary sinus in the pulmonary venous compartment. Even if such a patient has a CSSD that has eluded detection, it will not cause hemodynamic embarrassment.

H. Interrupted Inferior Vena Cava with Azygos Continuation

Although this anomaly is usually found in patients with heterotaxy syndrome, it can occasionally be found in isolation. Even when it appears at first glance to be an isolated finding, a careful search for signs of heterotaxy is warranted. On electrocardiogram, this may include abnormalities of atrial rate and p wave axis (and even third-degree atrioventricular block). On roentgenogram, there may be bilateral bi-lobed or tri-lobed lungs. On magnetic resonance imaging, there may be splenic abnormalities, bronchial symmetry, or abnormal bronchopulmonary artery relationships. (The morphological right bronchus usually lies above the pulmonary artery while the morphological left bronchus is below the pulmonary artery.)

On echocardiography, there may be bilaterally symmetric atrial appendages (e.g., bilateral morphological left atrial appendages).

The easiest way to detect this anomaly is to employ a transverse abdominal view.[17] The superior renal poles are identified and the whole transducer plane is then moved slightly cephalad. The spinal column is displayed with the abdominal aorta on its ventral surface. The liver is even further ventral. The inferior vena cava (IVC) lies within the liver in a characteristic location. In patients with interrupted IVC, there is no structure at this characteristic location; instead, an azygos vein *posterior* to the liver substance and posterior to the abdominal aorta is visualized (see Figure 1A of Chapter 20). The usual cranial angulation of the transducer from the starting transverse abdominal plane is not effective in displaying the more cephalad course of the azygos. A parasagittal plane is better (Figure 13). The azygos continues upward to join the ipsilateral, or less commonly the contralateral, superior vena cava (Figures 14 and 15).

References

1. Lenox CC, Zuberbuhler JR, Park SC, Neches WH, Mathews RA, Fricker FJ, Bahnson HT, Siewers RD. Absent right superior vena cava with persistent left superior vena cava: implications and management. *Am J Cardiol* 1980; 45:117–122.

2. Choi JY, Anderson RH, Macartney FJ. Absent right superior caval vein (vena cava) with normal atrial arrangement. *Br Heart J* 1987; 57:474–478.

3. Fujimoto K, Abe T, Kumabe T, Hayabuchi N, Nozaki Y. Anomalous left brachiocephalic (innominate vein): MR demonstration. *AJR* 1992; 159:479–480.

4. Smallhorn JF, Zielinsky P, Freedom RM, Rowe RD. Abnormal position of the brachiocephalic vein. *Am J Cardiol* 1985; 55:234–236.

5. Gerlis LM, Ho SY. Anomalous subaortic position of the brachiocephalic (innominate) vein: a review of published reports and report of three new cases. *Br Heart J* 1989; 61:540–545.

6. Choi JY, Jung MJ, Kim YH, Noh CI, Yun YS. Anomalous subaortic position of the brachiocephalic vein (innominate vein): an echocardiographic study. *Br Heart J* 1990; 64:385–387.

7. Vaquez-Perez J, Frontera-Izquierdo P. Anomalous drainage of the right superior vena cava into the left atrium as an isolated anomaly: rare case report. *Am Heart J* 1979; 97:89–91.

8. Kirsch WM, Carlsson E, Hartmann AF. A case of anomalous drainage of the superior vena cava into the left atrium. *J Thorac Cardiovasc Surg* 1961; 41:550–556.

9. Chin AJ. Subcostal two-dimensional echocardio-

graphic identification of right superior vena cava connecting to left atrium. *Am Heart J* 1994 (in press).

10. van der Horst RL, Winship WS, Gotsman MS. Drainage of left hepatic vein into coronary sinus associated with other systemic venous anomalies. *Br Heart J* 1971; 33:164–166.

11. Sanders SP. Anomalous hepatic venous connection to the coronary sinus diagnosed by two-dimensional echocardiography. *Am J Cardiol* 1984; 54:458–459.

12. Freedom RM, Culham JAG, Rowe RD. Left atrial to coronary sinus fenestration (partially unroofed coronary sinus). *Br Heart J* 1981; 46:63–68.

13. Mantini E, Grondin CM, Lillehei CW, Edwards JE. Congenital anomalies involving the coronary sinus. *Circulation* 1966; 33:317–327.

14. Quaegebeur J, Kirklin JW, Pacifico AD, Bargeron LM. Surgical experience with unroofed coronary sinus. *Ann Thorac Surg* 1979; 27:418–425.

15. Rumisek JD, Pigott JD, Weinberg PM, Norwood WI. Coronary sinus septal defect associated with tricuspid atresia. *J Thorac Cardiovasc Surg* 1986; 92:142–145.

16. Chin AJ, Murphy JD. Identification of coronary sinus septal defect (unroofed coronary sinus) by Doppler color flow imaging. *Am Heart J* 1992; 124:1655–1657.

17. Huhta JC, Smallhorn JF, Macartney FJ, Anderson RH, deLeval M. Cross-sectional echocardiographic diagnosis of systemic venous return. *Br Heart J* 1982; 48:388–403.

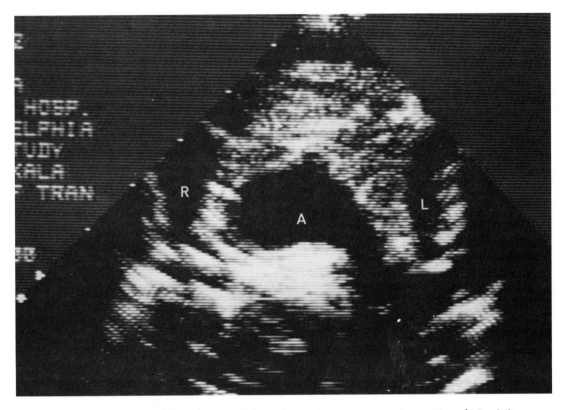

Figure 1: Suprasternal frontal view of bilateral superior vena cavae. A = aortic arch; L = left superior vena cava; R = right superior vena cava.

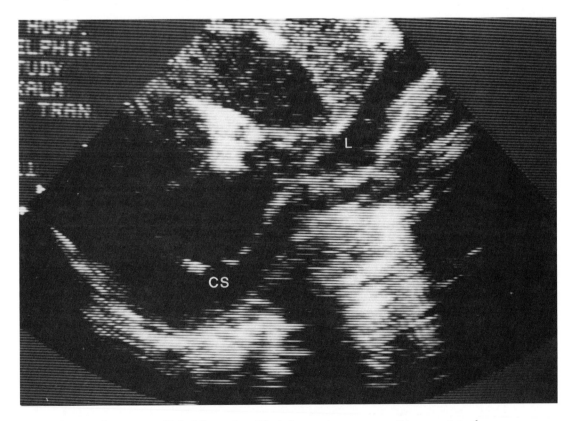

Figure 2: Suprasternal left oblique view. The left superior vena cava (L) connects to the coronary sinus (CS).

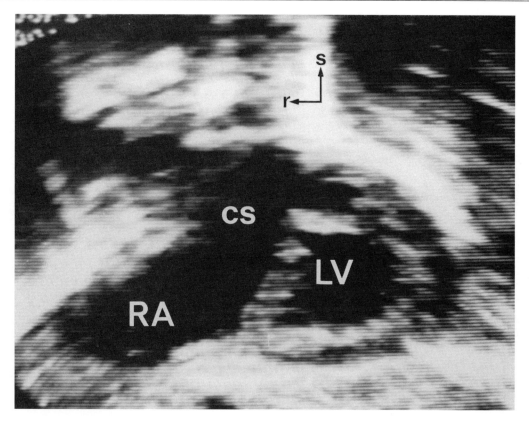

Figure 3: Subcostal frontal view. The coronary sinus (CS), an inferior structure, is dilated. RA = right atrium; LV = left ventricle.

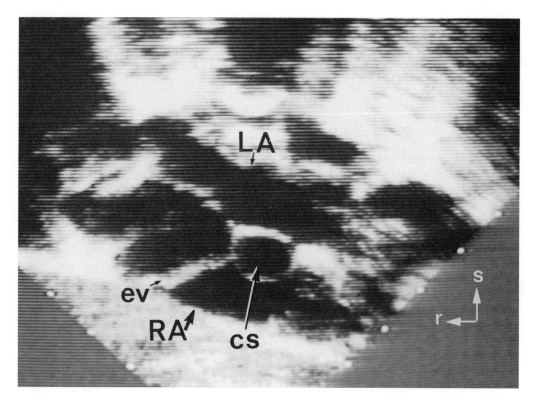

Figure 4: Subcostal frontal view, slightly superior to the plane of I 6-3. The mouth of coronary sinus (cs) is seen. The eustachian valve (ev) attaches to the rim of the coronary sinus. LA = left atrium; RA = right atrium.

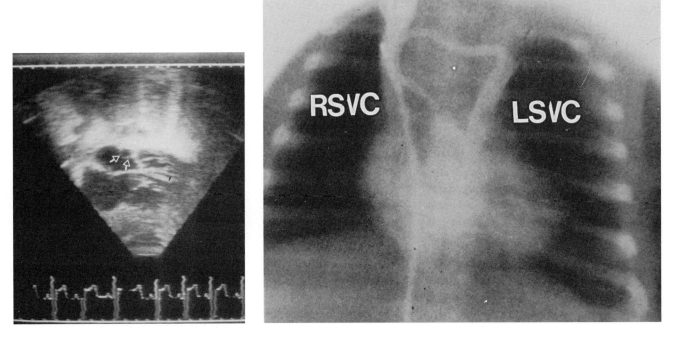

Figure 5: Subcostal frontal view, slightly superior to the plane of that shown in Figure 4. The junction of the left superior vena cava and the coronary sinus is seen as a circle (arrows).

Figure 6: Anteroposterior angiogram of a bridging vein. RSVC = right superior vena cava; LSVC = left superior vena cava.

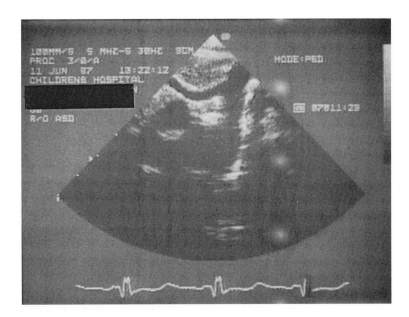

Figure 7: Suprasternal frontal view of bridging vein and left superior vena cava.

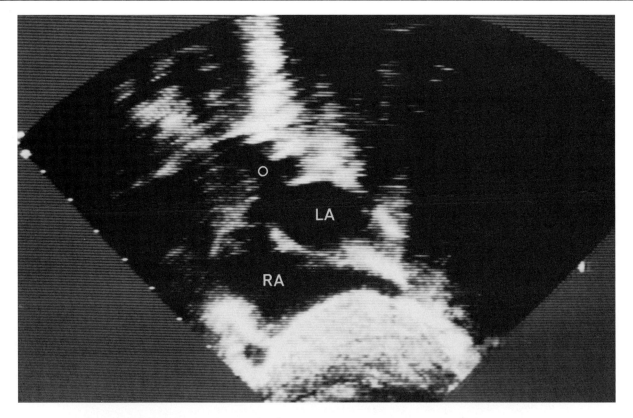

Figure 8: Subcostal sagittal view of right superior vena cava (open circle) to left atrium (LA). RA = right atrium.

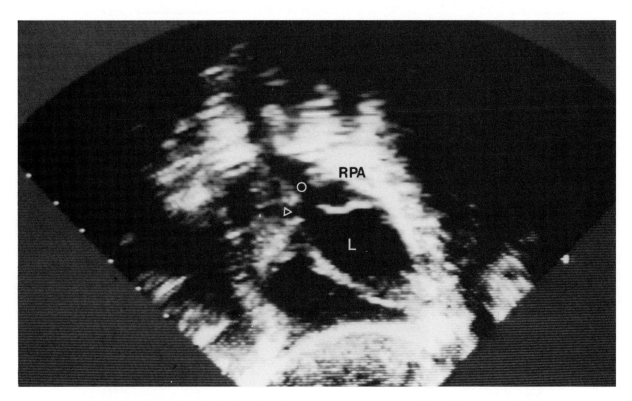

Figure 9: Subcostal sagittal view of right upper pulmonary vein (triangle) entering the left atrium (L) at the same point as the right superior vena cava (open circle). RPA = right pulmonary artery.

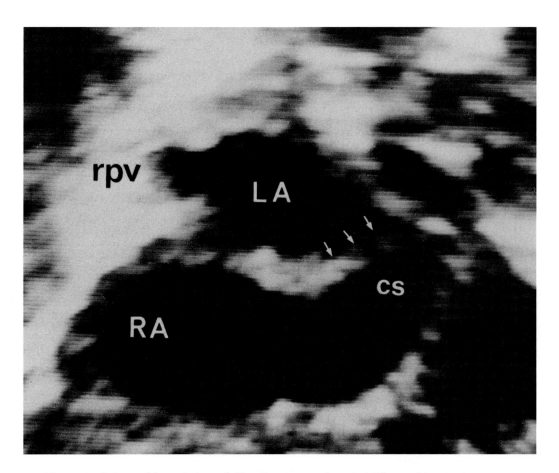

Figure 10: Subcostal frontal view of dilated coronary sinus (cs). The roof (arrows) appears intact. rpv = right pulmonary artery; LA = left atrium; RA = right atrium. Used with permission of American Heart Journal.

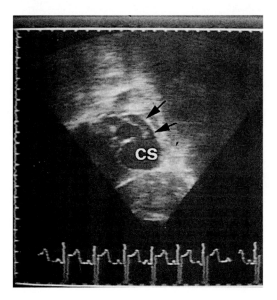

Figure 11: Subcostal sagittal view of the coronary sinus (cs, arrows). The roof has a small defect in it.

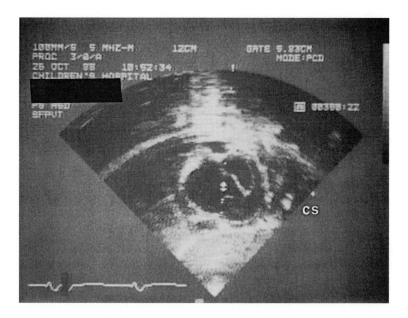

Figure 12: Subcostal left oblique view shows the roof and mouth of coronary sinus (cs) together with the septum primum, left atrium, and right atrium.

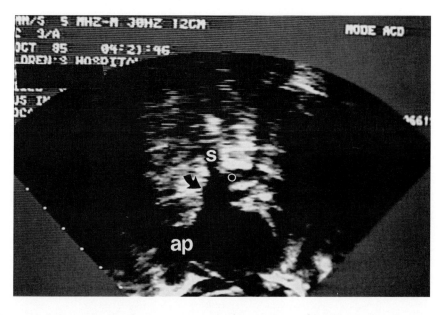

Figure 13: Subcostal sagittal view. Azygos (open circle) joins the left superior vena cava (s) just above the right pulmonary artery. Note that the caliber of the left superior vena cava enlarges (arrow) caudal to the azygos junction. The atrium has a left atrial appendage (ap).

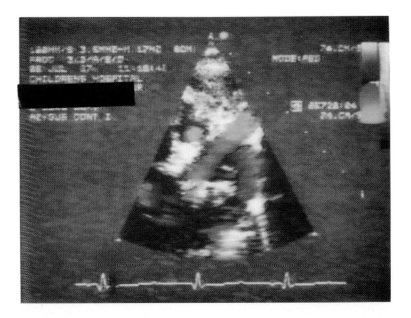

Figure 14: High parasternal sagittal view showing superior vena cava (blue).

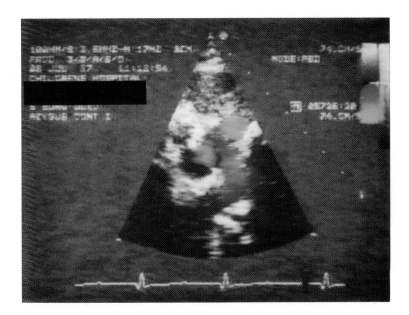

Figure 15: High parasternal sagittal view of patient shown in Figure 14. Azygos flow (red) joins the superior vena cava (blue).

Chapter 7

Pulmonary Veins

A. Total Anomalous Pulmonary Venous Connection

Lucas[1] has proposed the hypothesis that early atresia of the common pulmonary vein, together with persistence of connections of the splanchnic plexus to the cardinal, umbilical, or vitelline systems, leads to total anomalous pulmonary venous connection (TAPVC).

Beginning by displaying the abdominal great vessels in a transverse view (at approximately the T_{10} level), we can often visualize a descending vertical vein in cross-section (Figure 1). The aorta is the circular structure immediately adjacent to the vertebral column. (If there is an enlarged azygos vein, this structure is also typically adjacent to the vertebral column. In such cases, with two vascular structures *external* to the liver, the aorta is always the one closer to the midline.) The inferior vena cava, except in cases of interruption of the (intrahepatic) inferior vena cava, is more anterior (ventral) than the aorta and lies *within* the liver substance. Descending vertical veins (in infracardiac anomalous pulmonary venous connection) are virtually always circular in cross-section, presumably because of the high prevalence of obstruction "further downstream." If a descending vein is found, progressive cranial angulation[2] of the transducer allows tracking of the descending vein upward to the pulmonary venous connection (Figure 2). The descending vein can be traced to its junction with the portal vein (Figure 3) with caudal angulation or to its junction with the ductus venosus with cranial angulation. The ductus venosus lies between the caudate and left lobes of the liver.

If a descending vertical vein is not detected, the next step is to look for a pulmonary venous confluence posterior to the heart in the subcostal frontal view. Entrance sites of the individual pulmonary veins should be identified. Often the easiest way to identify a verti-

cal vein is to survey the entire superior aspect of the pulmonary venous confluence, from right hilum to left hilum. A vertical vein can often first be glimpsed as a "protuberance" from the superior aspect of the pulmonary venous confluence; it is *not* always midway between the right and left hila and bears no consistent relationship to the true midline. At any time during the surveillance of the pulmonary venous confluence, the examiner can always check that the structure being traced is indeed the pulmonary vein by momentarily angling more cranially. Since the branch pulmonary arteries are virtually always superior to the veins, the former should come into view (and eventually coalesce to form a main pulmonary artery).

If an ascending vein is detected (Figure 4), it is tracked until it connects to the systemic venous system (Figure 5). The course of the systemic vein back to the right side of the heart is examined (Figure 6).

If neither an ascending nor a descending vein is identified, we search for sites of more direct connection of the pulmonary venous confluence to the right superior vena cava, right atrium, or coronary sinus.

Parasagittal views are also useful (Figure 7). The examiner can, by aiming first to one side and then to the other, prove that four pulmonary veins connect to the confluence. Furthermore, the short connecting vein between a confluence and right superior vena (Figure 8) is often best seen in this view.

Unlike subcostal views, *suprasternal*[3,4] frontal and left oblique views sometimes allow the simultaneous display of all four pulmonary veins (Figure 9).

The most difficult variant of anomalous pulmonary venous connection to image is "mixed type." The two ways of minimizing failure in the recognition of mixed connection are: (1) never considering an exam complete until all four individual pulmonary veins have been identified, and (2) awareness of the fact that many variations of mixed connection do not have an easily discernible confluence. For example, in the case of right pulmonary veins to the coronary sinus and left pulmonary veins to an ascending vertical vein (to the innominate vein), the ascending vein may lie very lateral (i.e., adjacent to the medial surface of the left lung). It may be very difficult to display. In addition, there will be no true "confluence," and since the presence of two pulmonary veins draining into the coronary sinus is sufficient to enlarge the latter, the examiner may be tempted to assume that all four pulmonary veins connect to the coronary sinus. Occasional patients have a "dual type" connection[5,6] (Figure 10). Three, rather than two, right pulmonary veins can exist (Figures 11 and 12).

A potential pitfall in the echocardiographic assessment of *infracardiac* total anomalous pulmonary venous connection[7] is the failure to realize that one pulmonary vein enters the descending vein far from the entrance sites of the other three veins.

Finally, a helpful sign suggesting the presence of infracardiac total anomalous pulmonary venous connection is the inverted "Christmas tree" pattern[8,9]; the pulmonary veins tend to have a downward sloping trajectory (Figure 13).

Color Doppler echocardiography has greatly facilitated the tracing of individual pulmonary veins (Figure 14), especially in cases of heterotaxy syndrome. Heterotaxy syndrome is frequently associated with severe subpulmonary stenosis or pulmonary atresia, as part of an abnormality in ventriculoarterial alignment (transposition of the great arteries or double outlet right ventricle). The pulmonary veins in such patients are very small and thus difficult to resolve (Figure 15), even with 7.5 MHz transducers. Color Doppler imaging aids not only in the detection of pulmonary veins but also in allowing precise localization of the connection sites (Figure 16) vis-à-vis the atrial septal remnant.

B. Partial Anomalous Pulmonary Venous Connection

Early partial atresia of the common pulmonary vein may lead to partial anomalous pulmonary venous connection (PAPVC).[10]

1. Right Superior Pulmonary Vein to Right Superior Vena Cava

Since the entrance site is very lateral (i.e., next to the medial surface of the right lung), this anomaly is very difficult to identify. Occasionally a clue is that the

right superior vena cava inferior to the entrance site of the right superior pulmonary vein is slightly larger than the more cephalad portion of the right superior cava.

In the case of normally aligned great arteries and intact atrial septum, the presence of a dilated right ventricle should alert the examiner to the possibility of this anomaly.

In cases with abnormalities of ventriculoarterial alignment, there are frequently other reasons for the morphological right ventricle to appear dilated. In these circumstances, it is not infrequent for this pulmonary vein anomaly to escape unnoticed.

2. Left Superior Pulmonary Vein to Left Ascending Vertical Vein

While cases of *both* left pulmonary veins connecting to a left ascending vertical vein (to the innominate vein) are usually correctly identified because the examiner quickly notes the absence of *any* left pulmonary vein entrance site in the left atrium, cases in which only one left pulmonary vein connects anomalously are occasionally missed. Since the ascending vein lies in a lateral position (and can in fact be quite short), it can be quite difficult to display. Color Doppler imaging from the suprasternal window is probably the most reliable way to identify this anomaly.

C. Common Pulmonary Vein Atresia

The total atresia of the "bridge" to the pulmonary venous confluence[11-14] (*after* the connections between pulmonary veins and systemic veins have disappeared) yields the entity dubbed "common pulmonary vein atresia." Stenosis (Figure 16), rather than atresia, of the bridge appears to yield the entity dubbed cor triatriatum (see Chapter 5, section D).

Common pulmonary vein atresia always presents in the first few days of life. (Cor triatriatum usually presents in the first few months of life, but rare examples of individuals not presenting until adulthood have been reported.)

Common pulmonary vein atresia is displayed in the same way as total anomalous pulmonary venous connection except *no* connection to a large systemic or coronary vein is visible. Care must be taken to exclude cases of TAPVC with largely intraparenchymal connecting vein.[15]

References

1. Lucas RV, Woolfrey BF, Anderson RC, Lester RG, Edwards JE. Atresia of the common pulmonary vein. *Pediatrics* 1962; 29:729.

2. Chin AJ, Sanders SP, Sherman F, Lang P, Norwood WI, Castaneda AR. Accuracy of subcostal 2-dimensional echocardiography in prospective diagnosis of total anomalous pulmonary venous connection. *Am Heart J* 1987; 113:1153–1159.

3. Huhta JC, Gutgesell HP, Nihill MR. Cross sectional echocardiographic diagnosis of total anomalous pulmonary venous connection. *Br Heart J* 1985; 53:525–534.

4. Smallhorn JF, Sutherland GR, Tommasini G, Hunter S, Anderson RH, Macartney FJ. Assessment of total anomalous pulmonary venous connection by two-dimensional echocardiography. *Br Heart J* 1981; 46:613–623.

5. Kanjuh VI, Katkov H, Singh A, Franciosi RA, Helseth HK, Edwards JE. Atypical total anomalous pulmonary venous connection: two channels leading to infracardiac terminations. *Pediatr Cardiol* 1989; 10:115–120.

6. Arciprete P, McKay R, Watson GH, Hamilton DI, Wilkinson JL, Arnold RM. Double connections in total anomalous pulmonary venous connection. *J Thorac Cardiovasc Surg* 1986; 92:146–152.

7. Snider AR, Silverman NH, Turley K, Ebert PA. Evaluation of infradiaphragmatic total anomalous pulmonary venous connection with two-dimensional echocardiography. *Circulation* 1982; 66:1129–1132.

8. Kawashima Y, Matsuda H, Nakano S, Miyamoto K, Fujino M, Kozuka T, Manabe H. Tree-shaped pulmonary veins in infracardiac total anomalous pulmonary venous drainage. *Ann Thorac Surg* 1977; 23:436–441.

9. Delisle G, Ando M, Calder AL, Zuberbuhler JR, Rochenmacher S, Alday LE, Mangini O, Van Praagh S, Van Praagh R. Total anomalous pulmonary venous connection: report of 93 autopsied cases with emphasis on diagnostic and surgical considerations. *Am Heart J* 1976; 91:99–122.

10. Nakib A, Moller JH, Kanjuh VI, Edwards JE. Anomalies of the pulmonary veins. *Am J Cardiol* 1967; 20:77–90.

11. Ledbetter MK, Wells DH, Connors DM. Common pulmonary vein atresia. *Am Heart J* 1978; 96:580–586.

12. Hawker RE, Celermajer JM, Gengos DC, Cartmill TB, Bowdler JD. Common pulmonary vein atresia. *Circulation* 1972; 46:368–374.

13. Khonsari S, Saunders PW, Lees MH, Starr A. Common pulmonary vein atresia. *J Thorac Cardiovasc Surg* 1982; 83:443–448.

14. Deshpande JR, Kinare SG. Atresia of the common pulmonary vein. *Int J Cardiol* 1991; 30:221–226.

15. Matsui M, Arai T, Horikoshi S, Sugita Y, Hashimoto K, Morita K, Mochizuki Y. Successful repair of a rare type of total anomalous pulmonary venous drainage. *Ann Thorac Surg* 1991; 52:131–133.

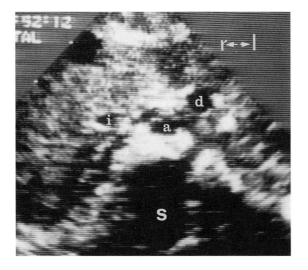

Figure 1: Transverse abdominal view. The inferior vena cava (i) is to the right of the spine (s). The aorta (a) is slightly to the left of the spine. A circular descending vein (d) is seen. Used with permission of American Heart Journal.

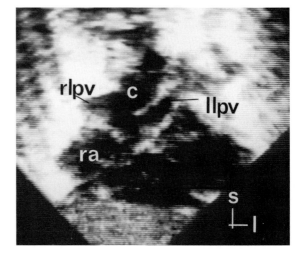

Figure 2: Two pulmonary veins can be seen. The left atrium is not visible. c = confluence; llpv = left lower pulmonary vein; ra = right atrium; rlpv = right lower pulmonary vein. Used with permission of American Heart Journal.

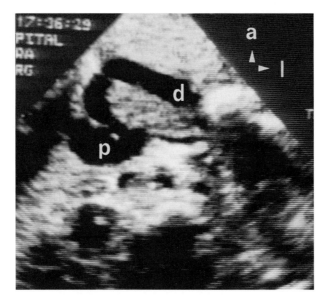

Figure 3: Caudal angulation from the plane in I 7-1 shows that the descending vein (d) connects with the portal vein (p). Used with permission of American Heart Journal.

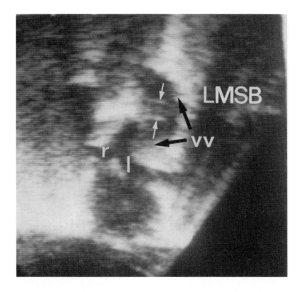

Figure 4: In supracardiac TAPVC to a left ascending vein (vv), the right pulmonary vein (r) is often more horizontal than the left pulmonary vein (l). LMSB = left mainstem bronchus. Used with permission of American Heart Journal.

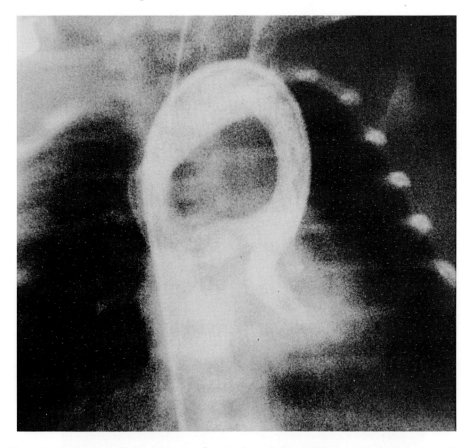

Figure 5: Anteroposterior angiogram shows a large left ascending vertical vein connecting to the innominate vein. Again note the horizontal orientation of the right pulmonary vein and the nearly vertical orientation of the left lower pulmonary vein.

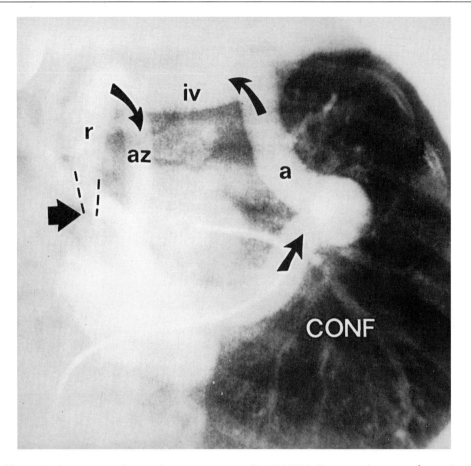

Figure 6: Anteroposterior angiogram, supracardiac TAPVC. For completeness, the entire course of the systemic vein back to the right heart should also be examined for sites of obstruction. This patient had a stenotic right (r) superior vena cava (broad arrow). Because of this obstruction, some pulmonary venous flow actually traveled down the azygos (az). a = ascending vein; CONF = confluence; iv = innominate vein.

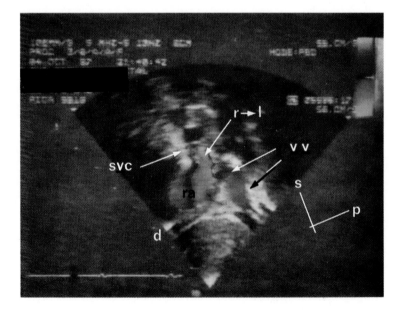

Figure 7: Subcostal view of infracardiac TAPVC. The descending vertical vein (vv) can be seen penetrating the diaphragm (d). Superior vena caval (svc) flow enters the right atrium (ra); flow transverses the atrial septum (r–l).

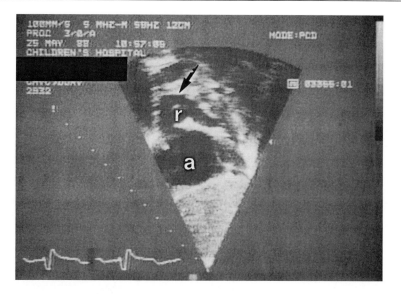

Figure 8: Subcostal sagittal view of TAPVC to the right superior vena cava. The short connecting vein (black arrow) is seen above the right pulmonary artery (r). a = right atrium.

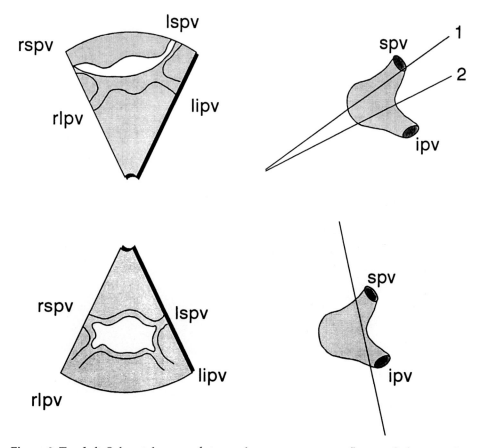

Figure 9: Top left: Subcostal approach to a pulmonary venous confluence. Only two veins can be seen simultaneously. rspv = right superior pulmonary vein; lspv = left superior pulmonary vein; lipv = left inferior pulmonary vein. **Top right:** To see the other two veins, the examiner must angle the transducer to plane 2. **Bottom left:** Suprasternal approach can frequently display all four veins simultaneously. **Bottom right:** The suprasternal plane allowing simultaneous visualization of all four veins.

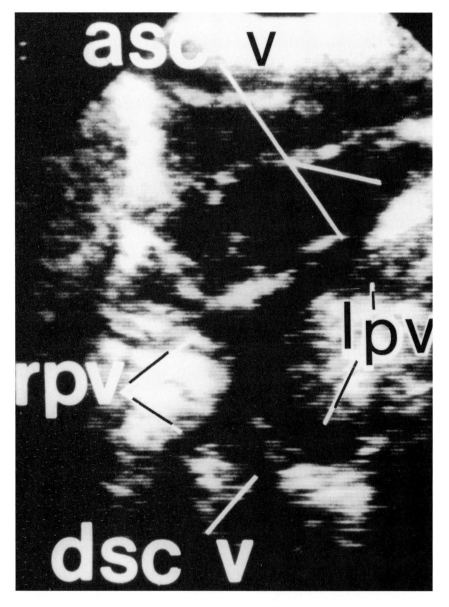

Figure 10: Suprasternal frontal view showing two right pulmonary veins (rpv), two left pulmonary veins (lpv), an ascending vein (asc v), and a descending vein (dsc v). Used with permission of Dr. S. P. Sanders.

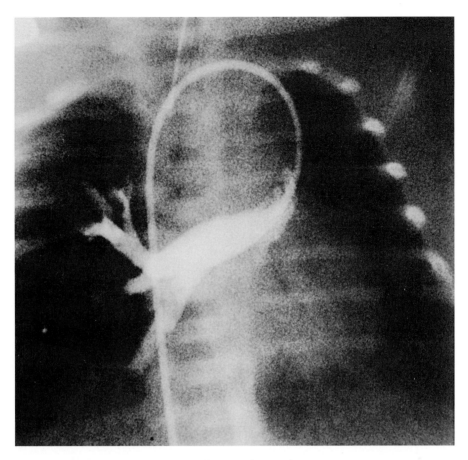

Figure 11: Anterioposterior angiogram showing three right pulmonary veins joining to form a common right pulmonary vein.

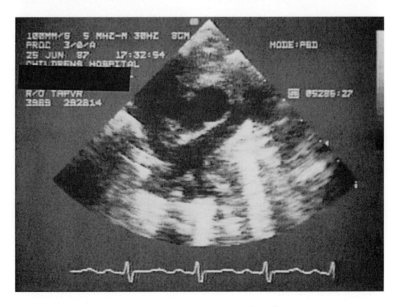

Figure 12: Suprasternal frontal view corresponding to that shown in Figure 11.

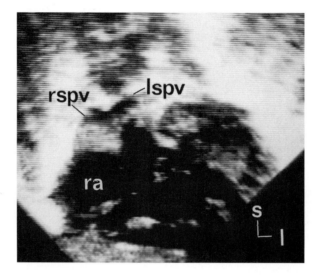

Figure 13: The subcostal approach; same patient as in Figure 2. Note the downward sloping trajectory of the right superior pulmonary vein (rspv) and the left superior pulmonary vein (lspv). Compare with Figure 12.

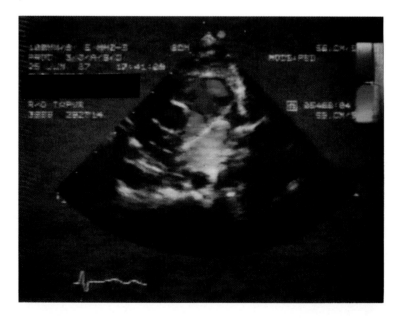

Figure 14: Color flow imaging of same patient as in Figure 12.

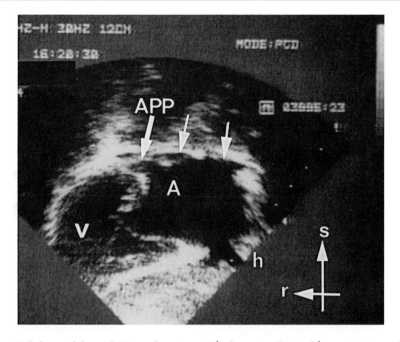

Figure 15: Subcostal frontal view of patient with dextrocardia and heterotaxy syndrome. The pulmonary veins (unlabeled arrows) connect to the middle of the posterior aspect of the common atrium (A). This patient had left atrial appendage isomerism. The right side of the common atrium has a morphological left atrial appendage (APP). h = hepatic veins; v = ventricle.

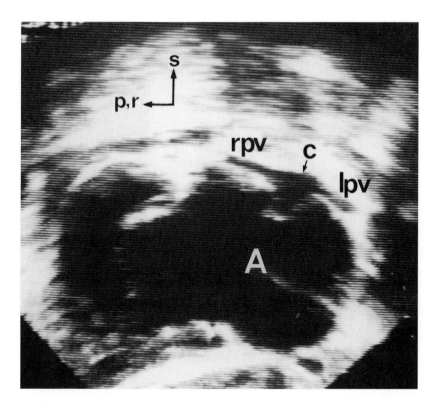

Figure 16: Subcostal right oblique view of a patient with dextrocardia and incomplete incorporation of the common pulmonary vein (c). The right pulmonary vein (rpv) and left pulmonary vein (lpv) connect to a pouch-like confluence that has penetrated the middle of the posterior aspect of the common atrium (A).

Chapter 8

Atrial Septum

A. Sinus Venosus Defect

There are two varieties of sinus venosus defect: superior vena caval type (Figure 1) and inferior vena caval type. The former is found immediately adjacent to the superior vena cava orifice (Figures 2 and 3), and the right upper pulmonary vein typically connects normally but drains (at least partially) anomalously.

The inferior vena caval type[1–5] is situated near the orifice of the inferior vena cava and usually associated with a right lower pulmonary vein (Figure 4) that connects normally but drains anomalously.[1,5] It is probable that many cases hitherto deemed "inferior vena cava-to-left atrium" are actually the inferior vena caval type of sinus venosus defect.

The posterior and inferior extent of the frontal sweep will display the sinus venosus defect of the inferior vena cava type (Figure 5); it is far to the right of the dilated mouth of the coronary sinus, which is a prominent feature of isolated coronary sinus septal defect (Figure 6) (see Chapter 6, section G, *Unroofed Coronary Sinus*). The more superior extent of the frontal sweep will display the sinus venosus defect of the superior vena cava type. The left oblique sweep is more effective for demonstrating it since the presence or absence of the superior limbic band is more easily discerned in a left oblique view (Figure 7).

The sagittal sweep can be used as a "cross-check." From the view in which the superior vena cava and the inferior vena cava are seen simultaneously, sweeping slightly to the patient's left (Figure 3) should display *either* type of sinus venosus defect.

B. Secundum Type

A defect in the thin flap tissue (termed *septum primum* by some) covering the fossa ovalis is called a secundum-type atrial septal defect. (There does not have to be complete deficiency in the flap.) Because of the possibility of transcatheter closure, sizing of such defects (Figure 8) is helpful. Many such defects are not circular; thus, echocardiographers need to remind themselves to image these defects in more than just the left oblique view (Figure 9). Initial defect size does correlate with prevalence of subsequent spontaneous closure;[6] defects >8 mm are unlikely to close spontaneously.

Malalignment of the septum secundum vis-à-vis the septum primum occurs in juxtaposition of the atrial appendages. The septum secundum is angled posteriorly in left-sided juxtaposition of the atrial appendages.[7]

C. Aneurysm of the Septum Primum

Although aneurysm of the septum primum can occur in patients without underdevelopment of one atrioventricular valve, the most common setting is atrioventricular valve atresia (Figure 10; see also Figure 8 in Chapter 6).[8–10] Since the importance of the display is to ascertain whether the aneurysm obstructs flow into the nonatretic atrioventricular valve, the best view is the left oblique one.

D. Leftward and Posterior Deviation of Superior Attachments of the Septum Primum

In patients with left atrioventricular valve underdevelopment, roughly 40–50% manifest a peculiar leftward and posterior deviation of the superior attachment of the septum primum (Figure 11). This phenomenon was first observed by van der Horst et al.[11] on postmortem specimens and subsequently confirmed by Weinberg.[12] It can be reliably demonstrated only with the sagittal and left oblique views (Figure 12). Use of only the frontal sweep can result in the diagnosis being missed, resulting in the mistaken impression that there is a large secundum-type atrial septal defect.[13]

The importance of recognizing this anomaly seems to be two-fold: interventional catheterization specialists need to be aware that the configuration of the atrial septum is different, and cardiac surgeons need to be aware that the superior extent of the atrial septum will be harder to visualize from the vantage point of a right atrial appendage incision (Figure 13).

References

1. Sturm JT, Ankeney JL. Surgical repair of inferior sinus venosus atrial septal defect. *J Thorac Cardiovasc Surg* 1979; 78:570–572.

2. Perna AM, Alajmo F. Partial anomalous pulmonary venous return of an uncommon type. *J Cardiovasc Surg* 1984; 25:563–565.

3. Ross DN. The sinus venosus type of atrial septal defect. *Guys Hosp Rep* 1956; 105:376–381.

4. McCormack RJM, Pickering D, Smith II. A rare type of atrial septal defect. *Thorax* 1968; 23:350–352.

5. Chin AJ, Murphy JD. Identification of coronary sinus septal defect by color Doppler echocardiography. *Am Heart J* 1992; 124:1655–1657.

6. Radzik D, Davignon A, von Doesburg N, Fournier A, Marchand T, Ducharme G. Predictive factors for spontaneous closure of atrial septal defects diagnosed in the first 3 months of life. *J Am Coll Cardiol* 1993; 22:851–853.

7. Chin AJ, Bierman FZ, Williams RG, Sanders SP, Lang P. Two-dimensional echocardiographic appearance of complete left-sided juxtaposition of the atrial appendages. *Am J Cardiol* 1983; 52:346–348.

8. Freedom RM, Rowe RD. Aneurysm of the atrial septum in tricuspid atresia: diagnosis during life and therapy. *Am J Cardiol* 1976; 38:265–267.

9. Casta A. Atrial septal aneurysm herniation across the mitral valve orifice in pulmonary atresia. *Am Heart J* 1988; 115:1136–1138.

10. Reder RF, Yeh HC, Steinfeld L. Aneurysm of the interatrial septum causing pulmonary venous obstruction in an infant with tricuspid atresia. *Am Heart J* 1981; 102:786–789.

11. van der Horst RL, Hastreiter AR, DuBrow IW, Eckner FAO. Pathologic measurements in aortic atresia. *Am Heart J* 1983; 106:1411–1415.

12. Weinberg PM, Chin AJ, Murphy JD, Pigott JD, Norwood WI. Postmortem echocardiography and tomographic anatomy of hypoplastic left heart syndrome after palliative surgery. *Am J Cardiol* 1986; 58:1228–1232.

13. Chin AJ, Weinberg PM, Barber G. Subcostal two-dimensional echocardiographic identification of anomalous attachment of septum primum in patients with left atrioventricular valve underdevelopment. *J Am Coll Cardiol* 1990; 15:678–681.

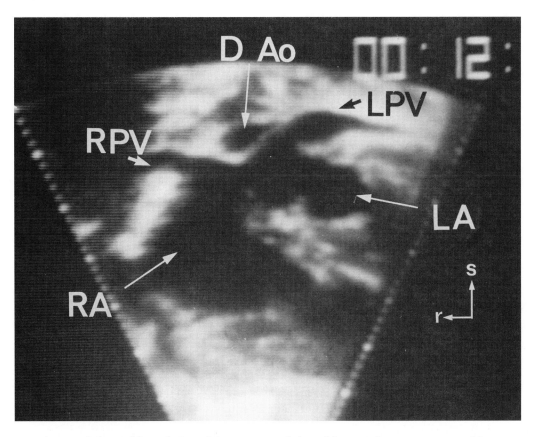

Figure 1: Subcostal frontal view of sinus venosus defect of the superior vena cava type. Note that a right pulmonary vein (RPV) is adjacent to the defect. D Ao = descending aorta; LA = left atrium; LPV = left pulmonary vein; RA = right atrium.

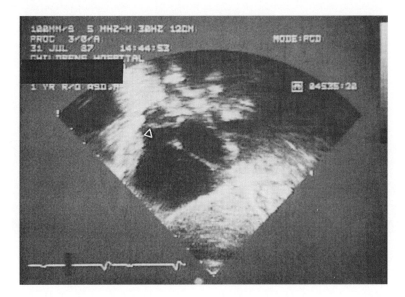

Figure 2: Subcostal left oblique view of sinus venosus defect of the superior vena cava type. The defect is adjacent to the superior vena caval orifice (triangle).

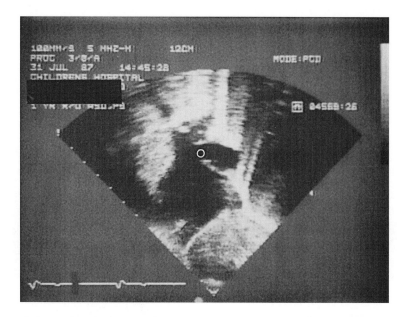

Figure 3: Subcostal sagittal view of same patient as in Figure 1. The defect (open circle) is an absence of the septum secundum. The septum primum (flap valve of the foramen ovale) is intact.

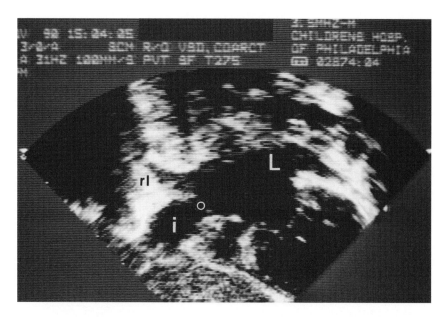

Figure 4: Subcostal right oblique view of sinus venosus defect of the inferior vena cava (i) type (open circle). Note that the defect is adjacent to the entrance site of the right lower (rl) pulmonary vein. L = left atrium.

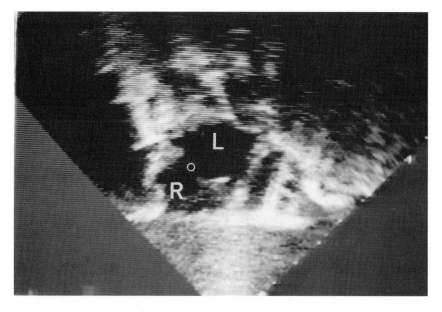

Figure 5: Inferior portion of the subcostal frontal sweep. The left atrium (L) and the very bottom of the right atrium (R) are seen. A large defect (open circle) is seen, representing the sinus venosus defect of the inferior vena cava type.

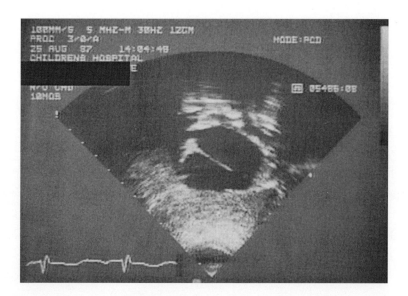

Figure 6: Subcostal frontal view of coronary sinus septal defect. The dropout in coronary sinus septal defect (unroofed coronary sinus) is far to the left of that in sinus venosus defect of the inferior vena cava type. The right pulmonary veins are distant.

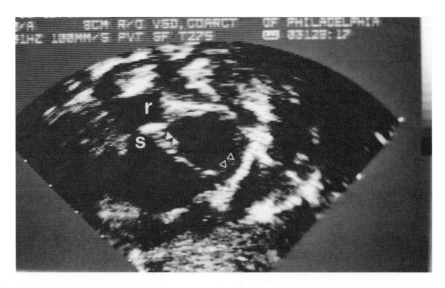

Figure 7: Subcostal left oblique view of same patient as in Figure 5. Note that sinus venosus defect of the superior vena cava (s) type is ruled out by the presence of septum secundum (closed arrowheads). The roof of the coronary sinus is intact (open arrowheads). r = right pulmonary artery.

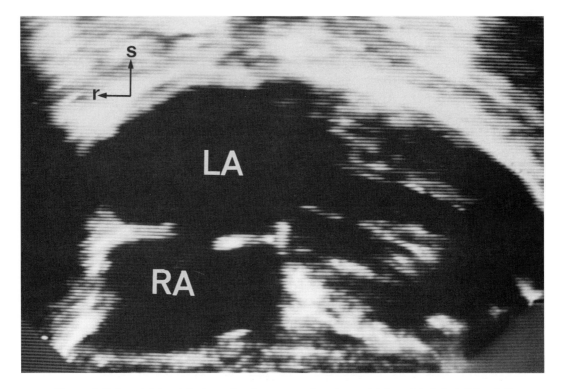

Figure 8: Subcostal frontal view of ostium secundum type atrial septal defect. LA = left atrium; RA = right atrium.

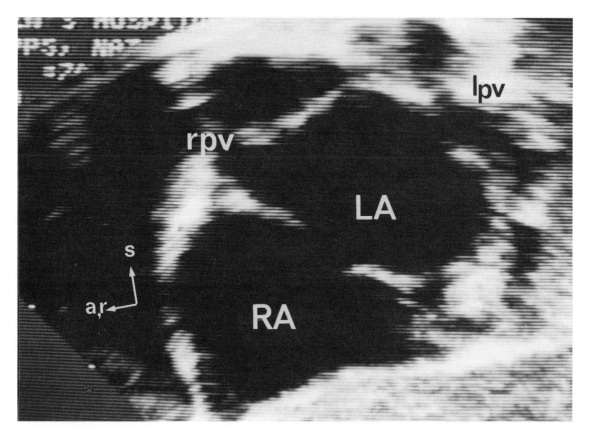

Figure 9: Subcostal left oblique view of ostium secundum type atrial septal defect. lpv = left pulmonary vein; rpv = right pulmonary vein. LA = left atrium; RA = right atrium.

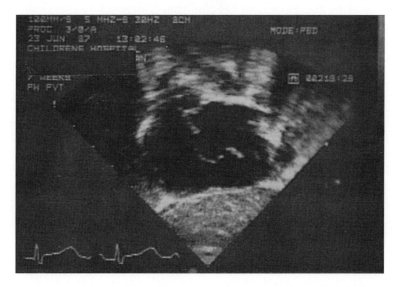

Figure 10: Subcostal left oblique view of aneurysm of septum primum.

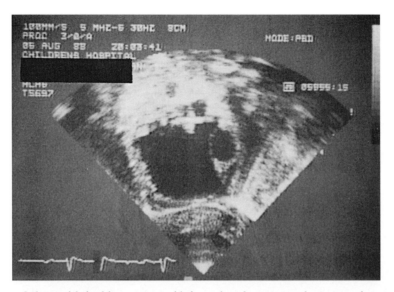

Figure 11: Subcostal left oblique view of leftward and posterior deviation of superior attachment of septum primum. Note that the septum primum attaches not to the left side of septum secundum but to the left atrial roof.

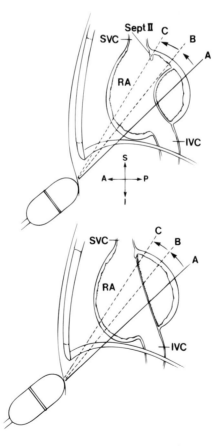

Figure 12: Top panel: Subcostal frontal sweep in patient shown in Figure 11 would travel from A to B to C. An atrial septal defect might be diagnosed mistakenly as the sector moves from B to C. **Bottom panel:** In a patient with a normal superior attachment of septum primum, such false dropout does not occur. Used with permission of Elsevier Science Publishing.

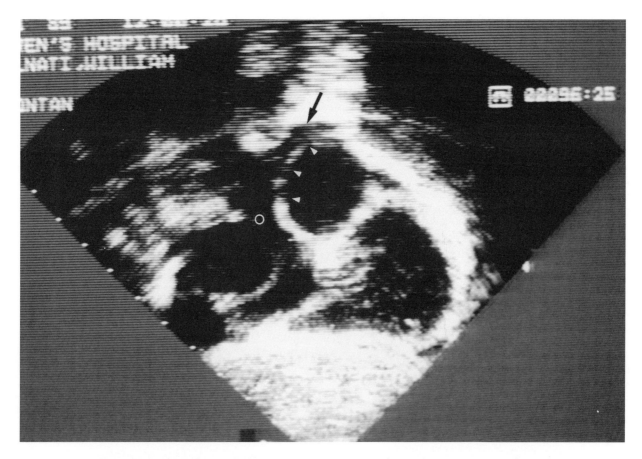

Figure 13: Because the atrial septum curves away from the vantage point of a right atriotomy, its attachment site can be difficult to identify. Thus, a surgeon may perceive the patient to have a large atrial septal defect. In extreme cases, the pulmonary veins (black arrow) can connect to the right of the septum primum (white arrowheads) attachment site. In this rare case, the atrial septal deviation was not recognized even at the time of Fontan operation. The atrial septal defect (open circle) was not critically restrictive; thus, no hemodynamic embarrassment resulted.

Chapter 9

Atria-to-Atrioventricular Valve Connections

A. Normal

1. Ebstein's Anomaly

Not only can this occur in a D-loop right ventricle, but it can also occur in a milder fashion in the L-loop right ventricle. Both stenosis and regurgitation can be present (see also Chapter 12). The "nondelamination" that is the central feature of Ebstein's anomaly causes stenosis in two ways: by narrowing the functional annulus size and by reducing interchordal spaces. Regurgitation is caused by inadequate coaptation.

The echocardiographic correlate of incomplete delamination is transposition of the "hinge points" to more apical positions (Figure 1) and to positions closer to the right ventricular outflow tract. The exact points of delamination can be identified with subcostal sweeps (Figures 2 and 3); the sagittal view (Figure 4) and right oblique view (Figure 5) are both helpful.

2. Unguarded Tricuspid Orifice

This extremely rare anomaly can also be termed absent tricuspid leaflets (Figure 6).

3. Isolated Tricuspid Stenosis

Isolated congenital tricuspid stenosis, unrelated to Ebstein's anomaly (Figure 7), is extremely rare (Figure 8).

4. Tricuspid Valve Dysplasia

Rare cases of knobbly-looking tricuspid valves (Figure 9) which leak (because of noncoaptation) have been seen. Trisomy 18 is frequently associated with "polyvalvar disease," of which tricuspid dysplasia is a part.[1]

5. "Ebstein's Anomaly" of the Mitral Valve

Rare[2-4] cases have been seen in which the posterior (lateral, mural) leaflet of the mitral valve (Figure 10) is not separated from the free wall of the morphological left ventricle.

6. Double-Orifice Mitral Valve

There are three basic types: orifices unequal in size with the larger orifice over the anterolateral papillary muscle (Figures 11–14); orifices unequal in size with the larger orifice over the posteromedial papillary muscle (Figures 15 and 16); and orifices roughly equal in size. The first two types are commonly, but not universally, associated with stenosis.

The best way of identifying the first two types is to always suspect double-orifice mitral valve (DOMV) when a patient appears on first glance to have a parachute valve. The patient may actually have a DOMV[5]; a careful sweep (from apex to base) will uncover the smaller second orifice.

7. Anomalous Arcade

One of the most difficult diagnoses to make by echocardiography is so-called arcade,[6] i.e., direct attachment of papillary muscles onto the leaflet (Figures 17 and 18), which may represent developmental arrest at day 70. It is difficult to resolve chordae tendineae in the infant (Figure 19).

8. Parachute Mitral Valve

Many, but not all, cases of parachute valve are associated with stenosis. A case with normal annulus diameter and normal interchordal spaces should not be stenotic. The more frequent variety has all attachments to the posteromedial papillary muscle (Figure 20). In common atrioventricular canal,[7] it is usually the anterolateral papillary muscle that is involved (Figure 21). The mitral valve normally appears parachute until day 70–80 of fetal development.

9. Isolated Cleft of the Mitral Valve

A surgically correctable etiology of mitral regurgitation, this anomaly is uncommon (Figure 22).

B. Common Atrioventricular Canal

There are three basic forms that differ only in the "ventricular" attachments of the common atrioventricular valve:

Partial = atrioventricular valve attachments to the ventricular septal crest are complete preventing any ventricular-level shunting.

Transitional = atrioventricular valve attachments to the ventricular septal crest are incomplete, allowing a small "ventricular septal defect."

Complete = relatively few atrioventricular attachments to the ventricular septal crest, allowing a large "VSD" (Figures 23–28).

The degree of *atrioventricular septal* deficiency is similar in these three forms. Many transitional cases have atrioventricular valve leaflet deficiency.[8] Approximately 10% of patients with common atrioventricular canal have a solitary left ventricular papillary muscle[7] (Figure 21). Only rarely is the anterolateral papillary muscle hypoplastic (Figures 29 and 30).

Lev[9] made the important observation that the alignment of the common atrioventricular valve vis-à-vis the ventricles is not always balanced (see Chapter 10, section B).

Horiuchi[10] has observed that the alignment of the septum primum vis-à-vis the common atrioventricular canal is not always balanced.[11] If the septum primum is far to the right, then *right atrial outlet stenosis or atresia* is present, resulting in functional double-outlet left atrium. If the septum primum is far to the left, *left atrial outlet stenosis or atresia* is present (Figure 31), yielding functional double-outlet right atrium. The former should be distinguished from right atrial outlet atresia with straddling left atrioventricular valve.[12]

C. Tricuspid Atresia

The vast majority of tricuspid atresia cases display complete lack of development of the right atrioventricular orifice, not so-called "imperforate" tricuspid valve. Although the morphological left ventricle looks grossly very similar to the morphological left ventricle in a normal heart, whether it is functionally similar is unproved. The right ventricle is hypoplastic (Figure 32) except if a large ventricular septal defect coexists when the right ventricle may approach normal in size. Subvalvar pulmonary stenosis with or without valvar stenosis is common.

D. Mitral Atresia

Nearly half of mitral atresia cases display leftward and posterior deviation of the superior attachment of the septum primum (Figure 33) (see Chapter 8, section D). This striking finding suggests one possible reason why mitral atresia (underdevelopment of left atrioventricular orifice) is so much more frequent than tricuspid atresia. "Imperforate" mitral valve is exceedingly rare.

E. Double-Outlet Atria

In rare[10,13–20] cases, one atrium can drain via two atrioventricular valves into two ventricles.

References

1. Van Praagh S, Truman T, Firpo A, Bano Rodrigo A, Fried R, McManus B, Engle MA, Van Praagh R. Cardiac malformations in trisomy 18: a study of 41 postmortem cases. *J Am Coll Cardiol* 1989; 13:1586–1597.

2. Dusmet M, Oberhaensli I, Cox JN. Ebstein's anomaly of the tricuspid and mitral valve in an otherwise normal heart. *Br Heart J* 1987; 58:400–404.

3. Jacob JL, da Silveira LC, Braile DM. Echocardiographic and angiographic diagnosis of Ebstein's anomaly of the mitral valve. *Br Heart J* 1991; 66:379–380.

4. Leung M, Rigby ML, Anderson RH, Wyse RK, Macartney FJ. Reversed offsetting of the septal attachments of the atrioventricular valves and Ebstein's malformation of the morphologically mitral valve. *Br Heart J* 1987; 57:184–187.

5. Trowitzsch E, Bano Rodrigo A, Burger BM, Colan SD, Sanders SP. Two-dimensional echocardiographic findings in double orifice mitral valve. *J Am Coll Cardiol* 1985; 6:383–387.

6. Matsushima AY, Park J, Szulc M, Poon E, Bierman FZ, Cooper RS, Ursell PC. Anomalous atrioventricular valve arcade. *Am Heart J* 1991; 121:1842–1846.

7. Chin AJ, Bierman FZ, Sanders SP, Williams RG, Norwood WI, Castaneda AR. Subxyphoid 2-dimensional echocardiographic identification of left ventricular papillary muscle anomalies in complete common atrioventricular canal. *Am J Cardiol* 1983; 51:1695–1699.

8. Bharati S, Lev M, McAllister HA, Kirklin JW. Surgical anatomy of the atrioventricular valve in the intermediate type of common atrioventricular orifice. *J Thorac Cardiovasc Surg* 1980; 79:884–889.

9. Bharati S, Lev M. The spectrum of common atrioventricular orifice (canal). *Am Heart J* 1973; 86:553–561.

10. Horiuchi T, Saji K, Osuka Y, Sato K, Okada Y. Successful correction of double outlet left atrium associated with complete atrioventricular canal and L-loop double outlet right ventricle with stenosis of the pulmonary artery. *J Cardiovasc Surg* 1976; 17:157–161.

11. Alivizatos P, Anderson RH, Macartney FJ, Zuberbuhler JR, Stark J. Atrioventricular septal defect with balanced ventricles and malaligned atrial septum: double-outlet right atrium. *J Thorac Cardiovasc Surg* 1985; 89:295–297.

12. Otero Coto E, Calabro R, Marsico F, Lopez Arranz JS. Right atrial outlet atresia with straddling left atrioventricular valve. *Br Heart J* 1981; 45:317–324.

13. Starc TJ, Bierman FZ, Bowman FO, Steeg CN, Wang NK, Krongrad E. Pulmonary venous obstruction and atrioventricular canal anomalies: role of cor triatriatum and double outlet right atrium. *J Am Coll Cardiol* 1987; 9:830–833.

14. Navarro-Lopez F, Marin Garcia J, Zomeno M, Llorian AR. Mitral atresia and occlusive left atrial thrombus. *Br Heart J* 1969; 31:649–652.

15. Suzuki Y, Hamada Y, Miura M, Haneda K, Horiuchi T, Ogata H. Double-outlet left atrium with intact ventricular septum. *Ann Thorac Surg* 1988; 45:332–334.

16. Westerman GR, Norton JB, Van Devanter SH. Double-outlet right atrium associated with tetralogy of Fallot and common atrioventricular valve. *J Thorac Cardiovasc Surg* 1986; 91:205–207.

17. Otero Coto E, Quero Jimenez M, Deverall PB. Rare anomalies of atrioventricular connection: hidden or super numerary valves with imperforate right atrioventricular connection. *Int J Cardiol* 1984; 6:149–156.

18. Gerlis LM, Anderson RH, Dickinson DF. Duplication of the left atrioventricular valve in double inlet left ventricle: a triple inlet ventricle? *Int J Cardiol* 1984; 6:157–161.

19. Nunez L, Aguado MG, Sanz E, Perez Martinez V. Surgical repair of double-outlet right atrium. *Ann Thorac Surg* 1984; 37:165–166.

20. Corwin RD, Singh AK, Karlson KE. Double-outlet right atrium: a rare endocardial cushion defect. *Am Heart J* 1983; 106:1156–1157.

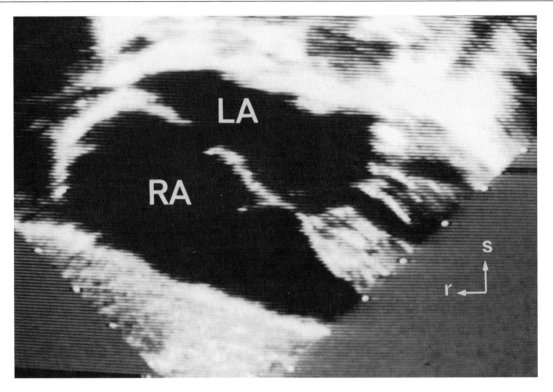

Figure 1: Subcostal frontal view of Ebstein's anomaly. The leaflet "hinge points" are not at the annulus but rather more apically situated. This produces the appearance of "downward displacement." LA = left atrium; RA = right atrium.

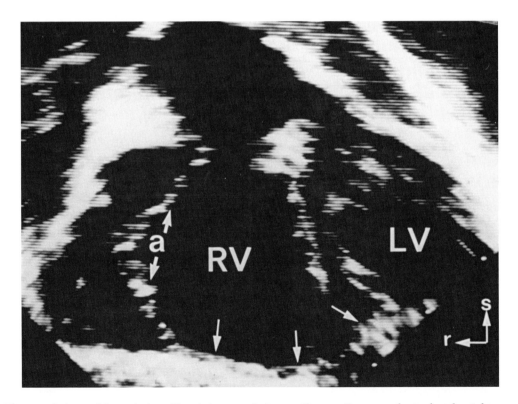

Figure 2: Subcostal frontal view. Ebstein's anomaly is actually a cardiomyopathy in that the right ventricular wall is malformed. The septal leaflet of the tricuspid valve is incompletely "delaminated" from the septum, and often the posterior (inferior) leaflet is incompletely delaminated from the diaphragmatic surface (unlabeled arrows). a = anterior leaflet; LV = left ventricle; RV = right ventricle.

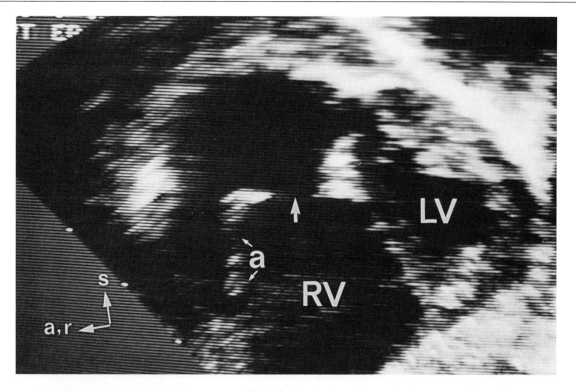

Figure 3: Subcostal left oblique view. This is the best view to assess the thickness of the right ventricular wall and septum. Compare the thickness of the inferior walls of the right (RV) and left ventricle (LV). The orientation of the functional orifice is superior in this case of Ebstein's. a = anterior leaflet.

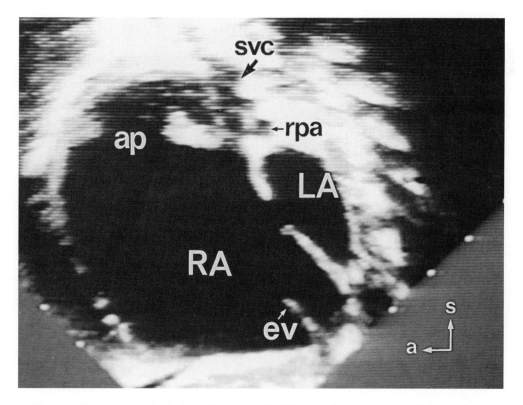

Figure 4: Subcostal sagittal view of a markedly dilated right atrium. ap = right atrial appendage; ev = eustachian valve; LA = left atrium; RA = right atrium; rpa = right pulmonary artery; svc = right superior vena cava.

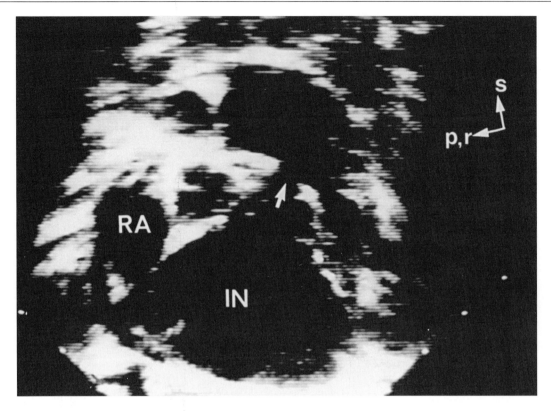

Figure 5: Subcostal right oblique view. The nondelamination has extended so far into the right ventricle in this case of Ebstein's anomaly that the functional orifice (arrow), instead of pointing to the apex of the right ventricular "inflow" (IN), actually points to the pulmonary valve! RA = right atrium.

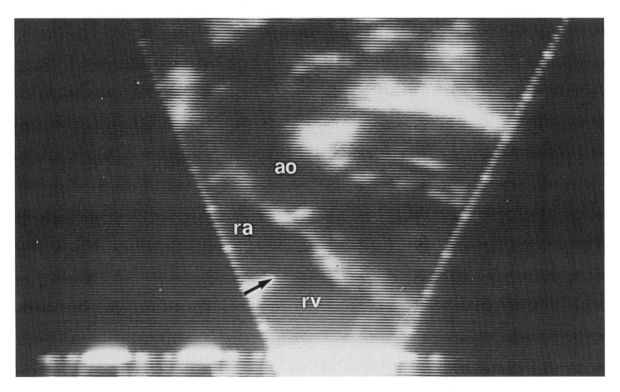

Figure 6: Subcostal frontal view of unguarded tricuspid orifice. At this plane, it is indistinguishable from Ebstein's anomaly; however, further scanning fails to identify any leaflets. ra = right atrium; rv = right ventricle; ao = aorta.

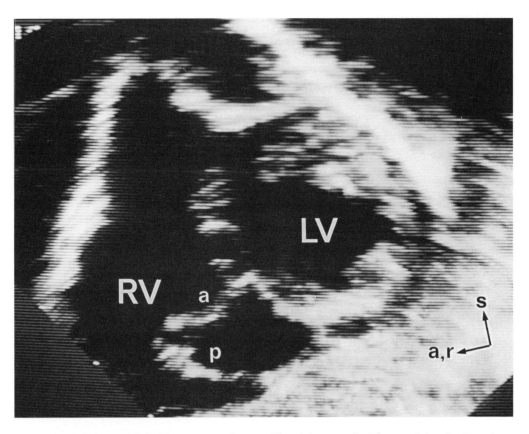

Figure 7: Subcostal left oblique view of severe Ebstein's anomaly. The nondelamination of most of the septal and posterior leaflets is creating a small functional orifice. a = anterior leaflet; p = posterior leaflet; RV = right ventricle; LV = left ventricle.

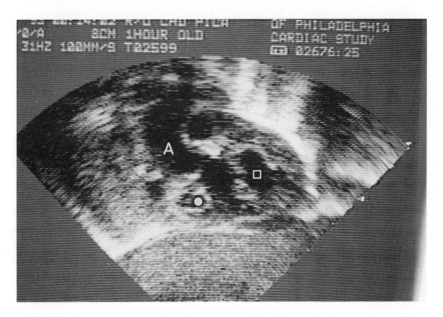

Figure 8: Subcostal left oblique view. This patient did not have Ebstein's anomaly; there was isolated tricuspid valve (circle) and right ventricular hypoplasia. The mitral valve (square) was slightly larger than normal. A = ascending aorta.

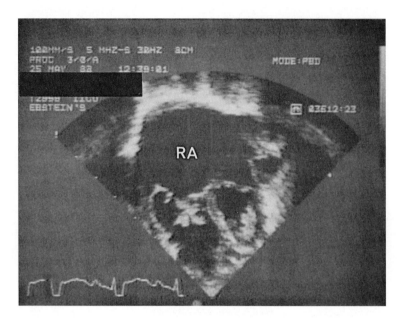

Figure 9: Apical view of malformed tricuspid valve. The leaflets appear knobbly; there was severe regurgitation. RA = right atrium.

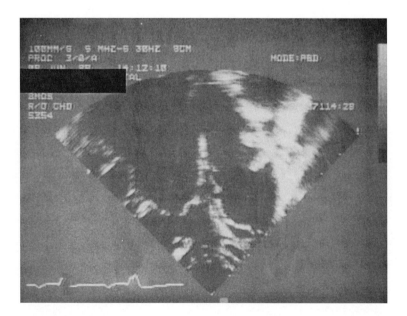

Figure 10: Apical four-chamber view of Ebstein's anomaly of the morphologically mitral valve. There is nondelamination of the lateral leaflet. This patient had D-ventricular loop.

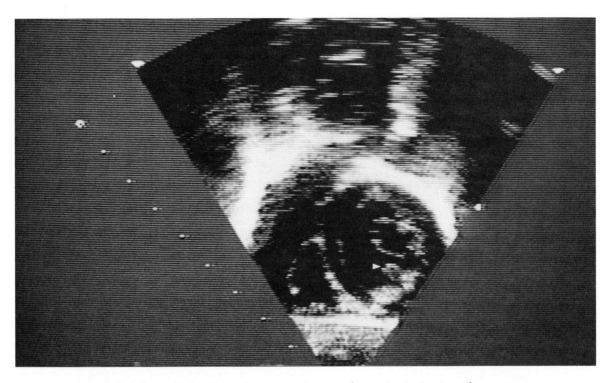

Figure 11: Subcostal left oblique view suggesting parachute mitral valve (see Chapter 9, section A, 8). The posteromedial papillary muscle (arrowhead) does not seem to have any valve attachments.

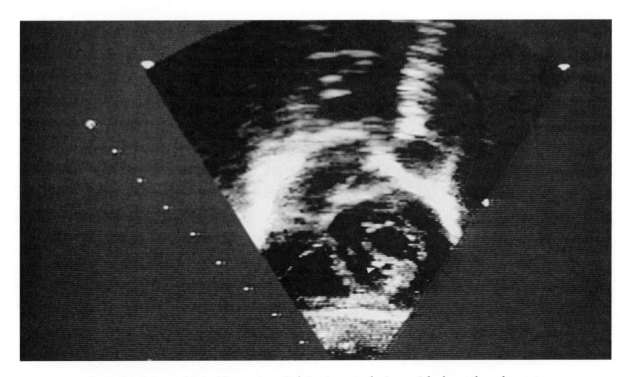

Figure 12: Subcostal left oblique view slightly closer to the base of the heart than shown in Figure 11. A small second orifice (arrowhead) is identified as attaching to the posteromedial papillary muscle.

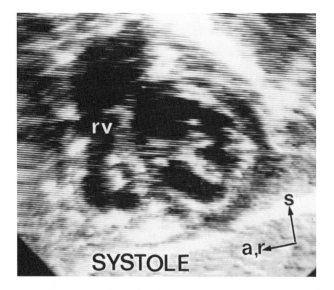

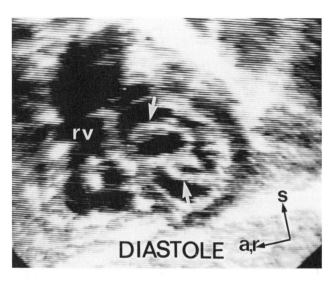

Figure 13: Subcostal left oblique view. In cases where the second orifice is only slightly smaller than the main orifice, the coaptation configuration can look "T-like." rv = right ventricle.

Figure 14: Subcostal left oblique view of the patient shown in Figure 13. The separate orifices are clearly visible (arrows). rv = right ventricle.

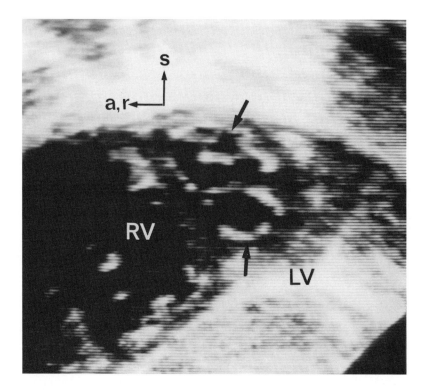

Figure 15: Subcostal left oblique view. The smaller orifice is situated over the anterolateral papillary muscle. RV = right ventricle; LV = left ventricle.

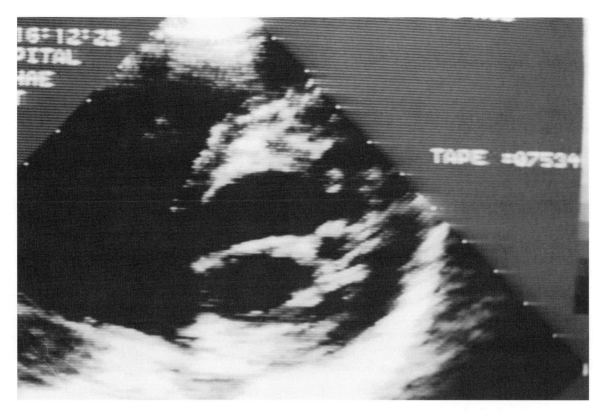

Figure 16: Parasternal short axis view. The smaller orifice is situated over the anterolateral papillary muscle.

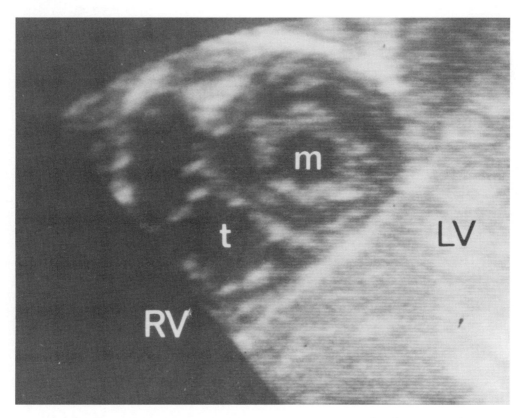

Figure 17: Subcostal left oblique view of anomalous arcade. Note that the edges of the mitral (m) leaflets appear thicker than those of the tricuspid (t) leaflets. RV = right ventricle.

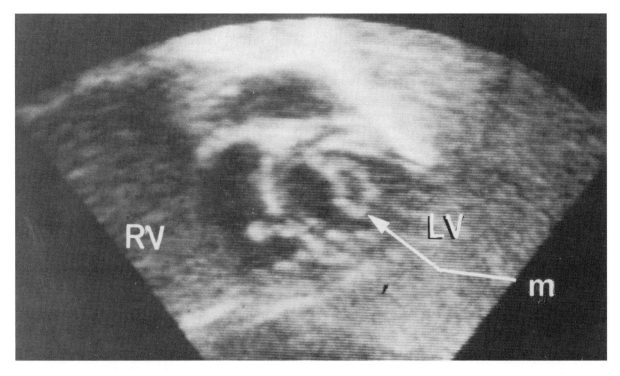

Figure 18: Subcostal left oblique view of patient shown in Figure 17. This plane is closer to the apex. Note the absence of any structures resembling chordae cut in cross-section. m = mitral; RV = right ventricle; LV = left ventricle.

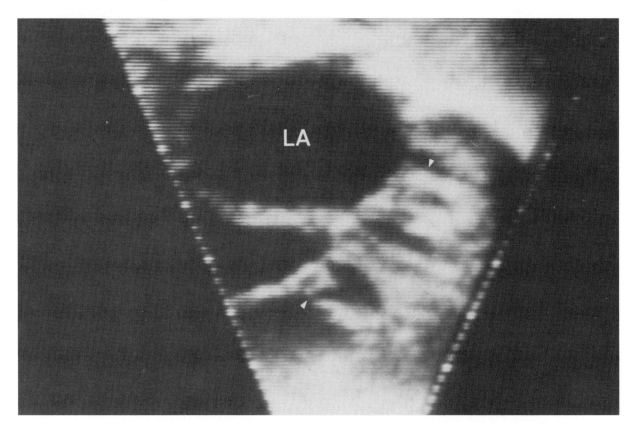

Figure 19: Subcostal frontal view of patient shown in Figure 18. Note an apparent difference in the thickness of the tensor apparatus of the mitral and tricuspid valves (arrowheads). LA = left atrium.

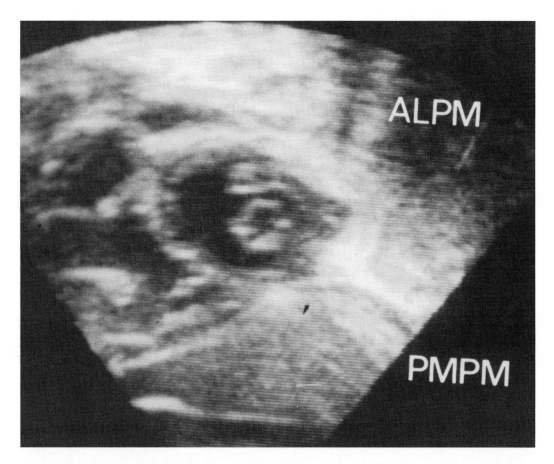

Figure 20: Subcostal left oblique view of parachute mitral valve. Note that in the non-atrioventricular canal patient, the valve typically attaches to the posteromedial papillary muscle (PMPM). ALPM = anterolateral papillary muscle.

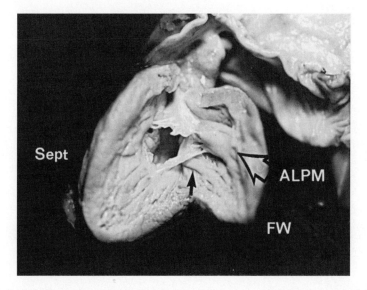

Figure 21: Postmortem view of the left ventricle in common atrioventricular canal. Note that the "mitral" valve attaches only to the anterolateral papillary muscle (ALPM), not the posteromedial papillary muscle (unlabeled arrow). FW = left ventricular free wall; Sept = septum.

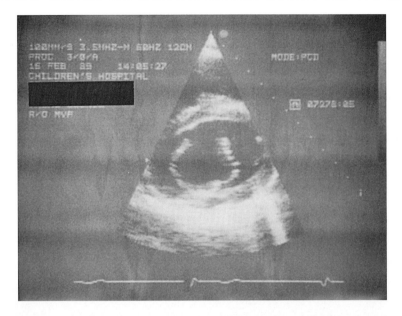

Figure 22: Parasternal short axis view of "isolated" mitral valve cleft. The orientation of the cleft points to the outflow tract. In common atrioventricular canal, the outflow tract is not "wedged" in between the atrioventricular orifices; thus, the mitral cleft (septal commissure) does not point to the outflow tract.

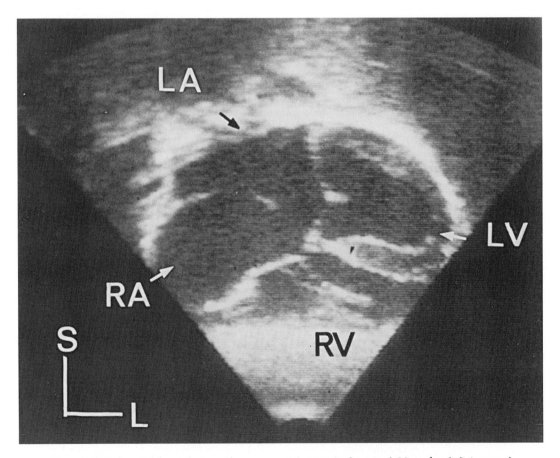

Figure 23: Subcostal frontal view of common atrioventricular canal. Note the deficiency of the atrioventricular septal area. There are relatively few attachments of the common atrioventricular valve to (the right side of) the ventricular septal crest, making this a "complete common atrioventricular canal." The valve has a radar-dish configuration.

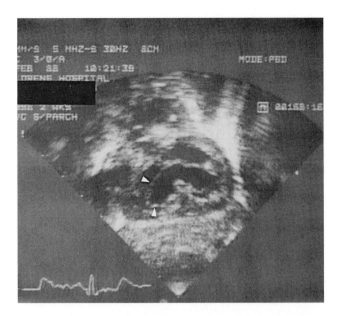

Figure 24: Subcostal left oblique view of the penta-leaflet common atrioventricular valve. The right superior leaflet and right lateral leaflet are shown by the arrowheads.

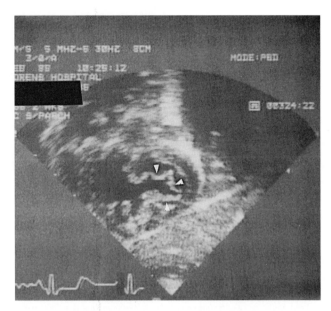

Figure 25: Subcostal left oblique view of the patient shown in Figure 24. The left superior leaflet, left lateral leaflet, and the inferior bridging leaflet are shown by the arrowheads.

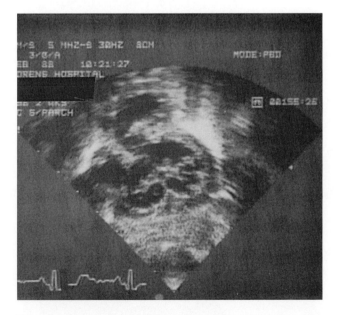

Figure 26: Subcostal left oblique view of the patient shown in Figure 24. The penta-leaflet configuration can also be recognized by studying the coaptation lines.

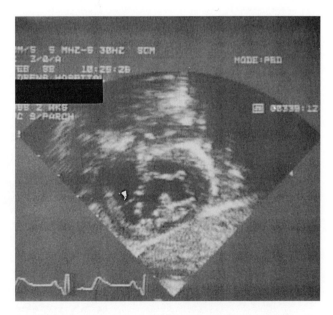

Figure 27: In neonates, even the chordae can often be displayed. The right superior leaflet attachment (arrowhead) in the patient shown in Figure 24 can be seen.

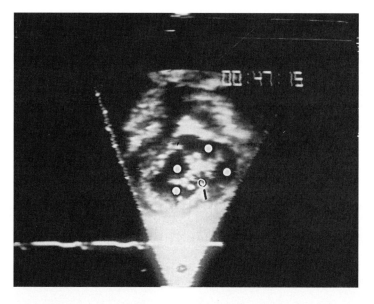

Figure 28: In so-called type A complete common atrioventricular canal, the right superior leaflet is well developed, and the left superior leaflet does not bridge the plane of the ventricular septum. The right superior, right lateral, left superior, and left lateral leaflets are shown by closed circles. The inferior leaflet (open circle) *does* bridge the plane of the ventricular septum (bold line).

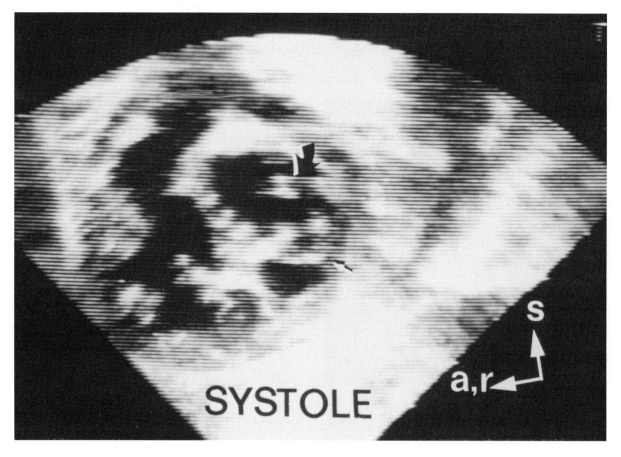

Figure 29: Subcostal left oblique view of rare case of common atrioventricular canal in which the anterolateral papillary muscle (large arrow) is hypoplastic. The valve attachment to the posteromedial papillary muscle (small arrowhead) is seen.

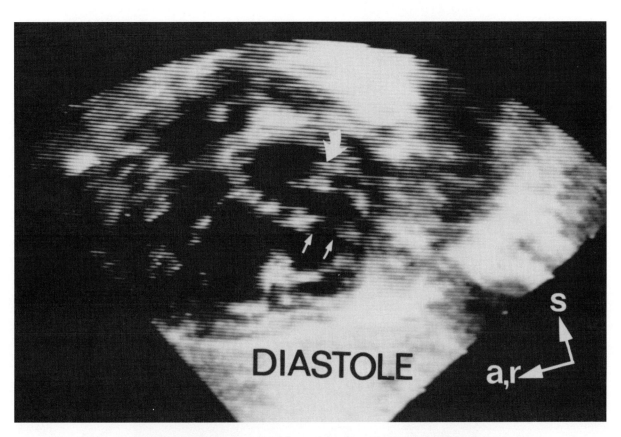

Figure 30: Subcostal left oblique view of the patient shown in Figure 29. The common atrioventricular valve attaches only to posteromedial papillary muscle (small arrows).

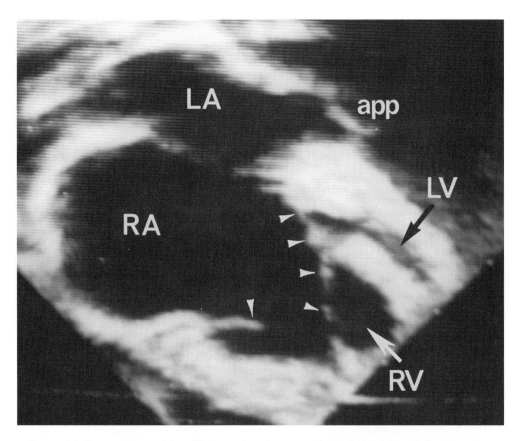

Figure 31: Postmortem echocardiogram showing not only malalignment of the common atrioventricular valve (arrowheads) vis-à-vis the ventricular septum, but also malalignment of the septum primum vis-à-vis the common atrioventricular valve. app = left atrial appendage; LA = left atrium; LV = left ventricle; RA = right atrium; RV = right ventricle.

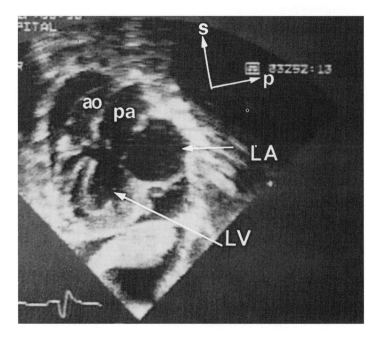

Figure 32: Subcostal sagittal view of tricuspid atresia. The right ventricle is tiny. Although this case was called transposition of the great arteries, note that it is very close to being double-outlet left ventricle.

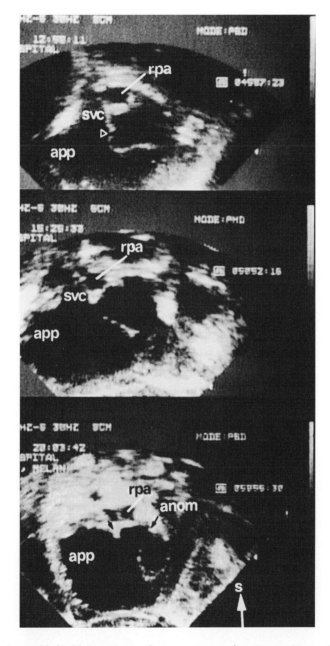

Figure 33: Subcostal left oblique views of an aneurysm of septum primum (top), high secundum-type atrial septal defect (middle), and leftward and posterior deviation of superior attachment of septum primum (bottom). Used with permission of Elsevier Publishing Co.

Chapter 10

Atrioventricular Valve-to-Two-Ventricle Connections

A. Two Atrioventricular Valves

1. Straddling Mitral Valve

This anomaly (Figure 1) is virtually always associated with a large malalignment-type ventricular septal defect (VSD) (Figures 2 and 3). Left ventricular hypoplasia, if present, is usually mild. A typical case is double-outlet right ventricle {S,D,D}, large subpulmonary malalignment-type VSD, and arch hypoplasia.[1–6] Were it not for the straddling mitral valve, the patient would be a candidate for arch repair, VSD closure, and arterial switch (Figure 4). Attempting this operation in the presence of straddling mitral valve risks the creation of left ventricular outflow obstruction (since the mitral valve sits partially underneath the native pulmonary valve).

The long axial oblique sweep is more helpful than the four-chamber view.[7]

2. Straddling Tricuspid Valve

This anomaly[5,6,8,9] is almost invariably associated with a large atrioventricular canal-type VSD (Figure 5). Common sites of attachment within the left ventricle are: the posteromedial papillary muscle (Figure 6) or an accessory papillary muscle (situated between the septum and the posteromedial papillary muscle). Right ventricular hypoplasia (Figure 7) is usually present and can be severe.

The long axial oblique and sagittal subcostal sweeps are best.

3. Straddling of Both Atrioventricular Valves

This extremely rare anomaly occurs when both straddling mitral valve and straddling tricuspid valve are present.

B. Common Atrioventricular Valve

1. Balanced

Lev[10] made the important observation that the alignment of the common atrioventricular valve vis-à-vis the ventricles was not always balanced. [In a balanced alignment, 50% of the diameter is above each ventricle (Figure 8)]. An abnormality of ventriculo-arterial alignment commonly coexists. For example, in double-outlet right ventricle, complete common atrioventricular canal can be associated with malalignment of the common atrioventricular valve towards the right ventricle.[11] In the case of tetralogy of Fallot, if malalignment of the common atrioventricular valve occurs, it tends to be toward the left ventricle.[11]

2. Malalignment Toward the Right Ventricle

The subcostal left oblique and sagittal sweeps are the best to use for alignment assessment (Figure 9). The attachment of the leftward aspect of the common atrioventricular valve "attenuates." In mild cases there is frequently attachment only to a normal anterolateral papillary muscle (Figure 10). In severe cases there is only attachment to the cephalad-most aspect of the left ventricle (Figure 11). This cannot be appreciated from the apical view (Figure 12).

3. Malalignment Toward the Left Ventricle

For unknown reasons, this type of malalignment is far less frequent than malalignment toward the right ventricle. Tetralogy of Fallot or double-outlet outlet chamber (single left ventricle with double-outlet right ventricle, see Chapter 11, section B) commonly coexist with this type of common atrioventricular canal. It occasionally occurs in patients with absolutely normal ventriculo-arterial alignment (Figure 13). The subcostal left oblique and sagittal sweeps facilitate its recognition.

References

1. Rice MJ, Seward JB, Edwards WD, Hagler DJ, Danielson GK, Puga FJ, Tajik AJ. Straddling atrioventricular valve: two-dimensional echocardiographic diagnosis, classification, and surgical implications. *Am J Cardiol* 1985; 55:505–513.

2. Kitamura N, Takao A, Ando M, Imai Y, Konno S. Taussig-Bing heart with mitral valve straddling. *Circulation* 1974; 49:761–767.

3. Muster AJ, Bharati S, Aziz KU, Idriss FS, Paul MH, Lev M, Carr I, et al. Taussig-Bing anomaly with straddling mitral valve. *J Thorac Cardiovasc Surg* 1979; 77:832–842.

4. Freedom RM, Bini R, Dische R, Rowe RD. The straddling mitral valve: morphological observations and clinical implications. *Eur J Cardiol* 1978; 8:27–50.

5. Milo S, Ho SY, Macartney FJ, Wilkinson JL, Becker AE, Wenink AC, Gittenberger-de Groot AC, et al. Straddling and overriding atrioventricular valves: morphology and classification. *Am J Cardiol* 1979; 44:1122–1134.

6. Wenink AC, Gittenberger-de Groot AC. Straddling mitral and tricuspid valves: morphologic differences and developmental backgrounds. *Am J Cardiol* 1982; 49:1959–1971.

7. Smallhorn JF, Tommasini G, Macartney FJ. Detection and assessment of straddling and overriding atrioventricular valves by two dimensional echocardiography. *Br Heart J* 1981; 46:254–262.

8. Rosenquist GC. Overriding right atrioventricular valve in association with mitral atresia. *Am Heart J* 1974; 87:26–32.

9. Ho SY, Milo S, Anderson RH, Macartney FJ, Goodwin A, Becker AE, Wenink ACG, et al. Straddling atrioventricular valve with absent atrioventricular connection. *Br Heart J* 1982; 47:344–352.

10. Bharati S, Lev M. The spectrum of common atrioventricular orifice (canal). *Am Heart J* 1973; 86:553–561.

11. Bharati S, Kirklin JW, McAllister HA, Lev M. The surgical anatomy of common atrioventricular orifice associated with tetralogy of Fallot, double outlet right ventricle, and complete regular transposition. *Circulation* 1980; 61:1142–1149.

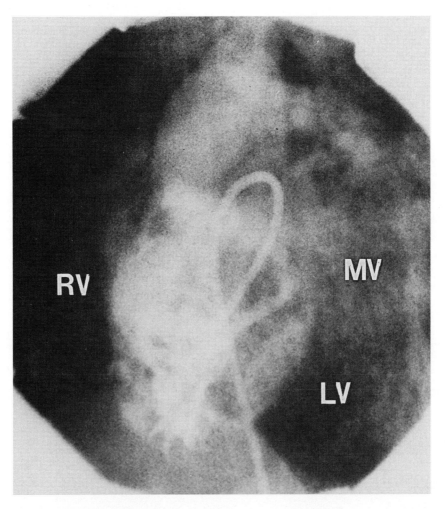

Figure 1: Lateral angiogram of mitral straddling. The annulus (MV) appears to be entirely above the right ventricle (RV). The ventricular septum, at its apical extent, deviates posteriorly resulting in this illusion. LV = left ventricle.

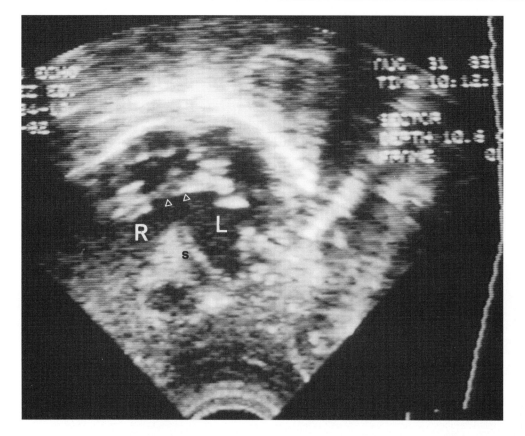

Figure 2: Subcostal left oblique view of straddling mitral valve (arrowheads). L = left ventricle; R = right ventricle; s = septum.

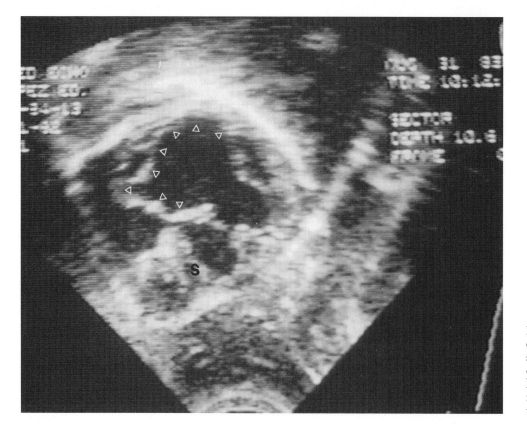

Figure 3: Subcostal left oblique view of patient shown in Figure 2. The straddling mitral valve (arrowheads) extends through a malalignment-type ventricular septal defect.

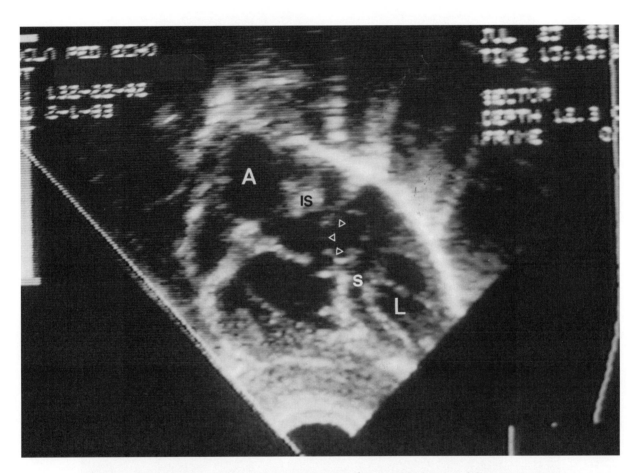

Figure 4: Subcostal frontal view of double-outlet right ventricle, large malalignment-type ventricular septal defect, and no valvar pulmonic stenosis. This patient would be a reasonable candidate for arterial repair and ventricular septal defect "closure," except that the straddling mitral valve (arrowheads) sits in the native subpulmonary region. A = aortic outflow; IS = infundibular septum; L = left ventricle; s = septum.

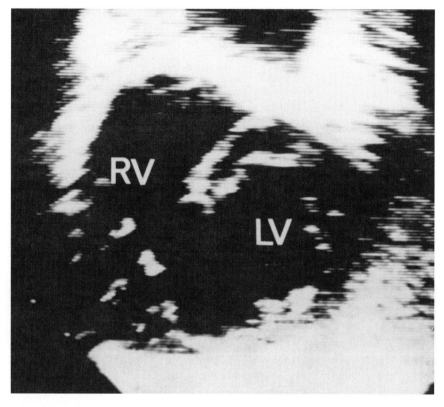

Figure 5: Subcostal left oblique view showing tricuspid valve chordae and large atrioventricular-type ventricular septal defect.

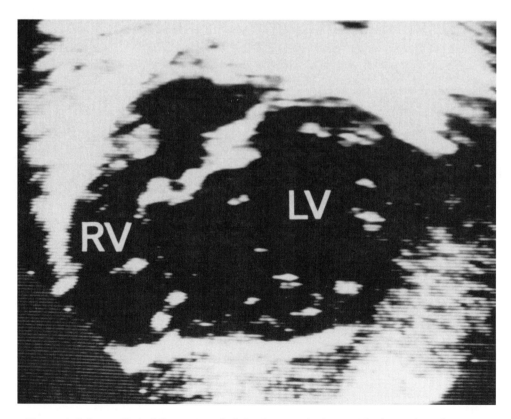

Figure 6: Subcostal left oblique view slightly closer to the base of the heart than shown in Figure 5. Leaflet tissue of the diamond-shaped tricuspid valve is now seen.

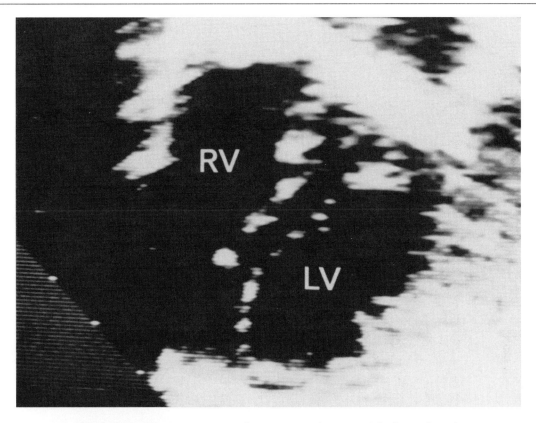

Figure 7: Subcostal left oblique view slightly closer to the apex of the heart than shown in Figure 5. The plane of the septum is now displayed. Note the right ventricular inflow is hypoplastic.

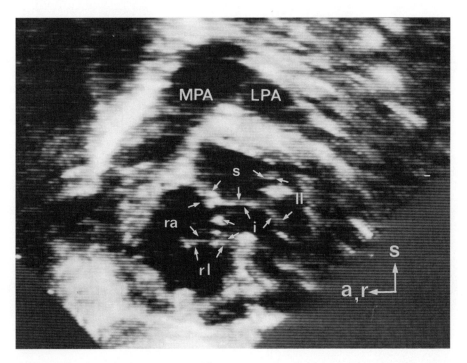

Figure 8: Subcostal left oblique view of the penta-leaflet common atrioventricular valve in type A complete common atrioventricular canal. Coaptation configuration allows analysis of the size of each leaflet. i = inferior bridging leaflet; ll = left lateral leaflet; LPA = left pulmonary artery; MPA = main pulmonary artery; ra = right superior leaflet; rl = right lateral leaflet; s = left superior leaflet.

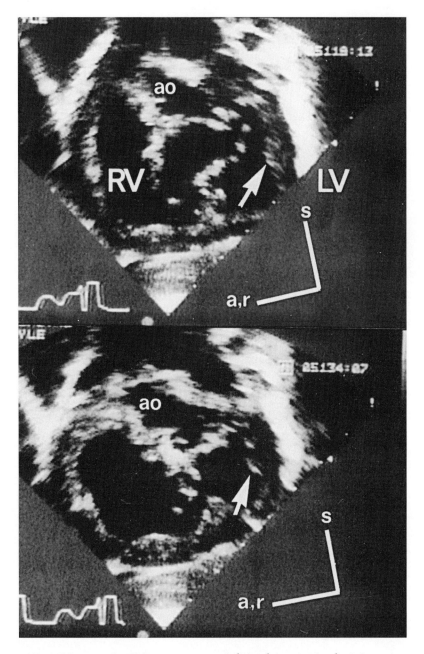

Figure 9: In mild cases of malalignment toward the right ventricle, the leftward aspect of the common atrioventricular valve attaches only to the anterolateral papillary muscle. (The arrow shows the posteromedial papillary muscle.)

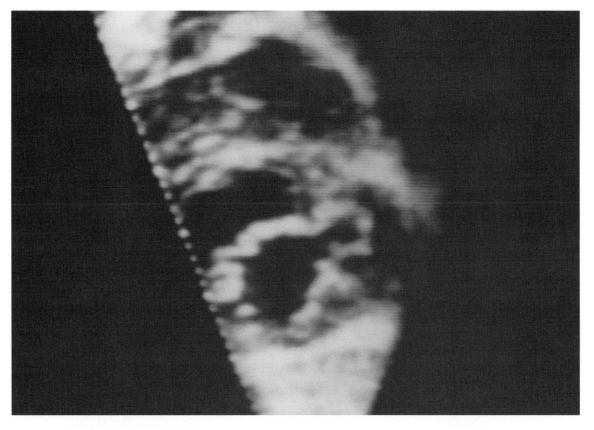

Figure 10: Subcostal left oblique view of a patient with more significant malalignment toward the right ventricle.

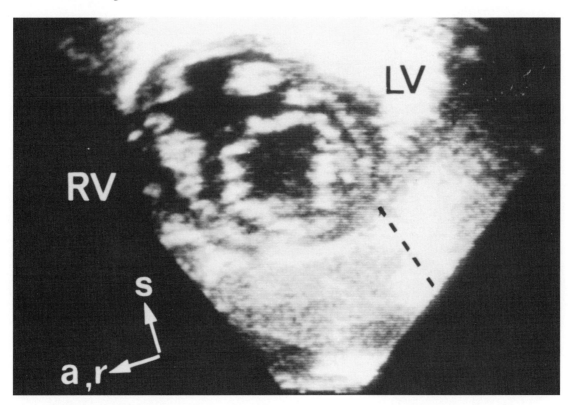

Figure 11: Subcostal left oblique view of severe malalignment toward the right ventricle (RV). The ventricular septal plane is shown by the dashed line. There is attachment to only the cephalad-most aspect of the left ventricle (LV).

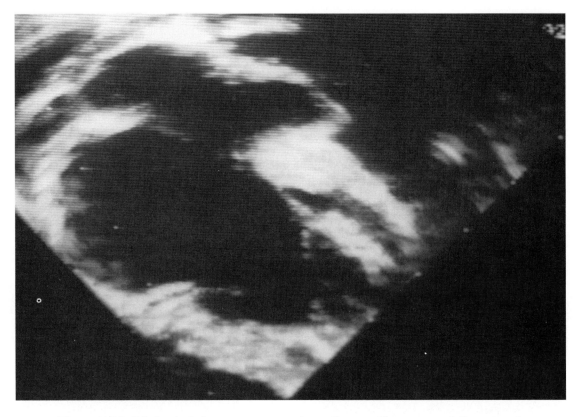

Figure 12: Modified apical view, postmortem echocardiogram. The severe malalignment of the common atrioventricular valve vis-à-vis the ventricles can be identified; however, the fact that the attachment involves only the *cephalad* portion of the left ventricle cannot be appreciated.

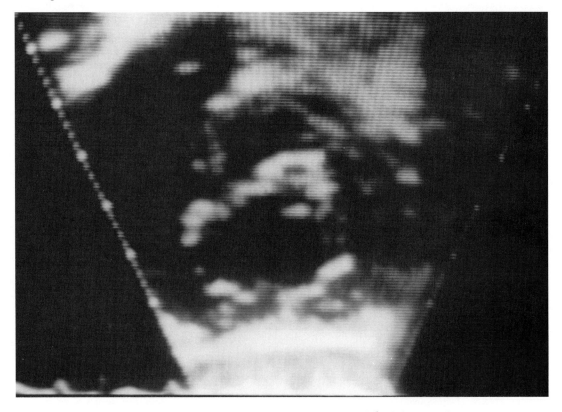

Figure 13: Subcostal left oblique view of malalignment toward the left ventricle.

Chapter 11

Atrioventricular Valve-to-One-Ventricle Connections

A. Double Inlet

1. Single Right Ventricle

Single right ventricle[1-4] is very much less common than single left ventricle, and the internal morphology is more variable. The two atrioventricular valves are usually approximately similar in size; if one is larger, it is the right. Both tend to be tri-leaflet.

2. Single Left Ventricle

The internal morphology of single left ventricle[5-8] is characterized by a smooth left septal surface. The two atrioventricular valves tend to be similar in size (Figure 1). In L-loop, if there is one that is larger, it is usually the right-sided one. Both tend to be bi-leaflet. In D-loop, if there is one that is larger, it is usually the left-sided one. The right-sided atrioventricular valve is usually tri-leaflet, while the left-sided one is bi-leaflet.

An "outlet chamber" is always present (Figures 2 and 3). The variation with {S,D,S} is termed Holmes heart.[9,10]

The *communication* between the left ventricle and the outlet chamber (called variously a ventricular septal defect, an outlet foramen, or a bulboventricular foramen) is usually small in patients with no pulmonary stenosis (Figure 4), and large in those with pulmonary stenosis (Figure 5). In L-loop, the left atrioventricular valve is closer to the outlet foramen; in D-loop, the right atrioventricular valve is closer to the outlet foramen (Figures 6 and 7). The outlet foramen may not be the smallest part of the pathway to the aorta (Figures 8 and 9).

Whether the myocytes in single ventricle are different in structure or in orientation and whether myocardial function is less efficient in single ventricle[11-13] is still unresolved (see also Chapter 31, section E).

3. Single Ventricle with Right Ventricle and Left Ventricle Components

Most of these cases are probably large ventricular septal defects with such deficiency in septal structure that is difficult to recognize any of the usual landmarks, e.g., septal band.

B. Common Inlet

1. Single Right Ventricle

This is by far the most common ventricular morphology in the common-inlet situation! Double-outlet right ventricle and heterotaxy syndrome frequently coexist.

2. Single Left Ventricle

Far less common than single right ventricle, common-inlet single left ventricle can coexist with transposition or with "double-outlet outlet chamber."

3. Single Ventricle with Right Ventricle and Left Ventricle Components

This is extremely rare.

References

1. Soto B, Bertranou EG, Bream PR, Souza A, Bargeron LM. Angiographic study of univentricular heart of right ventricular type. *Circulation* 1979; 60:1325–1334.

2. Quero Jimenez M, Perez Martinez VM, Maitre Azcarate MJ, Merino Batres G, Moreno Granados F. Exaggerated displacement of the atrioventricular canal towards the bulbus cordis. *Br Heart J* 1973; 35:65–74.

3. Wilkinson JL, Dickinson D, Smith A, Anderson RH. Conducting tissues in univentricular heart of right ventricular type with double or common inlet. *J Thorac Cardiovasc Surg* 1979; 77:691–698.

4. Keeton BR, Macartney FJ, Hunter S, Mortera C, Rees P, Shinebourne EA, Tynan M, Wilkinson JL, et al. Univentricular heart of right ventricular type with double or common inlet. *Circulation* 1979; 59:403–411.

5. Van Praagh R, Plett JA, Van Praagh S. Single ventricle. *Herz* 1979; 4:113–150.

6. Van Mierop LHS. Embryology of the univentricular heart. *Herz* 1979; 4:78–85.

7. Van Praagh R, David I, Van Praagh S. What is a ventricle? The single ventricle trap. *Pediatr Cardiol* 1982; 2:79–84.

8. Anderson RH, Arnold R, Thapar MK, Jones RS, Hamilton DI. Cardiac specialized tissue in hearts with an apparently single ventricular chamber (double inlet left ventricle). *Am J Cardiol* 1974; 33:95–106.

9. Holmes AF. A case of malformation of the heart. *Trans Med Chir Soc Edinburgh* 1824; 1:252–259.

10. Freedom RM, Rowe RD. Morphological and topographical variations of the outlet chamber in complex congenital heart disease: an angiocardiographic study. *Cath Cardiovasc Diag* 1978; 4:345–371.

11. Marcelletti C, Mazzera E, Olthof H, Sebel PS, Duren DR, Losekoot TG, Becker AE. Fontan's operation: an expanded horizon. *J Thorac Cardiovasc Surg* 1980; 80:764–769.

12. Gibson DG, Traill TA, Brown DJ. Abnormal ventricular function in patients with univentricular heart. *Herz* 1979; 4:226–231.

13. Sano T, Ogawa M, Taniguchi K, Matsuda H, Nakajima T, Arisawa J, Shimazaki Y, et al. Assessment of ventricular contractile state and function in patients with univentricular heart. *Circulation* 1989; 79:1247–1256.

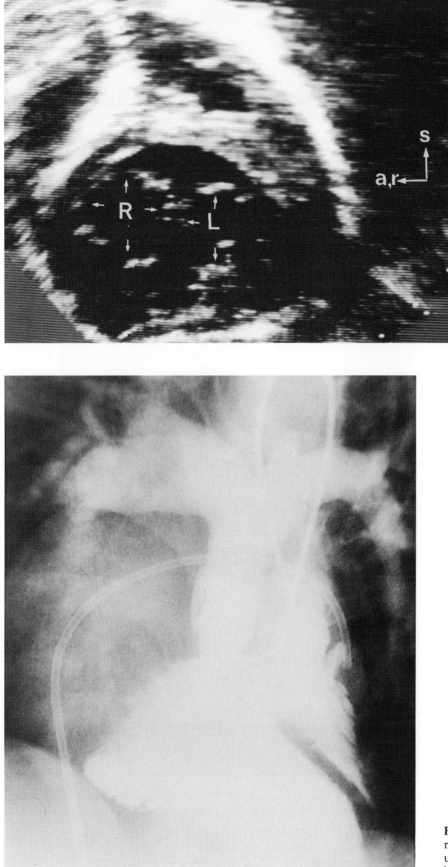

Figure 1: Subcostal left oblique view of single left ventricle with transposition of the great arteries {S,L,L}. Note the smooth left septal surface. The two atrioventricular valves (R and L) are roughly similar in diameter.

Figure 2: Cranially angled anteroposterior angiogram of same patient as in Figure 1. There is a left-sided outlet chamber.

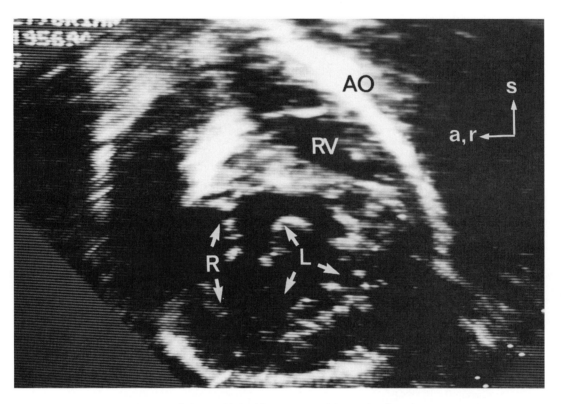

Figure 3: Subcostal left oblique view of the outlet chamber.

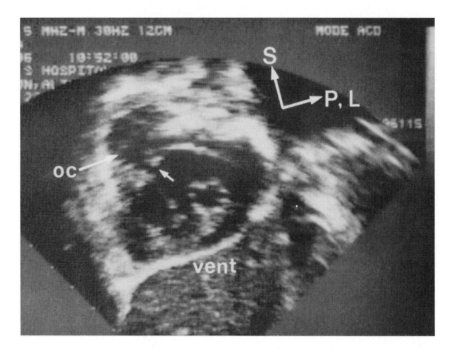

Figure 4: Subcostal left oblique view of single left ventricle with transposition of the great arteries {S,D,D} and no pulmonary stenosis. Note the small outlet foramen (unlabeled arrow). oc = outlet chamber; vent = left ventricle.

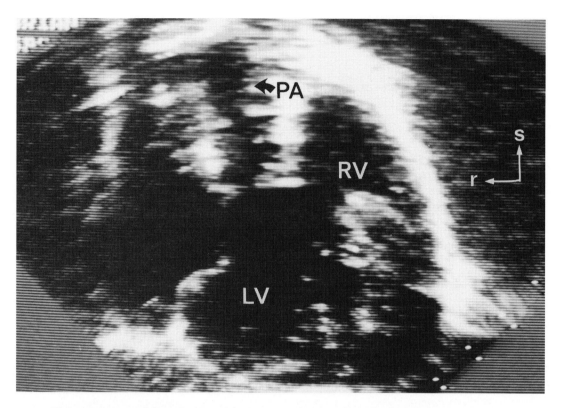

Figure 5: Subcostal frontal view of the large outlet foramen in the patient shown in Figure 1 with pulmonary stenosis.

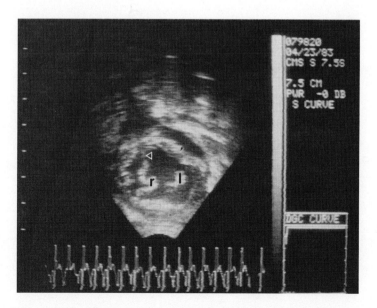

Figure 6: Subcostal left oblique view of single left ventricle with transposition of the great arteries {S,D,D}. Note the right (r) atrioventricular valve is closer than the left (l) atrioventricular valve to the outlet foramen. The triangle points to an attachment.

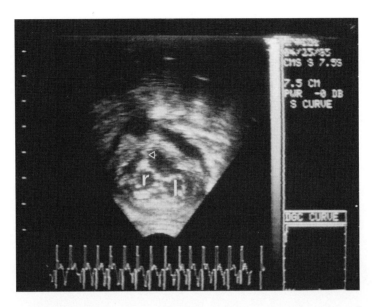

Figure 7: Subcostal left oblique view of the patient shown in Figure 6. The right atrioventricular valve (r) attaches (triangle) to the rim of the small outlet foramen.

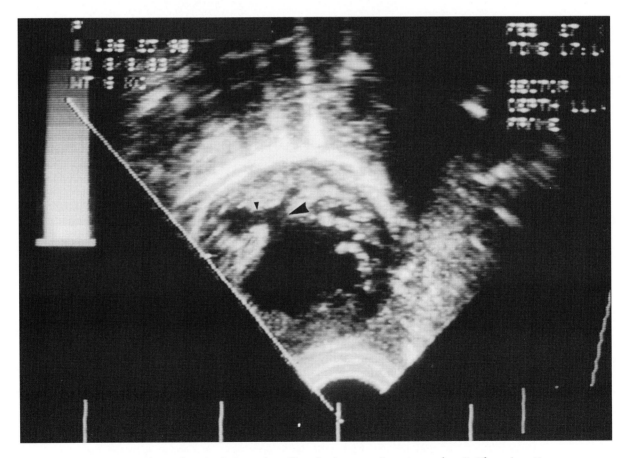

Figure 8: Subcostal sagittal view of small outlet foramen (large arrowhead). The subaortic infundibulum (small arrowhead) in diastole looks almost the same width.

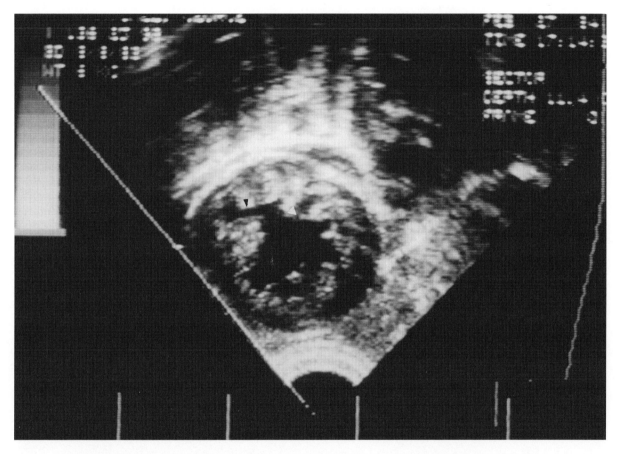

Figure 9: Subcostal sagittal view of small outlet foramen (white arrowhead). In systole, the width of the subaortic infundibulum (black arrowhead) has markedly decreased.

Chapter 12

Ventricles

A. Spongy Myocardium

This is a rare form of myopathy[1] that can be identified by two-dimensional echocardiography. Hemodynamically, it behaves as a dilated cardiomyopathy.

B. Ebstein's Anomaly

One of the most common cardiomyopathies is one that involves the septum and right ventricular free wall preferentially—Ebstein's anomaly[2-4] (see Chapter 9).

Although the first two-dimensional echocardiography studies suggested using the apical four-chamber cut[5] to identify Ebstein's, we have found that the subcostal left oblique sweep systemically uncovers all of the features. (Since Ebstein's anomaly is a cardiomyopathy, it is important to investigate all regions of the right ventricle.) The left oblique views also allow simultaneous visualization of all three leaflets of the tricuspid valve. We can appreciate the echocardiographic correlate of the "nondelamination" which is hypothesized to be the cardinal[6,7] feature in Ebstein's (Figure 1).

C. Uhl's Anomaly

Parchment right ventricle is termed Uhl's anomaly.[8-10] Just as with Ebstein's anomaly, the subcostal left oblique sweep is most reliable. This may well be the same disease as the "right ventricular dysplasia" reported in adults.

D. Isolated Ventricular Inversion ({S,L,S})

This uncommon isolated segmental discordance[11-13] is identified using the subcostal left oblique sweep.

E. Hypertrophic Cardiomyopathy

Many but not all families appear to have mutations[14] in the beta myosin heavy chain gene on chromosome 14. Some have mutations on other chromosomes. The extent of involvement (of both the septum and the left ventricular free wall) is best seen in the subcostal left oblique sweep. There is frequently left ventricular outflow tract obstruction. The two most common causes[15] are septal bulge and mitral valve systolic anterior motion (Figure 2).

Mitral regurgitation is a common coexisting problem. Although the subaortic stenosis is dynamic, some observers in adult laboratories have found the simplified Bernoulli formula to nevertheless yield close correlations with invasively measured gradients. This has yet to be confirmed in infants and in children.

F. Dilated Cardiomyopathy

A significant percentage are due not to myocarditis but to genetic alterations.[16,17] The "shortening fraction" of the left ventricle is the most commonly employed parameter, although individual end-diastolic and end-ejection dimensions may be just as helpful.

A relatively load-independent parameter of contractile state has been proposed by Colan et al.[18]—the end-systolic meridional wall stress versus corrected velocity of circumferential fiber shortening relationship.

It should allow the detection of abnormal ventricles whose shortening fraction has been "normalized" by a diminished afterload.

References

1. Chin TK, Perloff JK, Williams RG, Jue K, Mohrmann R. Isolated noncompaction of left ventricular myocardium: a study of eight cases. *Circulation* 1990; 82:507–513.

2. Anderson KR, Zuberbuhler JR, Anderson RH, Becker AE, Lie JT. Morphologic spectrum of Ebstein's anomaly of the heart. *Mayo Clin Proc* 1979; 54:174–180.

3. Anderson KR, Lie JT. The right ventricular myocardium in Ebstein's anomaly: a morphologic histopathologic study. *Mayo Clin Proc* 1979; 54:181–184.

4. Smith WM, Gallagher JJ, Kerr CR, Sealy WC, Kasell JH, Benson DW, Reiter MJ, et al. The electrophysiologic basis and management of symptomatic recurrent tachycardia in patients with Ebstein's anomaly of the tricuspid valve. *Am J Cardiol* 1982; 49:1223–1234.

5. Shiina A, Seward JB, Edwards WD, Hagler DJ, Tajik AJ. Two-dimensional echocardiographic spectrum of Ebstein's anomaly: detailed anatomic assessment. *J Am Coll Cardiol* 1984; 3:356–370.

6. Van Mierop LHS, Gessner IH. Pathologic mechanisms in congenital cardiovascular malformations. *Prog Cardiovasc Dis* 1972; 15:67–85.

7. Wenink ACG. Embryology of the ventricular septum: separate origin of its components. *Virchows Arch [Pathol Anat]* 1981; 390:71–79.

8. Uhl HSM. A previously undescribed congenital malformation of the heart: almost total absence of the myocardium of the right ventricle. *Bull Johns Hopkins Hosp* 1952; 91:197–205.

9. Segall HN. Parchment heart (Osler). *Am Heart J* 1950; 40:948–950.

10. Castleman B, Spraque HB. Case records of the Massachusetts General Hospital: weekly clinicopathological exercises. *N Engl J Med* 1952; 246:785–790.

11. Ostermeyer J, Bircks W, Krian A, Sievers G, Hilgenberg F. Isolated atrioventricular discordance. *J Thorac Cardiovasc Surg* 1983; 86:926–929.

12. Van Praagh R, Van Praagh S. Isolated ventricular inversion: a consideration of the morphogenesis, definition, and diagnosis of nontransposed and transposed great arteries. *Am J Cardiol* 1966; 17:396–406.

13. Snider AR, Enderlein MA, Teitel DF, Hirji M, Heymann MA. Isolated ventricular inversion: two-dimensional echocardiographic findings and a review of the literature. *Pediatr Cardiol* 1984; 5:27–33.

14. Hengstenberg C, Komajda M, Schwartz K. Genetics of familial hypertrophic cardiomyopathy: results and strategies. *Trends Cardiovasc Med* 1993; 3:115–118.

15. Rakowski H, Sasson Z, Wigle ED. Echocardiographic and Doppler assessment of hypertrophic cardiomyopathy. *J Am Soc Echo* 1988; 1:31–47.

16. Michels VV, Driscoll DJ, Miller FA. Familial aggregation of idiopathic dilated cardiomyopathy. *Am J Cardiol* 1985; 55:1232–1233.

17. Berko BA, Swift M. X-linked dilated cardiomyopathy. *N Engl J Med* 1987; 316:1186–1191.

18. Colan SD, Borow KM, Neumann A. Left ventricular end-systolic wall stress-velocity of fiber shortening relation: a load-independent index of myocardial contractility. *J Am Coll Cardiol* 1984; 4:715–724.

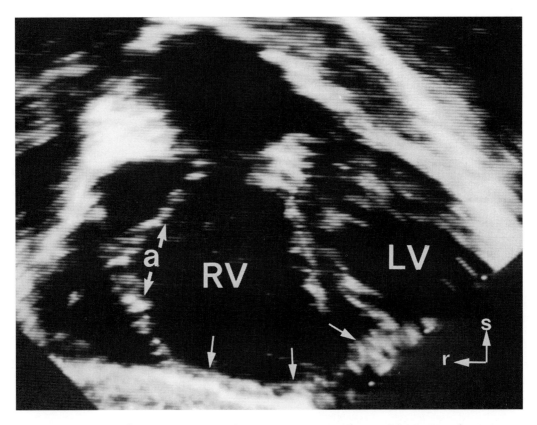

Figure 1: One of the strongest pieces of evidence supporting the nondelamination theory is the appearance of the leaflet tissue blending (arrows) into the wall (e.g., the diaphragmatic surface, in this case). a = anterior leaflet; LV = left ventricle; RV = right ventricle.

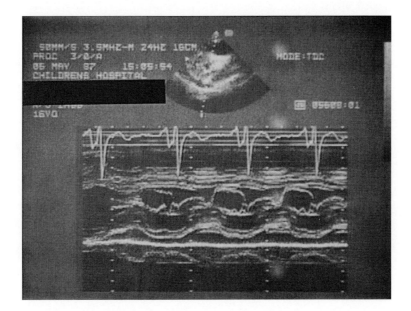

Figure 2: M-mode echocardiogram of systolic anterior motion of mitral leaflet in hypertrophic obstructive cardiomyopathy.

Chapter 13

Ventricular Septum

A. Perimembranous (sometimes called membranous or conoventricular) VSD

The most cephalad aspect of the atrioventricular canal is the membranous septum. In the case of normally aligned great arteries, this area lies immediately inferior (caudad) to the right coronary-noncoronary commissure of the aortic valve (Figure 1). From the right ventricular aspect, it lies immediately inferior to the most basal extent of the inferior limb of the "Y" of septal band. Since the "Y" of septal band (unlike the mid-portion) is rarely distinguishable by echocardiography, assignment of a ventricular septal defect (VSD) as perimembranous is unfortunately dependent on its position vis-à-vis the aortic valve (Figure 2); in the case of malalignment-type VSD, it is very difficult to be sure that such a VSD does not also extend to include the membranous septum.

There is frequently accessory tricuspid valve tissue attached to or near a perimembranous VSD (Figure 1). This phenomenon has made it difficult to judge the functional diameter of a perimembranous VSD preoperatively by two-dimensional echocardiography alone or even with Doppler color flow imaging. Thus, comparison of right ventricular systolic pressure with left ventricular systolic pressure is the most dependable way to assess whether a defect is small, moderate, or large.

In the first 2 months of age, the right ventricular pressure estimate may be misleading since the pulmonary vascular impedance may still be higher than its adult level; in such cases, a *combination* of color Doppler jet width and the right ventricular pressure estimate is probably the most reliable approach to judging size of VSD. In our experience, a 3 mm VSD is always restrictive while a 6 mm VSD is always nonrestrictive (large).

In cases of 4 mm or 5 mm jet width, if the right ventricular pressure estimate is equal to systemic, then re-evaluation after 2 months of age is necessary. If the right ventricular pressure estimate is more than 20 mm Hg lower than systemic, the VSD is "moderate" size.

The two ways of estimating right ventricular systolic pressure are to interrogate the VSD jet directly or to interrogate a tricuspid regurgitant jet if there is one. Some of the problems with the former approach are: difficulty aligning the continuous wave cursor with the VSD jet (Figures 3 and 4) and the temporal differences between the left ventricular and right ventricular pressure rise. If there is a phase difference, then there is a substantial difference between Doppler instantaneous gradient and catheter peak-to-peak gradient. In addition, it is important to remember not to neglect the velocity proximal to the VSD since it is often 1–2 m/sec.

One advantage of interrogating the tricuspid valve jet is that it is easier to align the continuous wave cursor with the jet. Another advantage is that since infants, even those in "heart failure," virtually always have right atrial pressures under 10 mm Hg, the pressure difference between right ventricle and the right atrium is almost always very similar to the absolute right ventricular systolic pressure. Thus, the error in this method is mostly due to cursor alignment. Given that tricuspid valve regurgitation can usually be displayed in three views (parasternal short axis, apical four-chamber, and subcostal frontal), it should be possible to obtain satisfactory alignment.

B. Malalignment Type VSD

The infundibular septum is the muscle that divides the arterial outflow tracts. In the normal heart, it lies snugly between the limbs of the "Y" of the septal band. In many malformations of the outflow tracts, it is displaced, or malaligned, vis-à-vis the "Y" of the septal band (Figures 5 and 6). Such a VSD is termed *malalignment-type*.[1]

C. Muscular VSD

These have been arbitrarily categorized by their location vis-à-vis the septal band and takeoff of moderator band. Those that are distal to the takeoff of the moderator band are termed *apical* (Figure 7). Those that are proximal to the moderator band takeoff but cephalad to the septal band are termed *anterior* (Figures 8 and 9). Those that are proximal to the moderator band takeoff but caudad to the septal band are termed *mid-muscular* (Figure 10). For defects closely related to but not contiguous with the atrioventricular valve annulus, the term *posterior* muscular (Figure 11) is used (see section E below).

D. Infundibular Septal Hypoplasia Type VSD

In some patients, the infundibular septum is not displaced vis-à-vis the "Y" of septal band; however, there are defects in it. A majority of these are nonrestrictive. As stated previously, the "Y" itself is not distinguishable; thus, the designation of a VSD as infundibular septal hypoplasia type depends on its contiguity with both arterial valves. In the case of normally aligned great arteries (or nearly normal great arteries, e.g., tetralogy of Fallot), the VSD should thus be not only near the aortic valve but also near the pulmonary valve. In the subcostal sagittal sweep, the VSD should be visible in the plane that displays the pulmonary valve (Figure 12).

Certain other ventriculo-arterial alignments frequently have coexistent infundibular septal hypopla-sia–double-outlet right ventricle and double-outlet left ventricle. The latter (see Chapter 15, section C) so frequently exhibits infundibular septal hypoplasia (and yet also commonly manifests short infundibular free walls) that complete infundibular hypoplasia seems to be a possible primary event in the malformation (Figures 13 and 14).

E. Atrioventricular Canal Type VSD

Inferior to the membranous septum is an area that has been termed *atrioventricular septum* or *atrioventricular canal septum*. It is missing in four types of atrioventricular canal (or atrioventricular septal defect): complete, transitional, partial, atrioventricular canal-type VSD. In the last type, the atrioventricular valves lie in their usual orientation; thus, there is no "gooseneck" deformity. (The atrioventricular valve plane in the other three types is distinctly abnormal. See Chapter 9, section B.)

The atrioventricular canal-type VSD is contiguous with the atrioventricular valve annulus. In roughly half the cases, there is a "cleft mitral valve." The subcostal sweeps are the best way of identifying this lesion (Figures 15 and 16). The apical four-chamber view can be misleading; many perimembranous VSDs can look like atrioventricular canal type in this cut.

F. Supero-Inferior Ventricles

Rarely the plane of the ventricular septum is horizontal.[2] The most common ventriculo-arterial alignments to exhibit this are double-outlet right ventricle and transposition of the great arteries. There is almost always a VSD of the malalignment type. The next most common type is a combination malalignment type and atrioventricular canal type.

References

1. Van Praagh R, Van Praagh S, Nebesar RA, Muster AJ, Sinha SN, Paul MH. Tetralogy of Fallot underdevelopment of the pulmonary infundibulum and its sequelae. *Am J Cardiol* 1970; 26:25–33.

2. Van Praagh S, LaCorte M, Fellows KE, Bossina K, Busch HJ, Keck EW, Weinberg PM, Van Praagh R. Supero-inferior ventricles: anatomic and angiocardiographic findings in ten postmortem cases. In: Van Praagh R, Takao A (eds). *Etiology and Morphogenesis of Congenital Heart Disease*. Futura Publishing Company, Mount Kisco, 1980, Chapter 17.

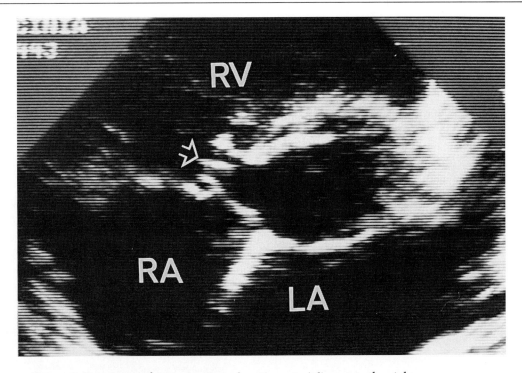

Figure 1: Parasternal short axis view of aortic root. Adjacent to the right coronary-non-coronary commissure is a perimembranous ventricular septal defect. Accessory tricuspid valve tissue (arrow) is situated near the defect. LA = left atrium; RA = right atrium; RV = right ventricle.

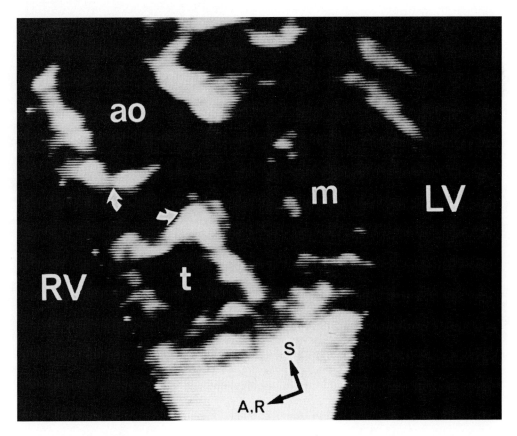

Figure 2: Subcostal left oblique view of large perimembranous ventricular septal defect (arrows), immediately adjacent to aortic cusps. m = mitral valve; t = tricuspid valve; RV = right ventricle; LV = left ventricle.

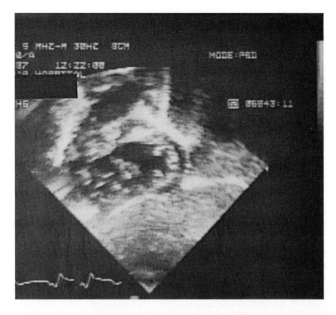

Figure 3: Subcostal left oblique view. Note that jet trajectory through a posterior muscular ventricular septal defect would be nearly at right angles to a Doppler cursor.

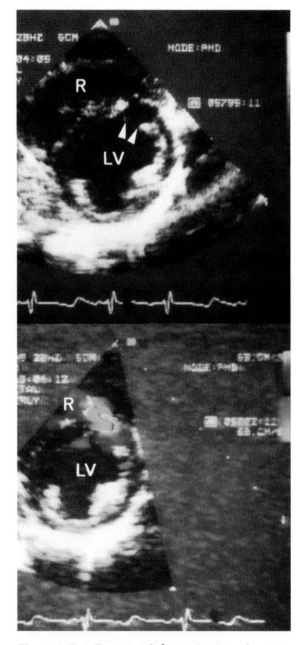

Figure 4: Top: Parasternal short axis view of anterior muscular ventricular septal defect. Arrows show the left ventricular (LV) aspect of the ventricular septal defect. Note that the defect takes a nearly right-angle course through the septum. **Bottom:** Color flow imaging of serpiginous path taken by ventricular septal defect jet.

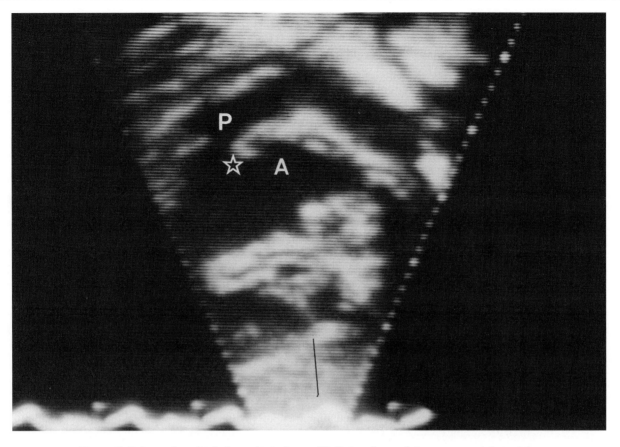

Figure 5: Subcostal sagittal view of tetralogy of Fallot and complete common atrioventricular canal. The infundibular septum (star) divides the aortic outflow from the subvalvar pulmonary (P) region and is malaligned anteriorly vis-à-vis the plane of the ventricular septum (black line).

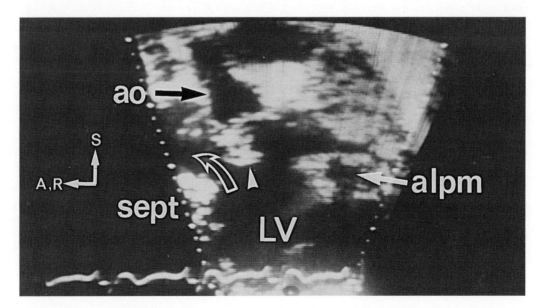

Figure 6: Subcostal left oblique view of subaortic stenosis and interrupted aortic arch. The infundibular septum (closed arrowhead) is malaligned posteriorly vis-à-vis the remainder of the ventricular septum (sept). The malalignment-type ventricular septal defect (open arrow) is 5 mm in diameter at its left ventricular end. alpm = anterolateral papillary muscle; ao = ascending aorta.

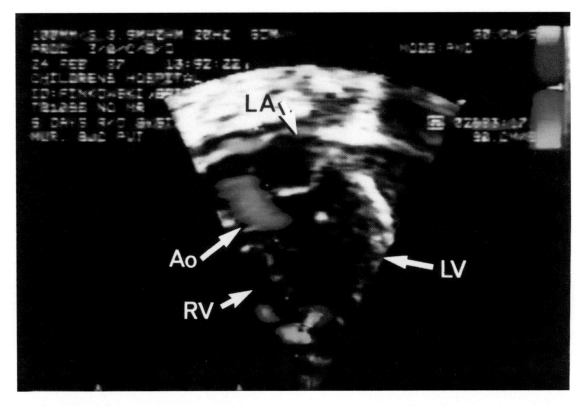

Figure 7: Apical view of apical muscular ventricular septal defect. LA = left atrium; Ao = aorta; RV = right ventricle; LV = left ventricle.

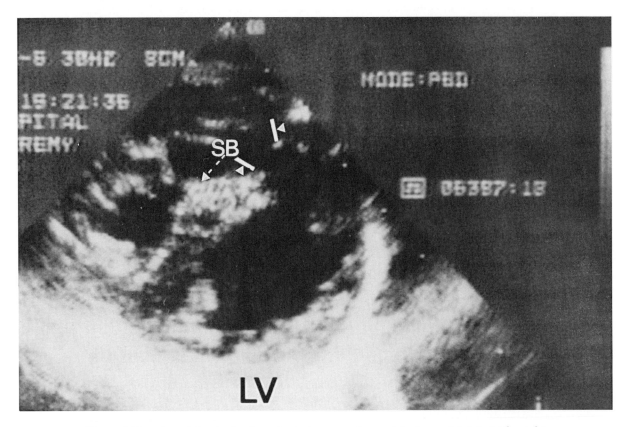

Figure 8: Parasternal short axis view of anterior muscular ventricular septal defect. The right ventricular aspect of the defect (unlabeled arrows) is cephalad to the septal band (SB).

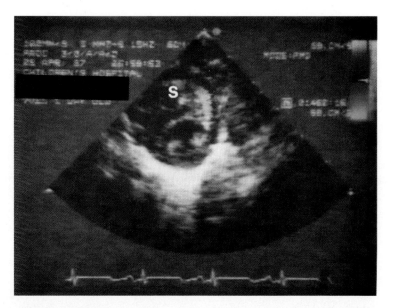

Figure 9: Color flow imaging of small anterior muscular ventricular septal defect cephalad to septal band (s).

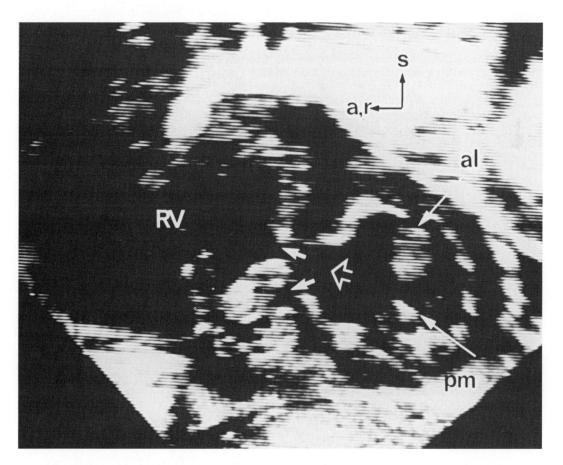

Figure 10: Subcostal left oblique view of mid-muscular ventricular septal defect. It appears as one defect (broad open arrow) from the left side and two defects (small unlabeled arrows) from the right side. al = anterolateral papillary muscle; pm = posteromedial papillary muscle.

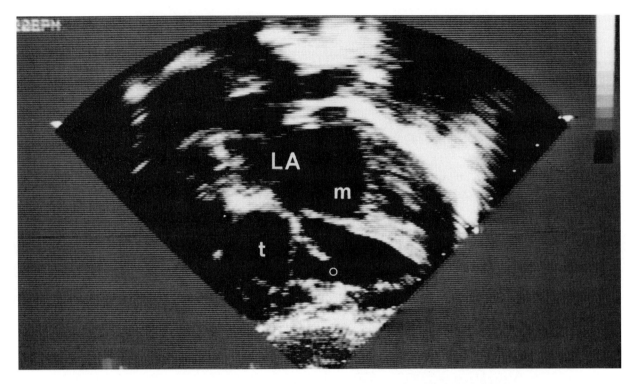

Figure 11: Subcostal frontal view of posterior muscular ventricular septal defect (open circle). LA = left atrium; m = mitral valve; t = tricuspid valve.

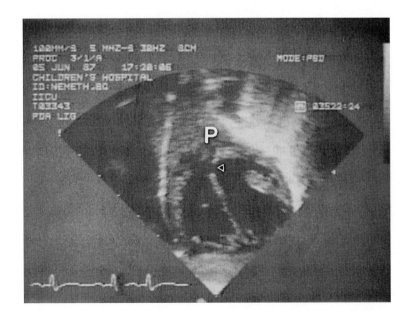

Figure 12: Subcostal sagittal view of severe infundibular septal hypoplasia (arrowhead) in the setting of normal ventriculo-arterial alignment. P = pulmonary root. Note that defect is contiguous with the pulmonary valve cusps.

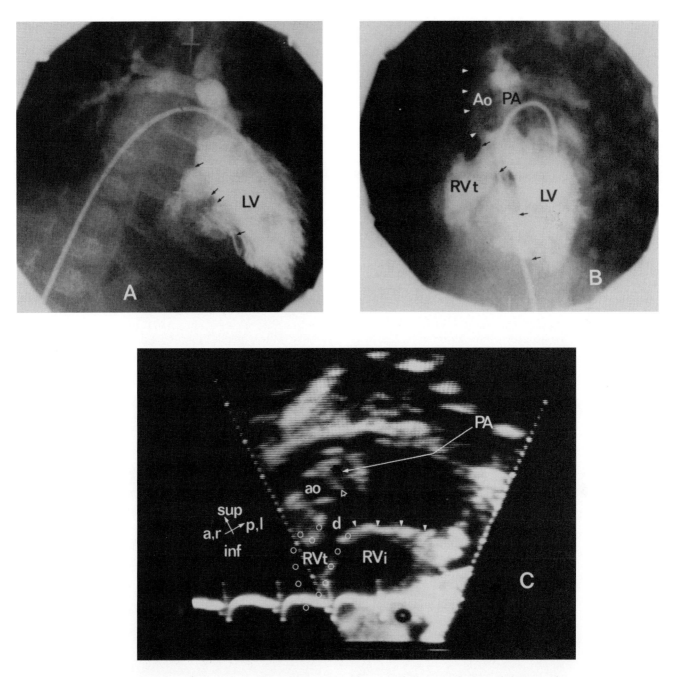

Figure 13: A: right anterior oblique view of double-outlet left ventricle. LV = left ventricle. **B:** long axial oblique view showing that both great arteries arise above the left ventricle (LV). Ao = aorta; PA = pulmonary artery ; RVt = trabecular portion of the right ventricle. **C:** subcostal long axial oblique view of same patient showing infundibular septal hypoplasia (open triangle). RVi = right ventricular inflow.

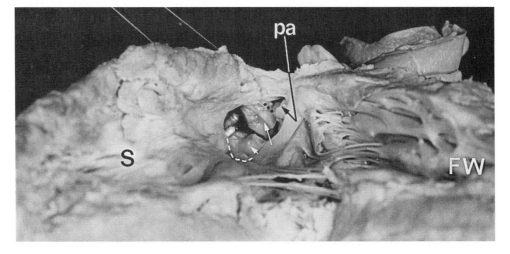

Figure 14: Postmortem view of left ventricular outflow tract of patient shown in Figure 3. White arrows show aortic cusps. The black dotted line is the hypoplastic infundibular septum. pa = pulmonary artery; s = septum; FW = free wall.

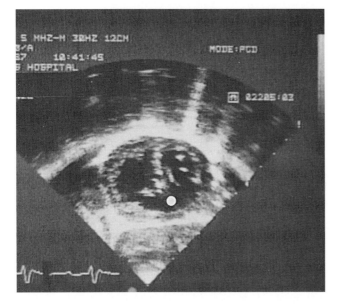

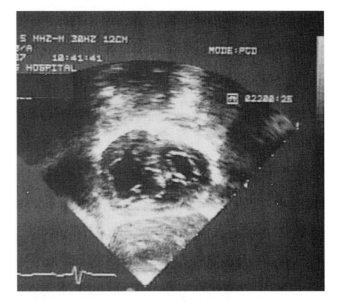

Figure 15: Subcostal left oblique view of rare case of double-outlet right ventricle with atrioventricular canal-type ventricular septal defect (closed circle). From this one part of the sweep, it is impossible to distinguish this from a posterior muscular ventricular septal defect.

Figure 16: Same patient as in Figure 13. A plane further toward the base of the heart shows the ventricular septal defect to be contiguous with the atrioventricular annuli.

Chapter 14

Criss-Cross Atrioventricular Relations

In the normal heart, the inflows to the two ventricles are arranged in a parallel configuration. Rare hearts have inflows that are nonparallel, or *criss-cross*. Pseudo criss-cross cases where there is the *illusion* of crossed inflows are fundamentally different from true criss-cross hearts.[1] The former can be "uncrossed" with rotation of the heart, whereas the latter can never be uncrossed no matter how the heart is rotated.

A. True Criss-Cross

When segmental diagnosis is "discordant" with the atrioventricular connections, the patient is said to have *true* criss-cross heart.[2] Examples are: a morphological right atrium (in situs solitus) connecting to a morphological right ventricle which is of L-loop topology (Figures 1–6), and a morphological right atrium (in situs solitus) connecting to a morphological left ventricle that is of D-loop topology.

B. Pseudo Criss-Cross

The more common so-called criss-cross heart is actually a *pseudo* criss-cross heart. The segmental anatomy is "concordant" with the atrioventricular connections. Examples are: a morphological right atrium in situs solitus connecting to a morphological right ventricle of D-loop morphology, and a morphological right atrium in situs solitus connecting to a morphological left ventricle of L-loop morphology.

References

1. Geva T, Sanders SP, Ayres NA, O'Laughlin MP, Parness IA. Two-dimensional echocardiographic anatomy of atrioventricular alignment discordance with situs concordance. *Am Heart J* 1993; 125:459–464.

2. Weinberg PM, Van Praagh R, Wagner HR, Cuaso CC. New form of criss-cross atrioventricular relations: an expanded view of the meaning of D and L-loops. In: *Abstract Book of World Congress of Paediatric Cardiology*. London, 1980, abstract no. 319.

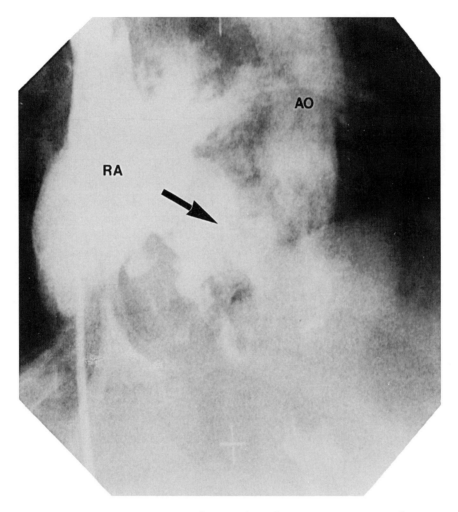

Figure 1: Anteroposterior angiogram showing the right atrium connecting to the left-sided right ventricle in a case of double-outlet right ventricle {S,L,L} with true criss-cross.

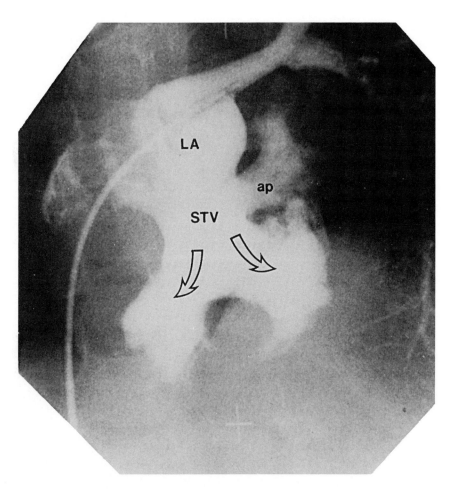

Figure 2: The left atrium connects to both ventricles through a straddling left-sided tricuspid valve (STV). ap = left atrial appendage; LA = left atrium.

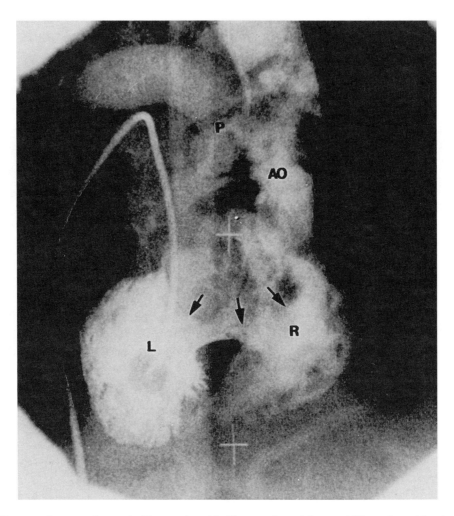

Figure 3: Same patient as in Figures 1 and 2. The annulus of the straddling tricuspid valve is seen. Ao = aorta.

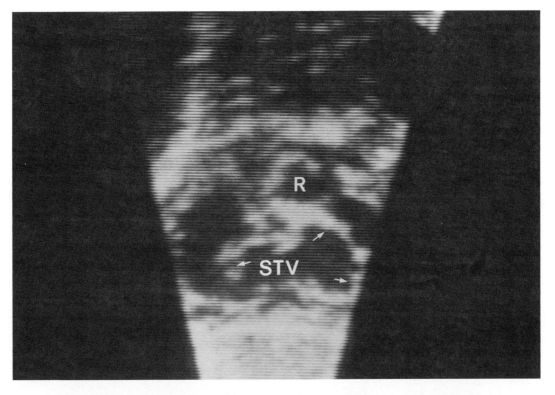

Figure 4: Subcostal frontal view of the same patient as in Figures 1–3. The right (R) atrioventricular valve is superior to the left-sided straddling tricuspid valve (STV).

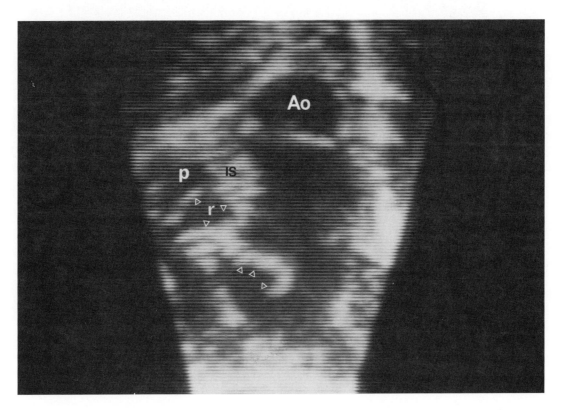

Figure 5: Same patient as in Figure 4. The right (r) atrioventricular valve is crowding the pulmonary outflow (P). IS = infundibular septum; Ao = aorta.

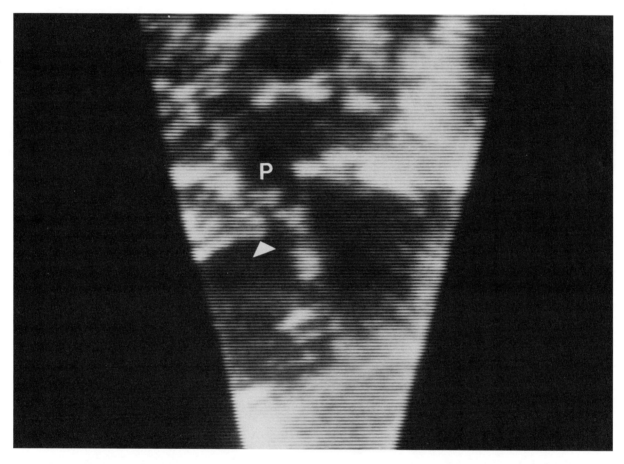

Figure 6: Subcostal sagittal view of same patient as in Figure 5. The right atrioventricular valve (arrow) is very close to the pulmonary (P) valve cusps.

Chapter 15

Ventriculo-Arterial Alignments

There are six ventriculo-arterial alignments: normal, inversus, double-outlet right ventricle, double-outlet left ventricle, transposition of the great arteries, and anatomically corrected malposition. Normal and inversus will be discussed under the same section.

All may have coexistent arch anomalies or branch pulmonary artery stenosis (or atresia).

A. Normal and Inversus (Inverted Normal)

The normal ventriculo-arterial alignment is the pulmonary artery above the right ventricle and the aorta above the left ventricle (with continuity of the aortic valve and mitral valve).

Examples of outflow tract anomalies that nevertheless maintain normal or near-normal alignment are: pulmonary outflow underdevelopment [tetralogy of Fallot[1-4] (Figures 1–4) and most types of truncus arteriosus[5-11]] and *aortic outflow underdevelopment*[12-17] [subaortic atresia (or stenosis) with ventricular septal defect (VSD) as well as the entity of truncus arteriosus with interrupted aortic arch (Figure 5)].

Subaortic stenosis (or atresia) with (malalignment-type) ventricular septal defect is a malformation that provides added circumstantial support for Van Praagh's hypothesis that the infundibular septum is formed separately from the "Y" of the septal band. In tetralogy of Fallot, the infundibular septum is found to be "displaced" anteriorly, superiorly, and leftward in relation to the "Y" of the septal band. In subaortic stenosis (or atresia) with ventricular septal defect, the infundibular septum is "displaced" posteriorly and rightward. In both types of infundibular septal displacement, the right oblique view is extremely helpful.

In malalignment-type VSD or conal septal hypoplasia VSD with arch interruption, the type of interruption is Type B in over 90% of cases.

B. Double-Outlet Right Ventricle (DORV)

1. Bilateral Infundibulum

Both great arteries are >50% above the right ventricle. The types of VSD[18-24] are malalignment-type, membranous, muscular, or combination malalignment-type and AVC-type. Isolated AVC-type is extremely rare (see Chapter 13, Figures 15 and 16).

Malalignment-type VSDs are by far the most common. The orientation (Figures 6–8) of the great arteries vis-à-vis the "Y" of septal band is one of the four determinants of the "position" of the VSD. The other three determinants are the length of the subvalvar infundibulum (Figure 7), the presence or absence of infundibular septum, and the tricuspid valve attachments (Figure 9). The VSD can thus be labeled subaortic, subpulmonary, noncommitted, or doubly committed in order to assist the surgeon in planning the repair.

Isolated membranous or muscular VSDs are rare in DORV. Presumably these are characterized by infundibular muscle (probably infundibular free wall) filling in the "Y" of septal band. Thus, the only egress from the left ventricle is through a defect in the remainder of the septum. Isolated membranous or muscular VSDs are noncommitted.

173

Combination malalignment-type and AVC type VSDs are usually noncommitted (see Chapter 13, Figure 15).

2. Unilateral Infundibulum

If the great artery arising from the infundibulum is >50% over the right ventricle and if the arterial root without infundibulum is in continuity with the atrioventricular valve lying within the right ventricle, this is also DORV. By far the more common variation of unilateral infundibulum in DORV is subpulmonary, i.e., pulmonary artery arising from infundibulum and aortic valve-to-tricuspid valve continuity.

Subaortic infundibulum with pulmonary valve-to-tricuspid valve continuity has been observed in postmortem series.[24]

3. Bilaterally Absent Infundibulum

Although theoretically possible, this type of DORV has not yet been reported.

C. Double-Outlet Left Ventricle (DOLV)

Three cases (bilateral infundibulum, unilateral infundibulum, and bilaterally absent infundibulum) analogous to the preceding discussion of double-outlet right ventricle also exist.[25–33] Since DOLV is far less prevalent than DORV, it is convenient to concentrate on the four most frequently seen variants (Figure 10).

1. Unilateral Subpulmonary Infundibulum with Pulmonary Stenosis[27,29] ("tetralogy-like") (Figures 11 and 12)

This was the first DOLV variant to be widely recognized by angiographers.

2. Unilateral Subaortic Infundibulum with Pulmonary Stenosis and Overriding Aorta ("TGA {S,D,L}-like") (Figures 13 and 14)

3. Unilateral Subaortic Infundibulum with Nearly Overriding Pulmonary Valve ("ACM {S,D,L}-like")

4. Unilateral Subpulmonary Infundibulum with Arch Hypoplasia or Coarctation

This was the original type of DOLV reported by Sakakibara.[33]

D. Transposition of the Great Arteries

Unilateral subaortic infundibulum[34–46] is by far the most common arrangement (Figure 15); however, bilateral infundibulum is seen in perhaps 2% and unilateral subpulmonary infundibulum[47–52] with aortic valve-to-tricuspid valve continuity is found in about 1% (Figures 16–18). Bilaterally absent infundibulum has not been reported.

In subaortic infundibulum, dynamic subpulmonary stenosis is gradually acquired (Figures 15 and 19). Fixed types of subpulmonary stenosis[53] have been described, of which one (accessory tricuspid valve tissue) can be easily dealt with (Figure 20) at the time of arterial repair.[54] Those who might otherwise be candidates for Rastelli repair[55–59] may have tricuspid attachments to the infundibular septum (Figure 21).

In L-loop, bilateral infundibulum is rare (Figures 22 and 23).

E. Anatomically Corrected Malposition (ACM)

Bilateral infundibulum (Figure 24) is the most common[60–66]; however, unilateral subaortic infundibulum (Figure 25) with pulmonary valve-to-tricuspid valve continuity has been reported (Figure 26). Bilaterally absent infundibulum has not been reported.

F. Cases with Main Pulmonary Artery Atresia

Obviously, if the main pulmonary artery cannot be identified (Figure 27), then assignment to one of the six ventriculo-arterial alignments cannot always be accomplished.[67–71] A simple convention has been suggested by Weinberg.[72]

If there is aortic-to-mitral continuity, the case is designated tetralogy of Fallot with pulmonary atresia. If the aorta arises above the left ventricle but without aortic-to-mitral continuity, the case is "left ventricular aorta with pulmonary atresia." If the aorta arises above the right ventricle without aortic-to-mitral continuity, the case is "right ventricular aorta with pulmonary atresia."

References

1. VanPraagh R, VanPraagh S, Nebesar RA, Muster AJ, Sinha SN, Paul MH. Tetralogy of Fallot: underdevelopment of the pulmonary infundibulum and its sequelae. *Am J Cardiol* 1970; 26:25–33.

2. Anderson RH, Allwork SP, Ho SY, Lenox CC, Zuberbuhler JR. Surgical anatomy of tetralogy of Fallot. *J Thorac Cardiovasc Surg* 1981; 81:887–896.

3. Fellows KE, Freed MD, Keane JF, VanPraagh R, Bernhard WF, Castaneda AR. Results of routine preopeative coronary angiography in tetralogy of Fallot. *Circulation* 1975; 51:561–566.

4. Partridge JB, Fiddler GI. Cineangiocardiography in tetralogy of Fallot. *Br Heart J* 1981; 45:112–121.

5. VanPraagh R. Classification of truncus arteriosus communis. *Am Heart J* 1976; 92:129–132.

6. Rice MJ, Seward JB, Hagler DJ, Mair DD, Tajik AJ. Definitive diagnosis of truncus arteriosus by two-dimensional echocardiography. *Mayo Clin Proc* 1982; 57:476–481.

7. Nishibatake M, Kirby ML, VanMierop LHS. Pathogenesis of persistent truncus arteriosus and dextroposed aorta in the chick embryo after neural crest ablation. *Circulation* 1987; 75:255–264.

8. Butto F, Lucas RV, Edwards JE. Persistent truncus arteriosus: pathologic anatomy in 54 cases. *Pediatr Cardiol* 1986; 7:95–101.

9. Bartelings MM, Gittenberger-deGroot AC. Morphogenetic considerations on congenital malformations of the outflow tract. *Int J Cardiol* 1991; 32:213–230.

10. dela Cruz MV, Cayre R, Angelini P, Noriega Ramos N, Sadowinski S. Coronary arteries in truncus arteriosus. *Am J Cardiol* 1990; 66:1482–1486.

11. Suzuki A, Ho SY, Anderson RH, Deanfield JE. Coronary arterial and sinusal anatomy in hearts with a common arterial trunk. *Ann Thorac Surg* 1989; 48:792–797.

12. DeLeon SY, Idriss FS, Ilbawi MN, Tin N, Berry T. Transmediastinal repair of complex coarctation and interrupted aortic arch. *J Thorac Cardiovasc Surg* 1981; 82:98–102.

13. Smallhorn JF, Anderson RH, Macartney FJ. Cross-sectional echocardiographic recognition of interruption of aortic arch between left carotid and subclavian arteries. *Br Heart J* 1982; 48:229–235.

14. Moulaert AH, Bruins CC, Oppenheimer-Dekker A. Anomalies of the aortic arch and ventricular septal defects. *Circulation* 1976; 53:1011–1015.

15. Rychik J, Murdison KA, Chin AJ, Norwood WI. Surgical management of severe aortic outflow obstruction in lesions other than hypoplastic left heart syndrome: use of a pulmonary artery-to-aorta anastomosis. *J Am Coll Cardiol* 1991; 18:809–816.

16. Austin EH, Jonas RA, Mayer JE, Castaneda AR. Aortic atresia with normal left ventricle. *J Thorac Cardiovasc Surg* 1989; 97:392–395.

17. Sell JE, Jonas RA, Mayer JE, Blackstone EH, Kirklin JW, Castaneda AR. The results of a surgical program for interrupted aortic arch. *J Thorac Cardiovasc Surg* 1988; 96:864–877.

18. Sridaromont S, Feldt RH, Ritter DG, Davis GD, Edwards JE. Double outlet right ventricle: hemodynamic and anatomic correlations. *Am J Cardiol* 1976; 38:85–94.

19. VanPraagh R, Perez-Trevino C, Reynolds JL, Moes CAF, Keith JD, Roy DL, Belcourt C, et al. Double outlet right ventricle {S,D,L} with subaortic ventricular septal defect and pulmonary stenosis. *Am J Cardiol* 1975; 35:42–53.

20. Thanopoulos BD, Dubrow IW, Fisher EA, Has treiter AR. Double outlet right ventricle with subvalvar aortic stenosis. *Br Heart J* 1979; 41:241–244.

21. Luber JM, Castaneda AR, Lang P, Norwood WI. Repair of double-outlet right ventricle: early and late results. *Circulation* 1983; 68(Suppl II):II144–II147.

22. Battistessa S, Soto B. Double outlet right ventricle with discordant atrioventricular connexion: an angiographic analysis of 19 cases. *Int J Cardiol* 1990; 27:253–263.

23. Kanter K, Anderson R, Lincoln C, Firmin R, Rigby M. Anatomic correction of double-outlet right ventricle with subpulmonary ventricular septal defect (the "Taussig-Bing" anomaly). *Ann Thorac Surg* 1986; 41:287–292.

24. VanPraagh S, Davidoff A, Chin AJ, Shiel F, Reynolds J, VanPraagh R. Double outlet right ventricle: anatomic types and developmental implications based on a study of 101 autopsied cases. *Coeur* 1982; 13:389–440.

25. Bharati S, Lev M, Stewart R, McAllister HA, Kirklin JW. The morphologic spectrum of double outlet left ventricle and its surgical significance. *Circulation* 1978; 58:558–565.

26. Otero Coto E, Quero Jimenez M, Anderson RH, Castaneda AR, Freedom RM, Attie F, Kreutzer E, et al. Double outlet left ventricle. In: Anderson RH, Macartney FJ, Shinebourne EA, et al. (eds). *Paediatric Cardiology 5.* Churchill Livingstone, Edinburgh, 1983, pp 451–465.

27. Pacifico AD, Kirklin JW, Bargeron LM, Soto B. Surgical treatment of double-outlet left ventricle. *Circulation* 1973; 47(Suppl III):III19–III23.

28. Otero Coto E, Quero Jimenez M, Castaneda AR, Rufilanchas J, Deverall PB. Double outlet from chambers of left ventricular morphology. *Br Heart J* 1979; 42:15–21.

29. Brandt PWT, Calder AL, Barratt-Boyes BG, Neutze JM. Double outlet left ventricle. *Am J Cardiol* 1976; 38:897–909.

30. Paul MH, Muster AJ, Sinha SN, Cole RB, Van-Praagh R. Double-outlet left ventricle with an intact ventricular septum. *Circulation* 1970; 41:120–139.

31. Subirana MT, DeLeval M, Somerville J. Double-outlet left ventricle with atrioventricular discordance. *Am J Cardiol* 1984; 54:1385–1388.

32. Beitzke A, Suppan C. Double outlet left ventricle with intact ventricular septum. *Int J Cardiol* 1984; 5:175–183.

33. Sakakibara S, Takao A, Arai T, Hashimoto A, Nogi M. Both great vessels arising from the left ventricle. *Bull Heart Inst Jpn* 1967, pp 66–86.

34. Moene RJ, Oppenheimer-Dekker A. Congenital mitral valve anomalies in transposition of the great arteries. *Am J Cardiol* 1982; 49:1972–1978.

35. Aziz KU, Paul MH, Muster AJ, Idriss FS. Positional abnormalities of atrioventricular valves in transposition of the great arteries including double outlet right ventricle, atrioventricular valve straddling and malattachment. *Am J Cardiol* 1979; 44:1135–1145.

36. Moene RJ, Oppenheimer-Dekker A, Bartelings MM. Anatomic obstruction of the right ventricular outflow tract in transposition of the great arteries. *Am J Cardiol* 1983; 51:1701–1704.

37. Deal BJ, Chin AJ, Sanders SP, Norwood WI, Castaneda AR. Subxiphoid two-dimensional echocardiographic identification of tricuspid valve abnormalities in transposition of the great arteries with ventricular septal defect. *Am J Cardiol* 1985; 55:1146–1151.

38. Pasquini L, Sanders SP, Parness IA, Colan SD. Diagnosis of coronary artery anatomy by two-dimensional echocardiography in patients with transposition of the great arteries. *Circulation* 1987; 75:557–564.

39. Yacoub MH, Radley-Smith R. Anatomy of the coronary arteries in transposition of the great arteries and methods for their transfer in anatomical correction. *Thorax* 1978; 33:418–424.

40. Rosenquist GC, Stark J, Taylor JFN. Congenital mitral valve disease in transposition of the great arteries. *Circulation* 1975; 51:731–737.

41. Layman TE, Edwards JE. Anomalies of the cardiac valves associated with complete transposition of the great vessels. *Am J Cardiol* 1967; 19:247–255.

42. van Doesburg NH, Bierman FZ, Williams RG. Left ventricular geometry in infants with d-transposition of the great arteries and intact ventricular septum. *Circulation* 1983; 68:733–739.

43. Gittenberger-de Groot AC, Sauer U, Oppenheimer-Dekker A, Quaegebeur J. Coronary arterial anatomy in transposition of the great arteries: a morphologic study. *Pediatr Cardiol* 1983; 4(Suppl I):15–24.

44. Gittenberger-de Groot AC, Sauer U, Quaegebeur J. Aortic intramural coronary artery in three hearts with transposition of the great arteries. *J Thorac Cardiovasc Surg* 1986; 91:566–571.

45. Bierman FZ, Williams RG. Prospective diagnosis of d-transposition of the great arteries in neonates by subxiphoid, two-dimensional echocardiography. *Circulation* 1979; 60:1496–1502.

46. Buchler JR, Bembom JC, Buchler RD. Transposition of the great arteries with posterior aorta and subaortic conus: anatomical and surgical correlation. *Int J Cardiol* 1984; 5:13–18.

47. Wilkinson JL, Arnold R, Anderson RH, Acerete F. Posterior transposition reconsidered. *Br Heart J* 1975; 37:757–766.

48. Van Praagh R, Perez-Trevino C, Lopez-Cuellar M, Baker FW, Zuberbuhler JR, Quero M, Perez VM, et al. Transposition of the great arteries with posterior aorta, anterior pulmonary artery, subpulmonary conus and fibrous continuity between aortic and atrioventricular valves. *Am J Cardiol* 1971; 28:621–631.

49. Virdi IS, Keeton BR, Monro JL. Complete transposition with posteriorly located aorta and multiple ventricular septal defects. *Int J Cardiol* 1988; 21:347–351.

50. Tam S, Murphy JD, Norwood WI. Transposition of the great arteries with posterior aorta: anatomic repair. *J Thorac Cardiovasc Surg* 1990; 100:441–444.

51. Chin AJ, Alboliras ET, Barber G, Murphy JD, Helton JG, Pigott JD, Norwood WI. Prospective detection by Doppler color flow imaging of additional defects in infants with a large ventricular septal defect. *J Am Coll Cardiol* 1990; 15:1637–1642.

52. Benatar A, Antunes MdJ, Levin SE. Posterior d-transposition of the great arteries with an unusual form of aortic obstruction. *Pediatr Cardiol* 1990; 11:170–172.

53. Chin AJ, Yeager SB, Sanders SP, Williams RG, Bierman FZ, Burger BM, Norwood WI, et al. Accuracy of prospective two-dimensional echocardiographic evaluation of left ventricular outflow tract in complete transposition of the great arteries. *Am J Cardiol* 1985; 55:759–764.

54. Riggs TW, Muster AJ, Aziz KU, Paul MH, Ilbawi M, Idriss FS. Two-dimensional echocardiographic and angiocardiographic diagnosis of subpulmonary stenosis due to tricuspid valve pouch in complete transposition of the great arteries. *J Am Coll Cardiol* 1983; 1:484–491.

55. Van Gils FAW, Moulaert AJ, Oppenheimer-Dekker A, Wenink ACG. Transposition of the great arteries with ventricular septal defect and pulmonary stenosis. *Br Heart J* 1978; 40:494–499.

56. Huhta JC, Edwards WD, Danielson GK, Feldt RH. Abnormalities of the tricuspid valve in complete transposition of the great arteries with ventricular septal defect. *J Thorac Cardiovasc Surg* 1982; 83:569–576.

57. Marcelletti C, Mair DD, McGoon DC, Wallace RB, Danielson GK. The Rastelli operation for transposition of the great arteries. *J Thorac Cardiovasc Surg* 1976; 72:427–434.

58. Villagra F, Quero-Jimenez M, Maitre-Azcarate MJ, Gutierrez J, Brito JM. Transposition of the great arteries with ventricular septal defects: surgical considerations concerning the Rastelli operation. *J Thorac Cardiovasc Surg* 1984; 88:1004–1011.

59. Imamura ES, Morikawa T, Tatsuno K, Konno S, Arai T, Sakakibara S. Surgical considerations of ventricular septal defect associated with complete transposition of the great arteries and pulmonary stenosis. *Circulation* 1971; 44:914–923.

60. Kirklin JW, Pacifico AD, Bargeron LM, Soto B. Cardiac repair in anatomically corrected malposition of the great arteries. *Circulation* 1973; 48:153–159.

61. VanPraagh R, Durnin RE, Jockin H, Wagner HR, Korns M, Garabedian H, Ando M, et al. Anatomically corrected malposition of the great arteries {S,D,L}. *Circulation* 1975; 51:20–31.

62. Arciprete P, Macartney FJ, deLeval M, Stark J. Mustard's operation for patients with ventriculo-arterial concordance. *Br Heart J* 1985; 53:443–450.

63. Anderson RH, Becker AE, Losekoot TG, Gerlis LM. Anatomically corrected malposition of great arteries. *Br Heart J* 1975; 37:993–1013.

64. Colli AM, deLeval M, Somerville J. Anatomically corrected malposition of the great arteries: diagnostic difficulties and surgical repair of associated lesions. *Am J Cardiol* 1985; 55:1367–1372.

65. Pasquini L, Sanders SP, Parness I, Colan S, Keane JF, Mayer JE, Kratz C, et al. Echocardiographic and anatomic findings in atrioventricular discordance with ventriculoarterial concordance. *Am J Cardiol* 1988; 62:1256–1262.

66. Zakheim R, Mattioli L, Vaseenon T, Edwards W. Anatomically corrected malposition of the great arteries {S,L,D}. *Chest* 1976; 69:101–104.

67. Macartney FJ. Pulmonary atresia with ventricular septal defect. *Modern Problems Paediat* 1983; 22: 186–201.

68. Liao PK, Edwards WD, Julsrud PR, Puga FJ, Danielson GK, Feldt RH. Pulmonary blood supply in patients with pulmonary atresia and ventricular septal defects. *J Am Coll Cardiol* 1985; 6:1343–1350.

69. Haworth SG, Rees PG, Taylor JFN, Macartney FJ, deLeval M, Stark J. Pulmonary atresia with ventricular septal defect and major aortopulmonary collateral arteries. *Br Heart J* 1981; 45:133–141.

70. Murphy DA, Sridhara KS, Nanton MA, Roy DL, Belcourt CL, Gillis DA. Surgical correction of pulmonary atresia with large systemic-pulmonary collaterals. *Ann Thorac Surg* 1979; 27:460–464.

71. Puga FJ, Leoni FE, Julsrud PR, Mair DD. Complete repair of pulmonary atresia, ventricular septal defect, and severe peripheral arborization abnormalities of the central pulmonary arteries: experience with preliminary unifocalization procedures in 38 patients. *J Thorac Cardiovasc Surg* 1989; 98:1018–1028.

72. Weinberg PM. Systemic approach to diagnosis and coding of pediatric cardiac disease. *Pediatr Cardiol* 1986; 7:35–48.

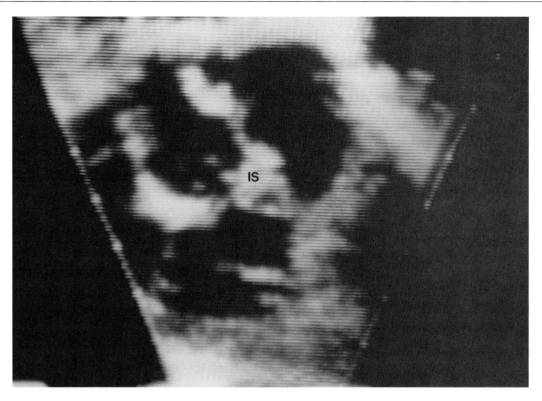

Figure 1: Subcostal frontal view of mild tetralogy of Fallot. The infundibular septum (IS) is leftward of and superior to its normal position.

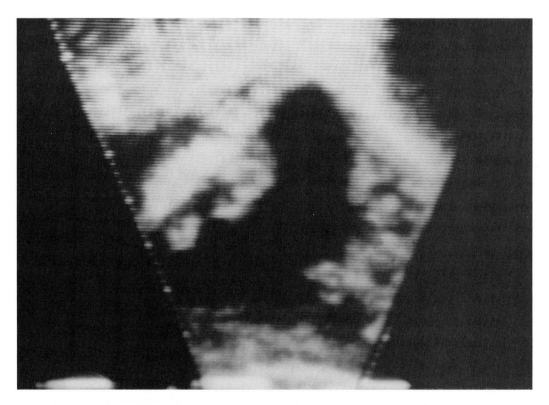

Figure 2: Subcostal frontal view, anterior to the plane shown in Figure 1. There is minimal subpulmonary stenosis. IS = infundibular septum.

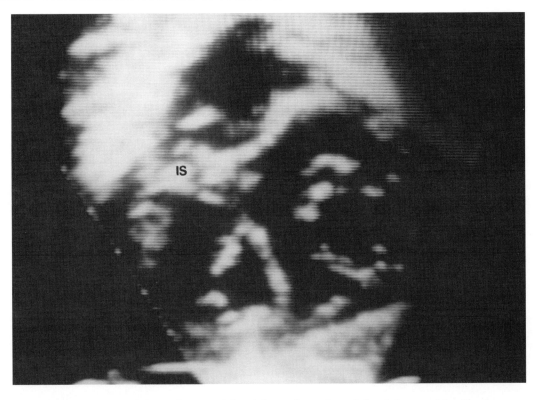

Figure 3: Subcostal sagittal view of the rightward portion of the right ventricle. The infundibular septum (IS) is displayed tangentially.

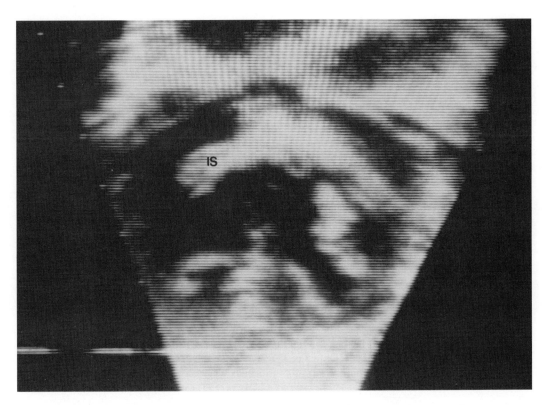

Figure 4: Subcostal sagittal view of the right ventricle, slightly left of the plane shown in Figure 3. The infundibular septum (IS) is superior to but only slightly anterior of its normal position.

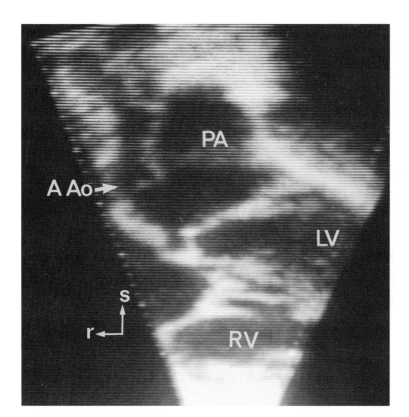

Figure 5: Subcostal frontal view of truncus arteriosus with interrupted aortic arch. Note the partitioning of the truncus such that the pulmonary artery component (PA) is much larger than the ascending aortic component (AAo). LV = left ventricle; RV = right ventricle.

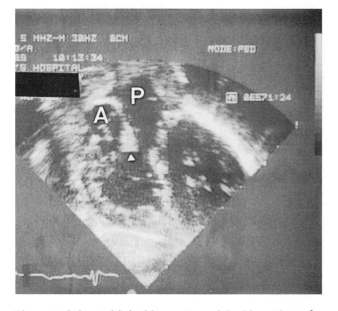

Figure 6: Subcostal left oblique view of double-outlet right ventricle. Early in the sweep, the aorta (A) is visualized as anterior and to the right of the pulmonary artery (P). The arrow shows the infundibular septum displaced anteriorly and to the right of its normal position.

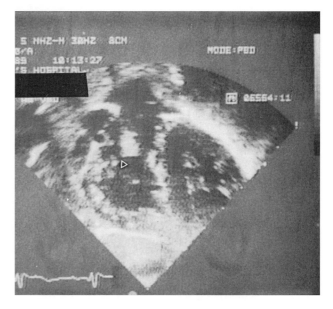

Figure 7: Subcostal left oblique view, slightly to the left of the view shown in Figure 6. The aortic outflow (arrowhead) is quite small. The subaortic infundibular free wall is shorter than the subpulmonary infundibular free wall, but the infundibular septum is quite large.

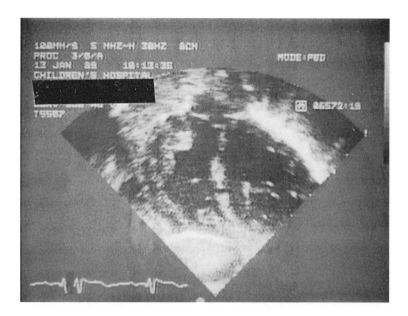

Figure 8: Subcostal left oblique view, slightly to the left of that shown in Figure 7. The aortic outflow is no longer visible. The pulmonary valve is quite high. This patient's malalignment-type ventricular septal defect was thus noncommitted.

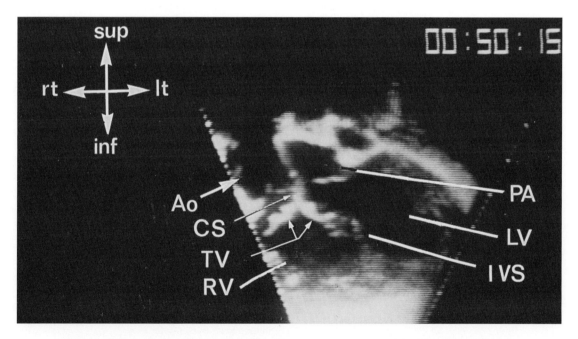

Figure 9: Subcostal frontal view of classical Taussig-Bing variant of double-outlet right ventricle, i.e., DORV {S,D,D} with side-by-side great arteries, no subpulmonary stenosis, malalignment-type ventricular septal defect. The ventricular septal defect is subpulmonary. The tricuspid valve (TV) attaches to the infundibular septum (CS). IVS = interventricular septum; Ao = aorta; PA = pulmonary artery; LV = left ventricle; RV = right ventricle.

Type I DOLV (Related to TOF, TGA with posterior aorta)

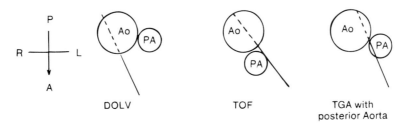

Type II DOLV (Related to TGA {S,D,A} or TGA {S,D,L})

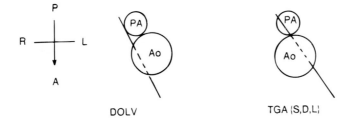

Type III DOLV (Related to Anatomically Corrected Malposition {S, D, L})

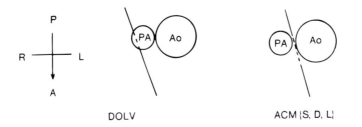

Type IV DOLV (Related to Infundibular Septal Defect)

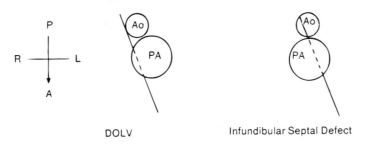

Figure 10: The four most commonly seen variants of double-outlet left ventricle. The solid line represents the plane of the trabecular portion of the ventricular septum. The dashed line represents the ventricular septal defect. Each type is similar to another malformation, shown in the right-hand column.

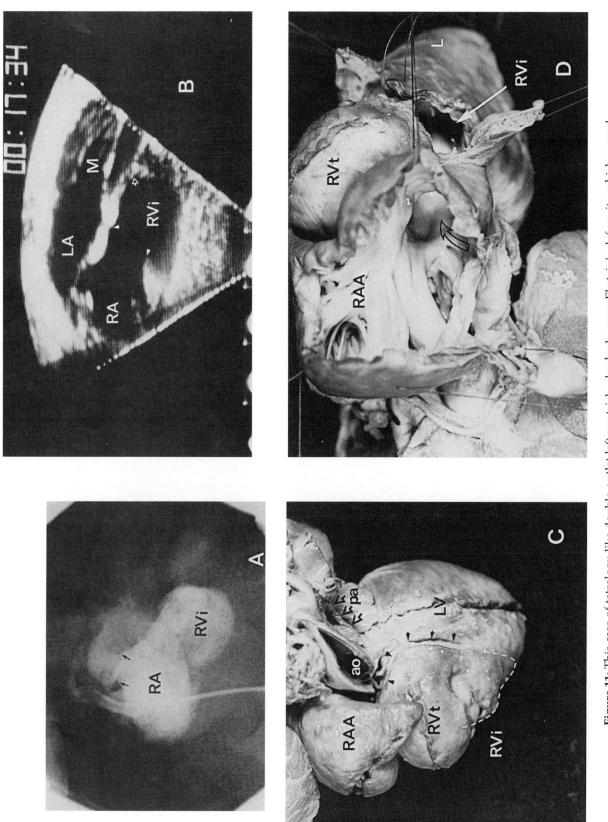

Figure 11: This case of tetralogy-like double-outlet left ventricle also had severe Ebstein's deformity which caused atresia of the tricuspid valve. **A:** Angiography demonstrating only the atrialized portion of the right ventricle (RVi). **B:** Subcostal frontal view showing Ebstein's anomaly. **C:** External view of postmortem specimen. **D:** Internal view of right atrioventricular orifice (black arrow). RVt = trabecular zone of the right ventricle; ao = aorta; pa = pulmonary artery; RAA = right atrial appendage.

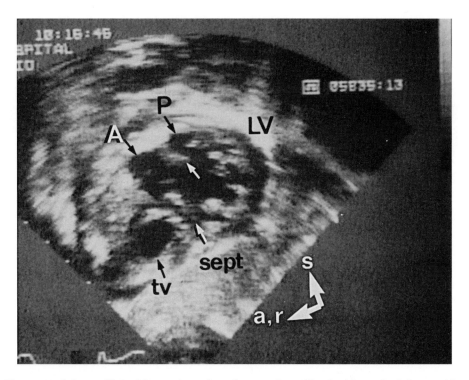

Figure 12: Subcostal left oblique view of another tetralogy-like double-outlet left ventricle. The infundibular septum (sept) is deviated so far leftward that the pulmonary artery (P) arises above the left ventricle (LV). tv = tricuspid valve.

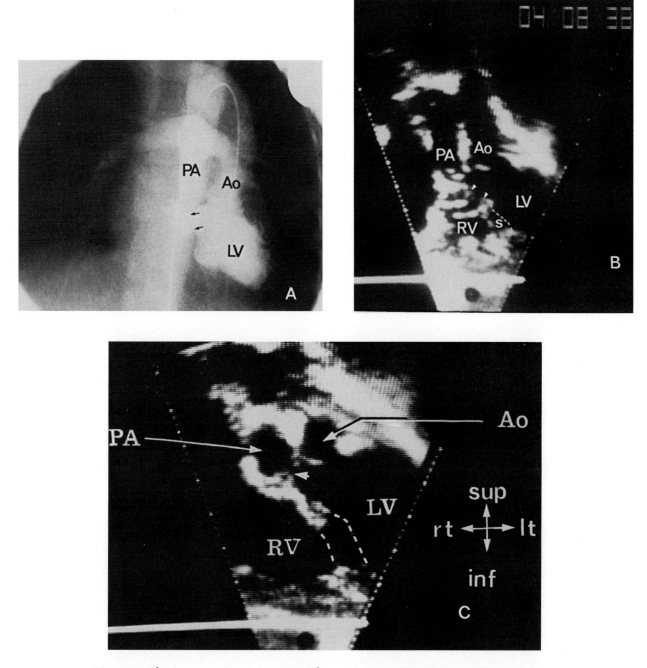

Figure 13: This is a case of transposition of the great arteries {S,D,L}-like DOLV. **A:** Antero-posterior angiogram. The aorta clearly arises above the left ventricle (LV). **B:** Subcostal frontal view showing the ventricular septal defect (unlabeled arrowheads). The pulmonary artery (PA) arises from the LV. s = septum. **C:** The infundibular septum is hypoplastic.

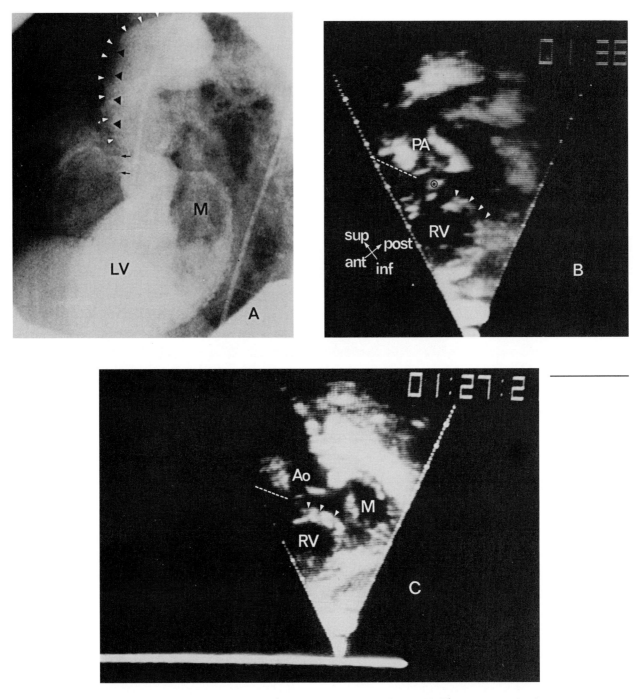

Figure 14: A: Lateral angiogram of the same patient as in Figure 13. The great arteries (arrowheads) both arise above the left ventricle (LV). M = mitral annulus. **B:** Subcostal sagittal view, confirming that the pulmonary artery (PA) arises above the left ventricle. RV = right ventricle. **C:** Subcostal sagittal view, slightly to the left of panel B. The aorta (Ao) arises above the left ventricle.

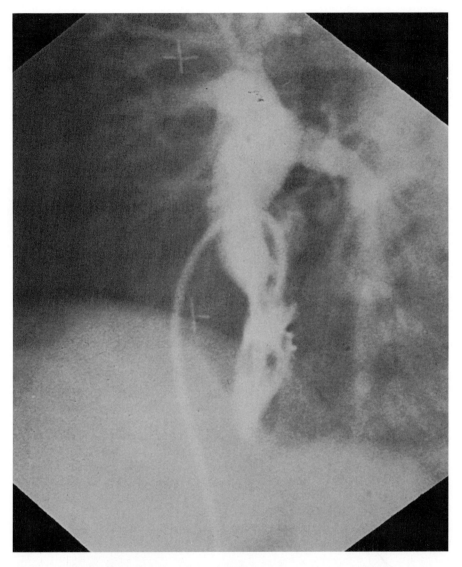

Figure 15: Long axial oblique view of the left ventricular outflow tract in transposition of the great arteries {S,D,D} with unilateral subaortic infundibulum. In systole, there is dynamic subpulmonary stenosis.

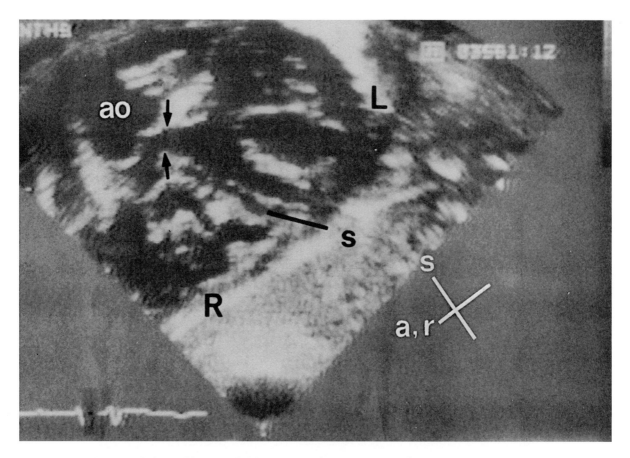

Figure 16: Subcostal long axial oblique view of transposition with unilateral subpulmonary infundibulum. Note the proximity of the aortic valve (ao) to the tricuspid valve. The arrows show a moderate-size perimembranous ventricular septal defect. s = septum.

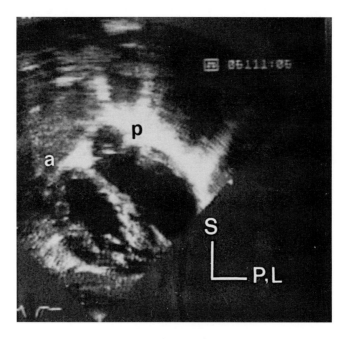

Figure 17: Subcostal left oblique view, slightly to the left of the view in Figure 16. The ascending aorta is not seen in this plane, but the pulmonary root (p) is visible.

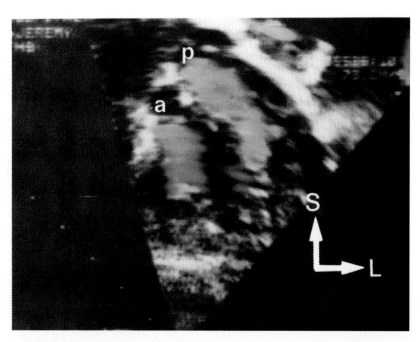

Figure 18: Subcostal frontal view showing a large anterior muscular ventricular septal defect. Used with permission of Elsevier Science Publishing.

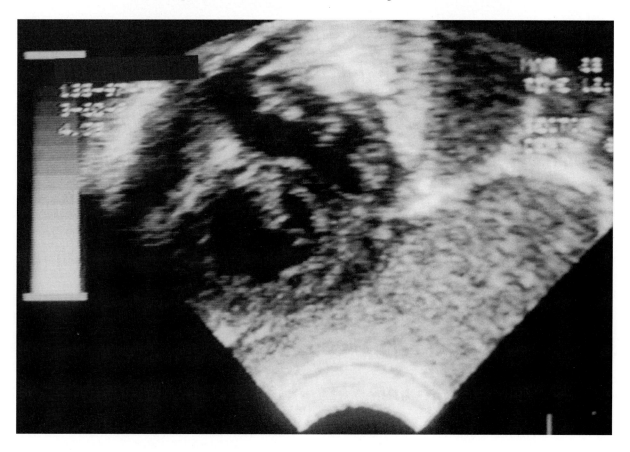

Figure 19: Subcostal long axial oblique view. To prove that stenosis is dynamic, one must see no obstruction in diastole.

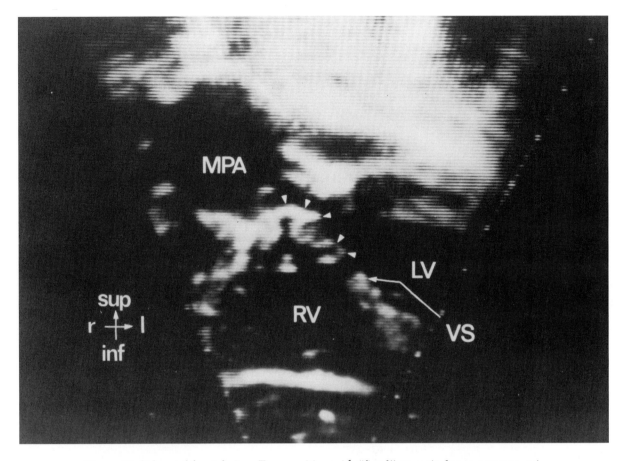

Figure 20: Subcostal frontal view. Transposition with "fixed" stenosis due to accessory tricuspid tissue (arrowheads). VS = ventricular septum; RV = right ventricle; LV = left ventricle; MPA = main pulmonary artery.

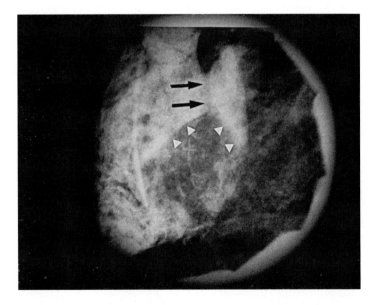

Figure 21: Subcostal long axial oblique view of the right ventricle. The tricuspid valve (white arrowheads) is seen, along with an attachment (black arrows) to the infundibular septum. Such attachments complicate attempts at a Rastelli repair and can be identified echocardiographically.

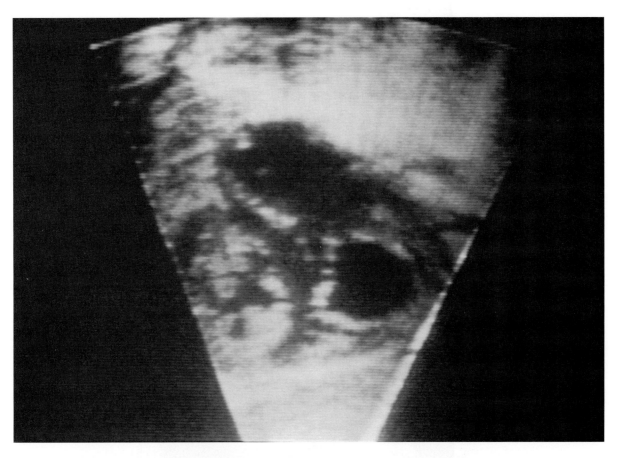

Figure 22: Subcostal left oblique view. In L-loop, virtually all patients with transposition of the great arteries have unilateral subaortic infundibulum.

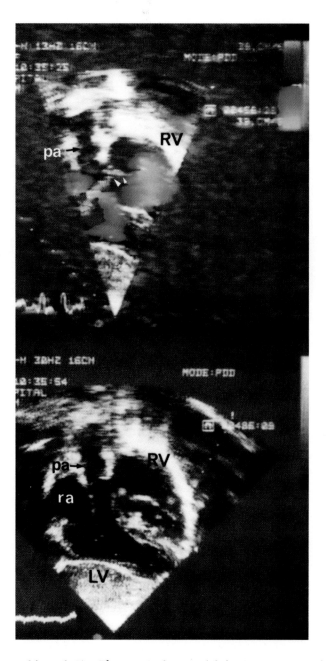

Figure 23: Subcostal frontal view. The ventricular septal defect jet trajectory is from the right ventricle (RV) to the left ventricle (LV). pa = pulmonary artery.

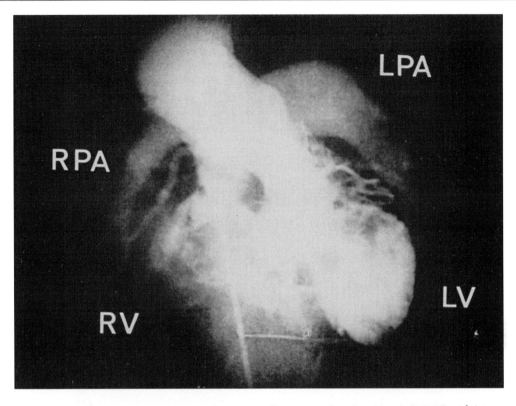

Figure 24: The most common type of anatomically corrected malposition is {S,D,L} with bilateral infundibulum. Note that there are trabeculations within the subaortic infundibulum. LPA = left pulmonary artery; RPA = right pulmonary artery; LV = left ventricle; RV = right ventricle.

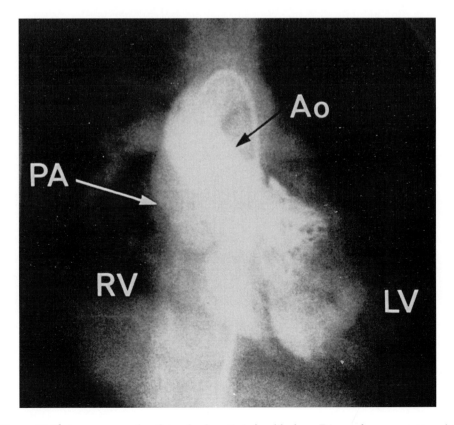

Figure 25: There are cases of unilateral subaortic infundibulum. PA = pulmonary artery; Ao = aorta; RV = right ventricle; LV = left ventricle.

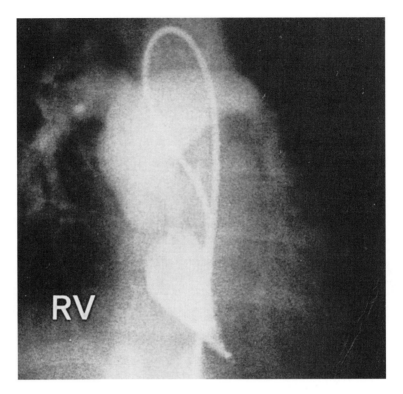

Figure 26: Anteroposterior angiogram. Note how low the pulmonary cusps are.

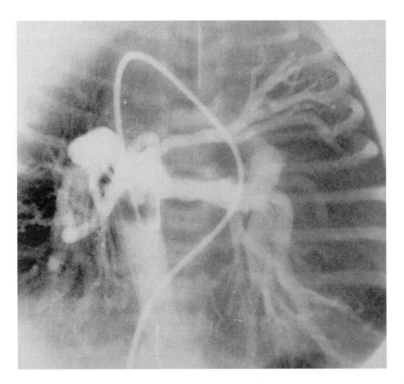

Figure 27: Anteroposterior angiogram of tetralogy of Fallot with pulmonary atresia. There was a right aortic arch and upper descending aorta. No main pulmonary artery could be seen. Numerous collaterals are displayed.

Chapter 16

Aortic Valve, Aortic Outflow, Truncal Valve

A. Aortic Stenosis

Approximately half of aortic stenosis patients have a normal size left ventricle (those with left ventricular hypoplasia resemble aortic atresia—see Chapter 16, section B). Most presenting in the neonatal period have uni-commissural valves. Rarely is the commissure between the noncoronary cusp and the left coronary cusp involved. Bicuspid nonstenotic aortic valves typically have a raphe. Bicuspid stenotic aortic valves have both a raphe and a fused commissure. Physiological subsets in the infant can be arbitrarily defined as follows:

Critical = poorly perfused when the ductus is closed or restrictive.

Severe, not well-compensated = well perfused with the ductus closed but showing diminished left ventricular shortening fraction.

Severe, well-compensated = well perfused with the ductus closed but showing normal or high left ventricular shortening fraction.

Ultrasound can thus play a central role in the initial management of aortic stenosis. There is general agreement that infants in the first two categories should have immediate relief of their obstruction either by surgery or by balloon dilatation. The optimal approach to the infant who presents with a nonrestrictive ductus in the setting of a transaortic gradient is still unresolved.

After infancy, physiological subsets have largely been demarcated using peak-to-peak catheter gradients, although catheter estimation of aortic valve area, peak instantaneous Doppler gradients, and Doppler estimates of valve area have also been used.

Although commissural fusion and the presence of a raphe may in some instances be visible, e.g., from the parasternal short axis view, prospective studies of sensitivity and specificity have not been reported in infants or in children. Anatomical features predicting poor outcome after surgical valvotomy or balloon dilatation[1] have not yet been identified, although intravascular ultrasound may eventually shed light on this issue.

Problems with assessing valve area by planimetry of two-dimensional echocardiograms arise from the difficulty in determining the apex of a dome (Figure 1) with any tomographic technique.

B. Aortic Atresia

Aortic atresia in the setting of normal or near-normal ventriculo-arterial alignment is associated with a normal size left ventricle perhaps 1–5% of the time.[2-4] Virtually all of these cases have a large malalignment-type ventricular septal defect (VSD). A rare case will have only a large muscular VSD (Figures 2 and 3).

The more common aortic atresia patient has an intact ventricular septum, hypoplasia of the left ventricle, hypoplasia and/or dysplasia of the mitral valve, and leftward and posterior deviation of the superior attachment of septum primum. The features of the atrial septal morphology have been discussed in Chapter 8, section D. All varieties of atrial-level shunting (including coronary sinus septal defect) have been reported except sinus venosus defects. Less than 5% have congenitally small (or closed) foramen ovale, defined arbitrarily as a diameter of 3 mm or less (Figure 4). Pulmonary venous connection anomalies have been described.[5] Cases with normal connection[5] but anomalous drainage are equally common.

The "string-like" ascending aorta is usually 2 mm in diameter. The suprasternal (or high right parasternal) left oblique view typically best displays the ascending aorta (Figure 5). Pulmonary valve stenosis[6] occurs in approximately 1% of cases of aortic atresia.

The presence of a patent mitral valve[7] does not appear to have prognostic significance for survival after reconstructive surgery. On the other hand, the function of the morphological tricuspid valve may be predictive.[8] Moderate or severe regurgitation correlates with significantly poorer survival following initial surgical palliation.

Occasionally, aortic atresia occurs with other ventriculo-arterial alignments[9] and with aortopulmonary window[10] or interrupted aortic arch.[3]

C. Absent Aortic Valve Leaflets

This exceedingly rare anomaly[11–13] is characterized by the absence of any aortic leaflet tissue. It is always associated with other malformations. Double-outlet right ventricle is the most frequently observed anomaly of ventriculo-arterial alignment. Abnormalities of the mitral valve include hypoplasia, double orifices, and atresia. Both pulmonary vein stenosis and total anomalous pulmonary venous connection have been observed. Ventricular myocardial morphology is usually abnormal, with one case demonstrating "spongy" myocardium.

The 2-D echocardiographic appearance rests on the recognition of absence of valve leaflets. There is usually no "post-stenotic dilatation" (as is seen in "absent" pulmonary valve), and the annulus size is usually normal. Color Doppler display of the free regurgitation renders the diagnosis simple. Pan-diastolic retrograde laminar flow should be observed in the left ventricular outflow tract, and interrogation of the upper descending aorta should likewise demonstrate pandiastolic reversal.

D. Subaortic Stenosis

The most common variety of subaortic stenosis is that due to "malalignment" of the infundibular septum, resulting in the arterial outflow tracts being disparate in size (see Chapter 13, section B, and Chapter 15, section A).

The other main variety of subaortic stenosis is discrete fibrous tissue. It is virtually never found at birth, so it is acquired rather than congenital. Though it may be found as an isolated lesion, it is frequent in cases of perimembranous VSD, with or without anomalous muscle bundle of the right ventricle. Distance from the aortic valve is variable (Figures 6 and 7).

Because of its size, it can be missed if only subcostal imaging is done. Even apical imaging can occasionally fail to display discrete subaortic stenosis. Parasternal (Figure 8) or transesophageal views (if transthoracic imaging is technically hampered) are necessary.

Rarer types of subaortic stenosis include accessory atrioventricular valve tissue[14] and anomalous attachments of atrioventricular valve (Figure 9).

In addition to left ventricular outflow tract obstruction, discrete subaortic stenosis also causes aortic regurgitation (Figures 10 and 11). The mechanism is still in dispute.

E. Truncal Valve Stenosis

Truncal valve stenosis is recognized to be a predictor of poorer survival following truncus arteriosus repair. Because the pulmonary/systemic flow ratio is usually much greater than 2, the proximal velocity cannot be neglected when employing the simplified Bernoulli formula to estimate peak instantaneous gradient.

References

1. Rupprath G, Neuhaus K-L. Percutaneous balloon valvoplasty for aortic valve stenosis in infancy. *Am J Cardiol* 1985; 55:1655–1656.

2. Freedom RM, Dische MR, Rowe RD. Conal anatomy in aortic atresia, ventricular septal defect, and normally developed left ventricle. *Am Heart J* 1977; 94:689–698.

3. Norwood WI, Stellin GJ. Aortic atresia with interrupted aortic arch. *J Thorac Cardiovasc Surg* 1981; 81:239–244.

4. Marino B, Sanders SP, Parness IA, Colan SD. Echocardiographic identification of aortic atresia with ventricular septal defect, normal left ventricle and mitral valve. *Am Heart J* 1987; 113:1521–1523.

5. Seliem MA, Chin AJ, Norwood WI. Patterns of anomalous pulmonary venous connection/drainage in hypoplastic left heart syndrome. *J Am Coll Cardiol* 1992; 19:135–141.

6. Bharati S, Nordenberg A, Brock RR, Lev M. Hypoplastic left heart syndrome with dysplastic pulmonary valve with stenosis. *Pediatr Cardiol* 1984; 5:127–130.

7. Murdison KA, Baffa JM, Farrell PE, Chang AC, Barber G, Norwood WI, Murphy JD. Hypoplastic left heart syndrome: outcome after initial reconstruction and before modified Fontan procedure. *Circulation* 1990; 82(Suppl. IV):IV-199–IV-207.

8. Barber G, Helton JG, Aglira BA, Chin AJ, Murphy JD, Pigott JD, Norwood WI. The significance of tricuspid valve regurgitation in hypoplastic left heart syndrome. *Am Heart J* 1988; 116:1563–1567.

9. McGarry KM, Taylor JFN, Macartney FJ. Aortic atresia occurring with complete transposition of great arteries. *Br Heart J* 1980; 44:711–713.

10. Rosenquist GC, Taylor JFN, Stark J. Aortopulmonary fenestration and aortic atresia. *Br Heart J* 1974; 36:1146–1148.

11. Lin AE, Chin AJ. Absent aortic valve. *Pediatr Cardiol* 1990; 11:195–198.

12. Hartwig NG, Vermeij-Keers C, DeVries HE, Gittenberger-DeGroot AC. Aplasia of semilunar valve leaflets: two case reports and developmental aspects. *Pediatr Cardiol* 1991; 12:114–117.

13. Bierman FZ, Yeh MN, Swersky S, Martin E, Wigger JH, Fox H. Absence of the aortic valve: antenatal and postnatal two-dimensional and Doppler echocardiographic features. *J Am Coll Cardiol* 1984; 3:833–837.

14. Sono J, McKay R, Arnold RM. Accessory mitral valve leaflet causing aortic regurgitation and left ventricular outflow tract obstruction. *Br Heart J* 1988; 59:491–497.

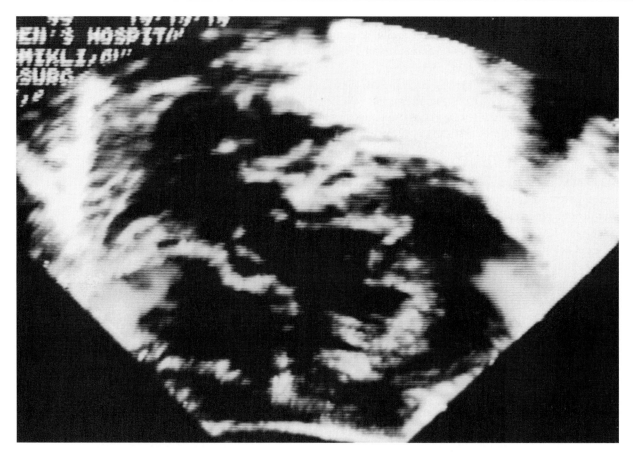

Figure 1: Subcostal left oblique view of valvar aortic stenosis with normal size left ventricle. The asymmetrical dome configuration shows how difficult it is to determine aortic valve area by planimetry.

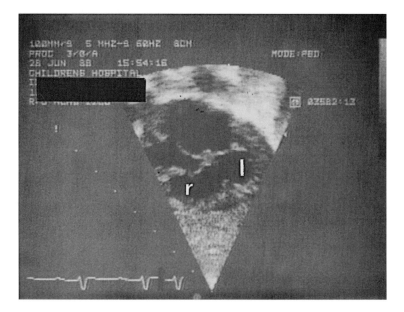

Figure 2: Subcostal frontal view of aortic atresia with normal size left ventricle (l) and mitral valve. There is a large posterior muscular ventricular septal defect. r = right ventricle.

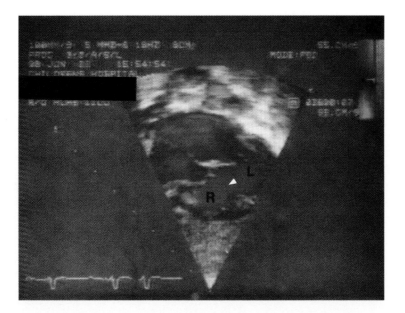

Figure 3: Color flow imaging of same patient as in Figure 2. The ventricular septal defect (arrowhead) is not contiguous with the atrioventricular annuli.

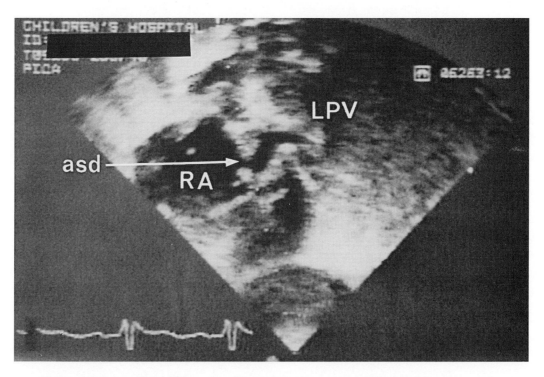

Figure 4: Subcostal left oblique view. Not only is there congenitally small foramen ovale, but there is a thick atrial septum. asd = atrial septal defect; LPV = left pulmonary vein; RA = right atrium.

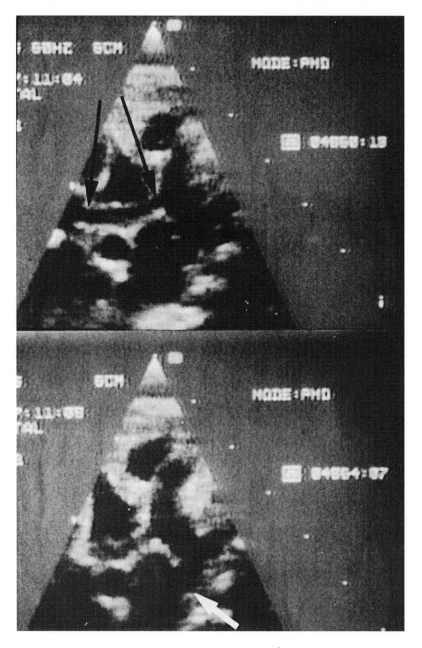

Figure 5: Suprasternal left oblique view of aortic atresia. The string-like ascending aorta is seen (top); the isthmus (bottom) resembles a branch off the ductus arteriosus.

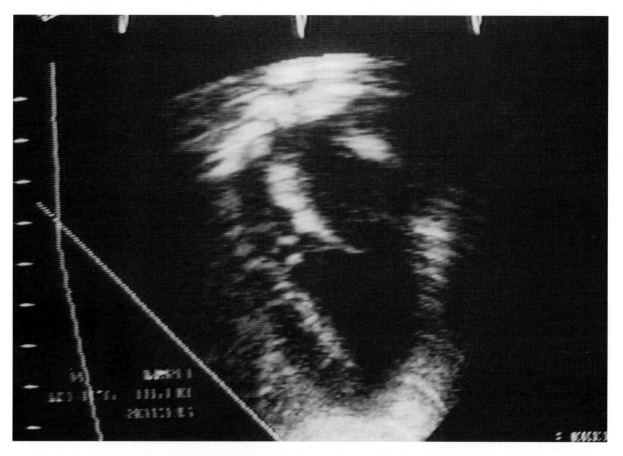

Figure 6: Apical view of discrete subaortic stenosis.

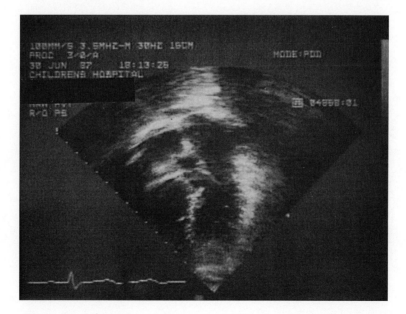

Figure 7: Apical view of discrete subaortic stenosis. The distance between the stenosis and the aortic valve is much larger than in Figure 6.

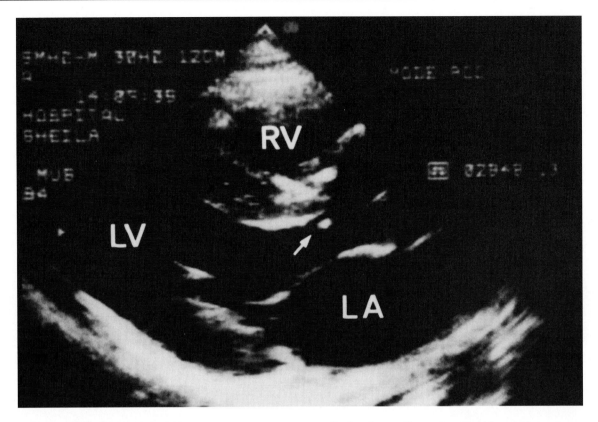

Figure 8: Parasternal long axis view is necessary to display the smallest subaortic ridges (arrow).

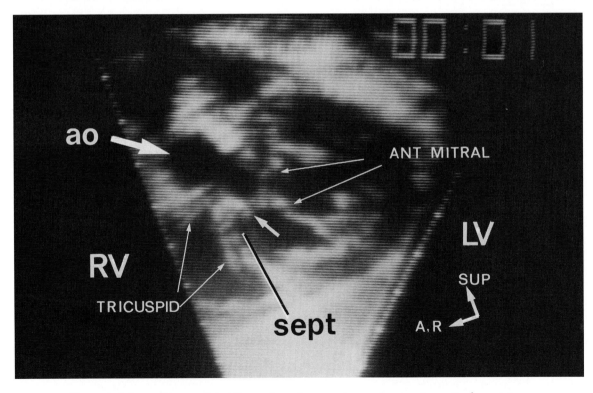

Figure 9: Subcostal long axial oblique view of unusual case of anomalous attachment (unlabeled arrow) of anterior leaflet of mitral valve. ant = anterior; ao = aortic; sept = ventricular septum.

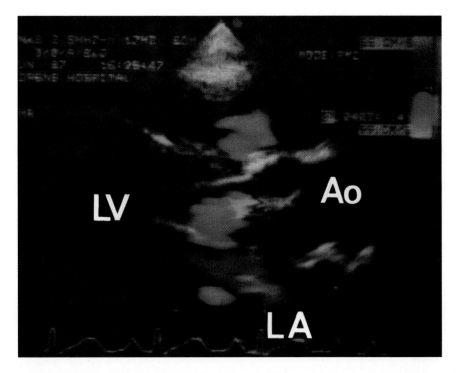

Figure 10: Parasternal long axis view of aortic regurgitation. LV = left ventricle; LA = left atrium; Ao = aorta.

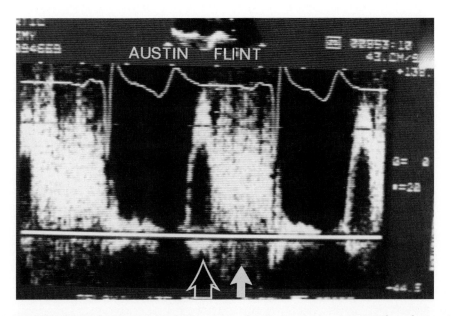

Figure 11: Pulsed Doppler interrogation of mitral inflow, apical window. When the aortic regurgitation jet strikes the anterior leaflet of the mitral valve, it causes turbulent inflow (solid white arrow) and an Austin-Flint murmur.

Chapter 17

Pulmonary Valve, Pulmonary Outflow

A. Valvar Pulmonary Stenosis

The two variations of stenotic pulmonary valves are: commissural fusion and dysplasia. It is impossible to consistently distinguish dysplasia from nondysplasia echocardiographically. Dysplasia is typically associated with little, if any, post-stenotic dilatation. The co-existence of Noonan's syndrome[1] in some patients with dysplasia can be suspected by the presence of concentric or asymmetric left ventricular hypertrophy.[2] Physiological subsets in the infant can be arbitrarily defined as follows:

> *Critical* = cyanosis accompanied by metabolic acidosis when the ductus is closed or restrictive.
> *Severe, not well-compensated* = cyanotic (but not acidotic) with the ductus closed.
> *Severe, well-compensated* = right ventricular pressure at or above systemic level; acyanotic.

Ultrasound can thus facilitate the initial management of pulmonic stenosis. There is general agreement that newborns in the first two categories should have immediate relief of their obstruction by balloon dilatation. For the third category, balloon dilatation does not need to be performed emergently in the first month of life.

Balloon dilatation of angiographically diagnosed dysplastic pulmonary valve may be less successful than that of commissural fusion. Since balloon diameter choices to some degree depend on annular diameter estimates, estimation of the latter, at the level of the bottom of the sinuses of Valsalva, is warranted during echocardiographic imaging.

In the neonate, subcostal imaging is a straightforward means of detecting the lesion and displaying the main pulmonary artery; sagittal (Figure 1) or right

oblique (Figure 2) views are the best. Image-directed continuous wave Doppler interrogation of the stenotic jet should be attempted from multiple windows [subcostal, multiple parasternal (Figure 3), apical]. Tricuspid valve hypoplasia or, occasionally, dysplasia can co-exist with valvar pulmonary stenosis and is obvious from the subcostal left oblique view. Right ventricular inflow hypoplasia invariably accompanies tricuspid valve hypoplasia, and its presence may be a relative contraindication for balloon dilatation.

B. Valvar Pulmonary Atresia

The variants of (valvar) pulmonary atresia continue to constitute a challenge to pediatric cardiac surgeons. The 30-day mortality rate is actually higher for this lesion than for (valvar) aortic atresia. Although the reasons for the difficulty in management of pulmonary atresia are still controversial, two which appear to dominate are: the relative rarity of the malformation and the wide diversity in anatomical features. For unknown reasons, the prevalence of aortic atresia is at least three-fold higher than pulmonary atresia. Of the anatomical features, the most important seems to be the presence and type of coronary artery abnormality. Freedom[3] and associates have reported on the absence of coronary artery anomalies in the uncommon Ebstein's variant, which is associated with thin right ventricular myocardium; however, in 60% of the remaining types of valvar pulmonary atresia, either coronary arterial stenosis, interruption, or sinusoid formation can be identified.[4]

Tricuspid valve hypoplasia or dysplasia usually coexists with pulmonary valve atresia. Judgment of severity of tricuspid stenosis is difficult[5] using Doppler interrogation since there is always a large atrial septal defect, allowing blood to enter the left atrium and by-pass the tricuspid orifice; morphology appears to be a more reliable means of detecting stenosis. Right ventricular volume can be estimated using various formulae or by measuring tricuspid annulus diameter.

Subcostal left oblique and right oblique views are very useful.[6]

Coronary artery abnormalities can occasionally be detected using color Doppler echocardiography; however, cardiac catheterization is superior for this purpose.

C. "Absent" Pulmonary Valve

An extreme form of dysplasia[7,8] has been termed "absent" pulmonary valve, although rudimentary leaflets are always visible. By contrast, leaflets are indeed absent in the absent aortic valve malformation (see Chapter 16, section C). While the right ventricle and main pulmonary artery are markedly dilated, the pulmonary annular size is normal or slightly small. The right pulmonary artery is typically enormous, and often the left pulmonary artery is markedly enlarged as well. Rabinovitch[9] reported the extension of the dilation phenomenon into the peripheral pulmonary vessels as well. The most frequent associated malformation[10] is a malalignment-type ventricular septal defect. Alpert[11] reported a case with a patent ductus arteriosus and without branch pulmonary artery dilatation. Spin echo MRI and three-dimensional reconstruction can display the vascular impingement on the airways. The advantage is that MRI can display the vascular and bronchial morphology simultaneously with equivalent resolution. Ultrasonic display of trachea and bronchi is difficult.

The color Doppler display of the pulmonary regurgitant jet is most straightforward from the parasternal window. Aliasing is minimized because the distance to target is reduced.

D. Anomalous Muscle Bundle of the Right Ventricle

There are numerous sites for "anomalous" muscle bundles[12,13] within the morphological right ventricle (Figures 4–6). The two most common are: an abnormally high takeoff of the moderator band from the septal band (Figure 7) and the proximal subpulmonary infundibular free wall.

The differentiation between tetralogy of Fallot and large perimembranous ventricular septal defect associated with right ventricular anomalous muscle bundle is frequently difficult on angiography. The right oblique view (Figure 8) facilitates this differentiation: in tetralogy, the angle of the infundibular septum vis-à-vis the diaphragm is more horizontal. In anomalous muscle bundle of the right ventricle, the infundibular septum is in its normal position, nearly vertical (Figure 9). The muscle bundle can be seen on the subpulmonary infundibular free wall.

E. Dynamic Subpulmonic Stenosis

Dynamic left ventricular outflow tract obstruction occurs only in hypertrophic cardiomyopathy and in transposition of the great arteries with intact, or virtually intact, ventricular septum. In the latter, it is a geometry-related problem since it is not present at birth, emerges at several months of age, and *disappears* after arterial switch surgery. The right ventricle–left ventricle pressure difference appears to affect the configuration of the left ventricular outflow tract sufficiently to bring it into close proximity with the mitral valve (see Chapter 15, Figure 15). The subpulmonic stenosis results from a combination of septal bulge and systolic anterior motion of the anterior mitral leaflet (see Chapter 12, Figure 2). Following arterial switch surgery, the left ventricular pressure exceeds right ventricular pressure, and the configuration of the outflow tract reverts to normal.

The subcostal long axial oblique equivalent view is best for distinguishing this from anatomical (fixed) types of obstruction.[14]

References

1. Pearl W. Cardiovascular anomalies in Noonan's syndrome. *Chest* 1977; 71:677–679.
2. Green CE, Elliott LP, Coghlan HC. Improved cineangiographic evaluation of hypertrophic cardiomyopathy by caudocranial left anterior oblique view. *Am Heart J* 1981; 102:1015–1021.
3. Coles JG, Freedom RM, Lightfoot NE, Dasmahapatra HK, Williams WG, Trusler GA, Burrows PE. Long-term results in neonates with pulmonary atresia and intact ventricular septum. *Ann Thorac Surg* 1989; 47:213–217.
4. Gittenberger-de Groot AC, Sauer U, Bindl L, Babic R, Essed CE, Buhlmeyer K. Competition of coronary arteries and ventriculo-coronary arterial com-

munications in pulmonary atresia with intact ventricular septum. *Int J Cardiol* 1988; 18:243–258.

5. Bass JL, Fuhrman BP, Lock JE. Balloon occlusion of atrial septal defect to assess right ventricular capability in hypoplastic right heart syndrome. *Circulation* 1983; 68:1081–1086.

6. Marino B, Franceschini E, Ballerini L, Marcelletti C, Thiene G. Anatomical-echocardiographic correlations in pulmonary atresia with intact ventricular septum: use of subcostal views. *Int J Cardiol* 1986; 11:103–109.

7. Lakier JB, Stanger P, Heymann MA, Hoffman JIE, Rudolph AM. Tetralogy of Fallot with absent pulmonary valve. *Circulation* 1974; 50:167–174.

8. Stellin G, Jonas RA, Goh TH, Brawn WJ, Venables AW, Mee RBB. Surgical treatment of absent pulmonary valve syndrome in infants: relief of bronchial obstruction. *Ann Thorac Surg* 1983; 36: 468–475.

9. Rabinovitch M, Grady S, David I, Van Praagh R, Sauer U, Buhlmeyer K, Castaneda AR, et al. Compression of intrapulmonary bronchi by abnormally branching pulmonary arteries associated with absent pulmonary valves. *Am J Cardiol* 1982; 50: 804–813.

10. Tenorio de Albuquerque AM, Ortiz J, De Moraes AV, Atik E, Ebaid M, Del Nero E, Pileggi F. Cross-sectional echocardiographic features of "absent" pulmonary valve. *Int J Cardiol* 1984; 5:155–161.

11. Alpert BS, Moore HV. "Absent" pulmonary valve with atrial septal defect and patent ductus arteriosus. *Pediatr Cardiol* 1985; 6:107–112.

12. Matina D, Van Doesburg NH, Fouron J-C, Guerin R, Davignon A. Subxiphoid two-dimensional echocardiographic diagnosis of double-chambered right ventricle. *Circulation* 1983; 67:885–888.

13. Pongiglione G, Freedom RM, Cook D, Rowe RD. Mechanism of acquired right ventricular outflow tract obstruction in patients with ventricular septal defect: an angiocardiographic study. *Am J Cardiol* 1982; 50:776–780.

14. Chin AJ, Yeager SB, Sanders SP, Williams RG, Bierman FZ, Burger BM, Norwood WI, et al. Accuracy of prospective 2-dimensional evaluation of the left ventricular outflow tract in complete transposition of the great arteries. *Am J Cardiol* 1985; 55:759–764.

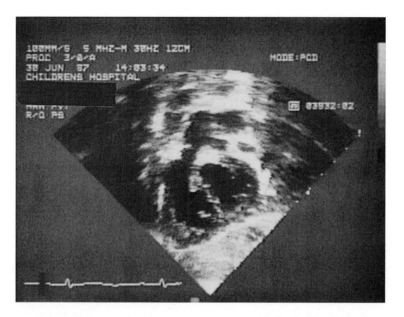

Figure 1: Subcostal sagittal view of valvar pulmonic stenosis and post-stenotic dilatation.

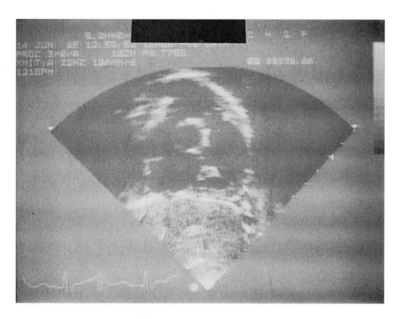

Figure 2: Subcostal right oblique view of valvar pulmonic stenosis.

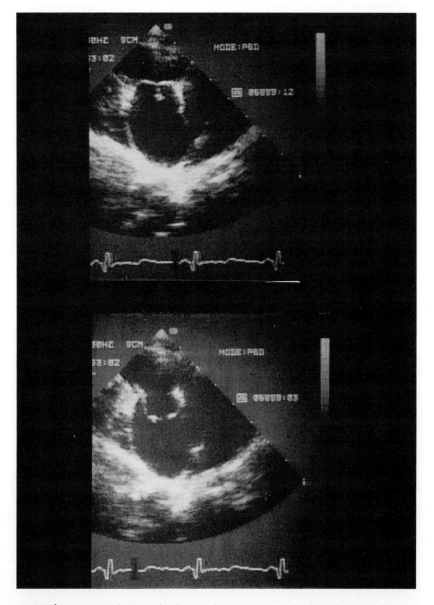

Figure 3: High parasternal view of valvar pulmonic stenosis in diastole (top) and in systole (bottom). This patient had commissural fusion.

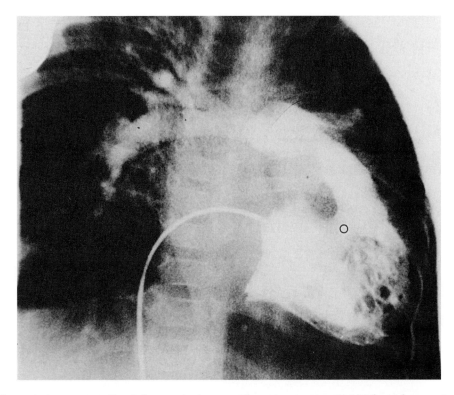

Figure 4: Anteroposterior right ventriculogram. The narrowest portion of the right ventricular outflow tract (open circle) is caused by a muscle bundle, not by infundibular septal deviation.

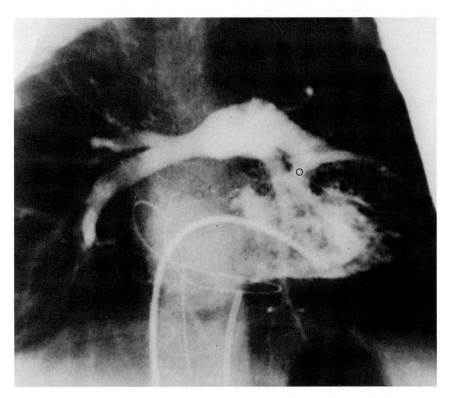

Figure 5: Anteroposterior right ventriculogram. Note how this patient's muscle bundle is *higher* than that in Figure 4. The infundibular septum is not deviated. The open circle denotes the narrowest portion of the outflow.

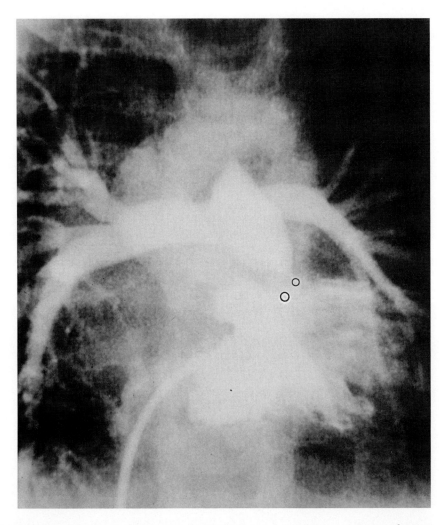

Figure 6: Anteroposterior angiogram. Anomalous muscle bundle can coexist with tetralogy of Fallot. The muscle bundle causes significant obstruction (large open circle). The infundibular septum, however, is deviated far to the left, causing severe stenosis (small open circle).

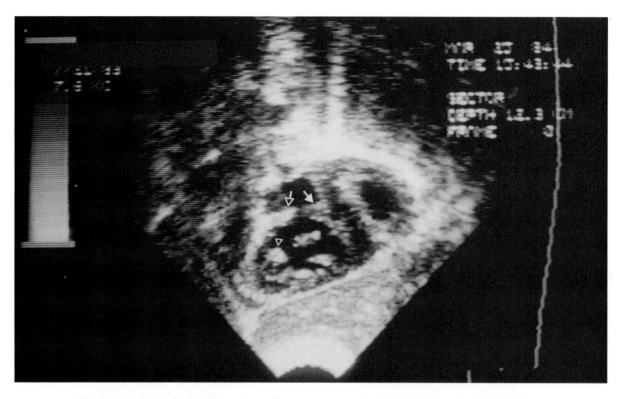

Figure 7: Subcostal left oblique view of anomalous muscle bundle (open arrow). closed arrow = septal band; open arrowhead = anterior papillary muscle.

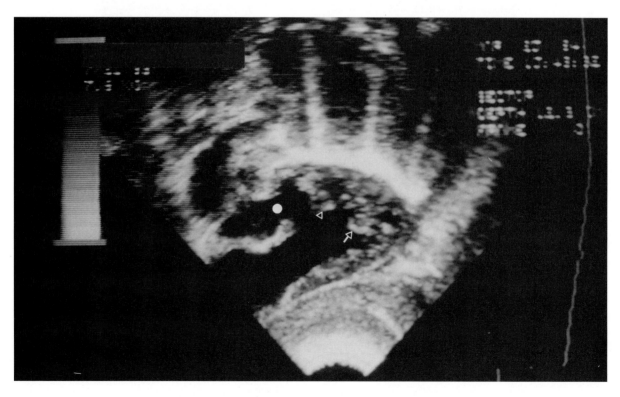

Figure 8: Subcostal right oblique view of anomalous muscle bundle (open arrowhead). closed circle = ventricular septal defect.

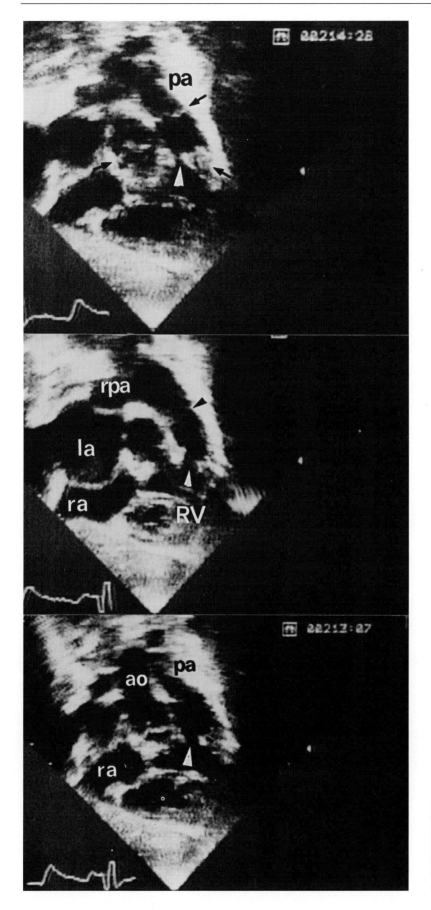

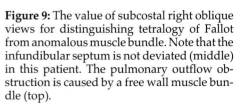

Figure 9: The value of subcostal right oblique views for distinguishing tetralogy of Fallot from anomalous muscle bundle. Note that the infundibular septum is not deviated (middle) in this patient. The pulmonary outflow obstruction is caused by a free wall muscle bundle (top).

Chapter 18

Aorta, Aortic Arch, Pulmonary Artery, and Ductus Arteriosus

Introduction

A brief review of the suprasternal technique discussed in Chapter 2 follows.

The patient's shoulders are elevated so that the neck is hyperextended to approximately 30°. The transducer is positioned in the suprasternal notch or a high parasternal window, and a frontal "reference" view showing the right superior vena cava, or bilateral venae cavae, is obtained (Figure 1). The transducer plane is then angled anteriorly until the arterial outflow tracts are visualized. From this point, the transducer is slowly swept posteriorly, so that the ascending aorta is displayed in the central region of the sector. This sweep is continued until the first branch of the ascending aorta is visualized.

Particular attention is paid to the lateralization of this vessel, in order to assign arch sidedness. If the first vessel courses to the right, the arch is identified as left-sided, and vice versa. Very rare exceptions to this rule have been reported.[1] Since airways are usually difficult to identify with ultrasound, the tracheobronchial structures, which are customarily used as radiographic landmarks to determine arch sidedness, cannot be used routinely in ultrasound imaging. The first branch is followed superiorly and laterally in search of a point where the vessel bifurcates into two vessels of equal or nearly equal caliber. If such a bifurcation is demonstrable, then the vessel is considered to be an innominate artery. Although the innominate artery (if present) is usually larger at its origin than the other brachiocephalic vessels arising from the arch, a vessel's size

cannot be used as a sufficient criterion to judge it as an innominate artery. In the case of either left arch and normal branching or right arch with mirror-image branching, a bifurcation point can be found; however, in cases of aberrant subclavian artery, such a bifurcation does not exist, since the aberrant subclavian artery arises from the upper descending aorta. Double aortic arch (with or without atresia of one arch), will also not have a bifurcation point in the first arch branch. Finally, cases of *isolation* of a subclavian artery will not have a bifurcation point.

The sweep is then continued until the second branch is identified. Its sidedness and course are also noted.

The third branch and the upper descending aorta are then displayed as the sweep is completed posteriorly. It is important to verify that the third branch courses *laterally* instead of directly cephalad, in order to distinguish the subclavian artery from the case in which the third vessel is actually a *vertebral* artery arising directly from the arch. Aberrant subclavian arteries and diverticulae (persistent dorsal aortae) are searched for. Isolated subclavian artery should be suspected any time the proximal portion of an "aberrant" subclavian is hard to display.

Sidedness of the upper descending aorta is noted with the transducer oriented in the frontal plane, centered in the suprasternal notch, and directed just anterior to the most posterior angulation of the sweep. In this position, the proximal portion of the upper descending aorta is visualized as a continuation of the distal aortic arch just imaged. If the descending aorta continues on the same side of the spine as the distal arch, that portion of the upper descending aorta appears as a short cylindrical structure oriented in a cephalad-caudad direction (Figure 2). If, however, the upper descending aorta descends on the opposite side from the distal aortic arch, it is visualized as a more elongated cylinder which is oriented in an oblique direction, from the side of the distal aortic arch to the side of the upper descending aorta.

Imaging of the entire arch in a single plane is also attempted. The transducer face is placed over the *apex of the arch* (in a left arch, this is usually either the high right parasternal window or the suprasternal notch). It is then rotated counterclockwise and angled toward the left hemithorax to bring the arch into view in a "candy-cane" or left oblique configuration. In a right arch, the apex of the arch is usually in the suprasternal notch region, and a parasagittal plane can be used, with the transducer angled slightly toward the right chest. This configuration allows the examiner to completely interrogate the arch and upper descending aorta with color, pulsed wave (and if necessary 2D-guided continuous wave) Doppler. It also allows the examiner to rule out the presence of a persistant fifth arch.

After imaging and Doppler ultrasound assessment of the arch[3] is satisfactorily completed, imaging of the ductus arteriosi is performed again starting from the suprasternal frontal view (Figure 2). When the arch is left-sided, a left patent ductus arteriosus is well seen from the high left parasternal window, in a parasagittal plane (Figure 3). This is accomplished by first imaging the distal main pulmonary artery in the near-field, with the upper descending aorta in the posterior sector. Ideally, the image should demonstrate both the origin of the right pulmonary artery from the underside of the distal main pulmonary artery and the proximal left pulmonary artery. The patent ductus arteriosus, when present, would appear as a "third branch," originating slightly higher on the distal main pulmonary artery (just cephalad to the origin of the left pulmonary artery) and coursing toward the descending aorta, which would lie just posterior to the branch point (Figure 4). The origin of the right pulmonary artery, proximal left pulmonary artery, and ductus arteriosus can sometimes be seen simultaneously. Pulsed wave and color Doppler interrogation of the ductus should be performed (Figure 5); diligence is imperative to ensure that erroneous sampling from the left pulmonary artery does not occur.

A. Aortopulmonary Window

Aortopulmonary window and truncus arteriosus are probably pathogenetically unrelated.[2]

The parasternal short axis views demonstrate the deficiency in the aortopulmonary septum[4]; however, since many normal patients exhibit echo dropout in this view, it is necessary to utilize more than one view in order to avoid a false-positive diagnosis. The advent of color Doppler echocardiography has also aided the diagnosis of this lesion[5]; flow should be demonstrated moving from ascending aorta *across* the area of dropout into the pulmonary arteries. Furthermore, in the suprasternal left oblique view, diastolic reversal of flow should extend far proximal to the region of ductus arteriosus since the site of "run-off" is far "upstream."

B. "Hemitruncus" (Anomalous Origin of a Pulmonary Artery From the Aorta)

The anomalous pulmonary artery tends to be on the side opposite the arch. Thus, since left aortic arch is far more common, most examples of "hemitruncus" are anomalous origin of the right pulmonary artery from the aorta.

This rare anomaly is relatively easy to miss when the takeoff of the right pulmonary artery is from the *posterior* aspect of the aorta rather than the rightward aspect. (On subcostal imaging of the normal heart, care must be taken to visualize the right pulmonary artery actually merging with the left pulmonary artery as the transducer is angled progressively anteriorly.)

Parasternal short axis scans reveal the anomaly since the pulmonary bifurcation is not present.

C. Left Aortic Arch, Right Upper Descending Aorta

A rare anomaly, forming a vascular ring. There may or may not be an aberrant right subclavian artery. Although it can be identified by echocardiography, magnetic resonance imaging is probably superior.

D. Left Aortic Arch, Left Upper Descending Aorta, Aberrant Right Subclavian Artery

1. Without Right Ductus Arteriosus/ Ligamentum

This is not a vascular ring, even if there is a left ductus or ligamentum. As discussed in the introduction to this chapter, the most likely initial clue to this diagnosis is the failure of the first arch vessel to bifurcate.

2. With Right Ductus Arteriosus/ Ligamentum

This is a vascular ring. When there is only a ligamentum, the only clue to its existence may be identification of the diverticulum of Kommerell (right dorsal aortic root).

E. Right Aortic Arch with Mirror-Image Branching, Right Upper Descending Aorta

1. With Left Ductus Arteriosus/Ligamentum

Although intuitively one might predict by symmetry argument that this constellation would be less common than right arch + right upper descending aorta + right ductus, it turns out to be far more common! In one variant, the left ductus arises from the (subclavian portion of the) innominate artery. This origin can be seen in the suprasternal frontal view while following the course of the left innominate artery toward the left arm. This is not a vascular ring.

In the other variant, the left ductus arises from the (persistent) left dorsal aortic root. This causes a vascular ring. Presumably, the aortic arch between the left subclavian artery and the left ductus is the segment that has regressed. This malformation is much more common than left arch, normal branching, right ductus from right dorsal aortic root. Right arch, mirror-image branching, and left ductus must be distinguished from two other anomalies: right arch, aberrant left subclavian artery, and left ductus; and double aortic arch with atresia of the left arch between the origins of the left carotid and left subclavian arteries.

2. With Right Ductus Arteriosus/ Ligamentum

The right ductus arises from the descending aorta and connects to the right pulmonary artery–main pulmonary artery junction (Figure 6). This is not a vascular ring. A parasagittal view is most helpful; usually the high right parasternal window is best (Figure 7).

F. Right Aortic Arch, Left Upper Descending Aorta

A rare anomaly (Figure 8), it forms a vascular ring whether or not there is an aberrant left subclavian artery (Figure 9). Although it can be identified by echocardiography, magnetic resonance imaging is probably better.

G. Right Aortic Arch, Right Upper Descending Aorta, Aberrant Left Subclavian Artery

1. Without Left Ductus/Ligamentum

This is not a vascular ring, even with a *right* ductus or ligamentum. The first vessel from the arch fails to bifurcate.

2. With Left Ductus/Ligamentum

This is a vascular ring. The usual origin of the left ductus (ligamentum) is from a diverticulum of Kommerell which presumably represents persistent (left) dorsal aorta, but the origin can be from the right descending aorta itself. If the origin is more lateral on the left subclavian artery, there may be little, if any, airway compression.

H. Double Aortic Arch

The ascending aorta bifurcates into two vessels, each of which gives off a carotid artery (Figures 10–12) and a subclavian artery (Figures 10–12). In the most posterior angulation from the frontal view, *four* circular or oval structures will be seen, representing the cross-sections of the brachiocephalic vessels (Figure 13). An attempt should be made to visualize the entire ring at once (Figure 14). Commonly, the right arch is slightly larger than the left arch. It is rare for the left arch to be larger than the right arch. This entity can be ruled out if an innominate artery is identified. Although theoretically the ductus may be on either side or there may be bilateral ductus arteriosi, most commonly there is only a left ductus arteriosus. The upper descending aorta may be on either side.

The variants of double aortic arch with atresia of the left arch between the carotid and subclavian arteries are sometimes difficult to distinguish from right arch + aberrant left subclavian artery + left ligamentum, even with Doppler color flow imaging. (Atresia can occur distal to a carotid or distal to a subclavian.) Stenosis, rather than atresia, is easier to identify (Figures 15 and 16).

I. Cervical Aortic Arch

In rare cases, the apex of the arch is actually high in the neck. For unknown reasons, this occurs more frequently in right aortic arch. The technique for display of cervical arch is largely the same as described above, except the footprint of the transducer must be placed cephalad to the high right parasternal window.

J. Aortic Arch Hypoplasia

The most common narrow site in the arch is the segment between the left subclavian artery and the ductus (see section K, *Coarctation*). The second most common is the segment of the arch between the left carotid and the left subclavian takeoffs (Figure 17); because such narrowings are typically long-segment, the designation "arch hypoplasia" is used, instead of "coarctation." The least common site of arch narrowing is between the innominate artery and the left carotid origins.

The suprasternal left oblique view is overwhelmingly the most useful. It is particularly important to examine the region immediately distal to the left carotid artery (Figure 18); occasionally a severe discrete narrowing there *coexists* with hypoplasia of the rest of the segment between the left carotid and left subclavian.

K. Coarctation

The diagnosis of coarctation is straightforward in any age group if the ductus is closed (Figures 19 and 20). Pulsed Doppler interrogation proximal to a putative narrowing reveals continuous, laminar, low-velocity flow. Distal to the narrowing there is continuous, turbulent, high-velocity flow ["sawtooth" pattern (Figure 21)].

In the presence of a persistently patent ductus (Figure 22), the Doppler findings are different. Recently, diagnostic criteria focused more on morphologic measurement have been proposed for the full-term newborn.[6] Isthmus size ≤3 mm in the suprasternal

sagittal view appears to be associated with coarctation, whereas isthmus ≥5 mm is never seen in coarctation. In cases with intermediate isthmus size, the Doppler findings of continuous flow in the isthmus appear to correlate with coarctation. Diagnostic criteria utilizing measurements in the orthogonal plane have yet to be reported.

L. Interruption of the (Left) Aortic Arch

Aortic arch (Figure 23) interruptions are far more common in left arch patients. The surgical outcome appears to depend on the size of the subaortic region (Figure 24). The right oblique view is helpful in showing malalignment of the infundibular septum.

1. Type A

In type A, the interruption occurs between the left subclavian and the ductus site (Figure 25). The suprasternal left oblique view allows the examiner to distinguish this from coarctation.

2. Type B

By far the most common type of interruption, type B interruption, occurs between the left carotid and the left subclavian origins. It appears to be particularly frequent in cases of diGeorge syndrome, a phenotype that is associated with deletions[7,8] of a segment of chromosome 22. It can also occur in CHARGE association.[9]

The suprasternal[10] left oblique sweep will fail to display arch continuity. Aberrant right subclavian artery and isolation of the right subclavian artery should be searched for.

3. Type C

Extremely rare, this interruption occurs between the innominate artery and the left carotid artery takeoffs.

M. Anomalous Origin of the Left Pulmonary Artery from the Right Pulmonary Artery

Also termed "pulmonary artery sling," this anomaly manifests the same clinical symptoms as a vascular ring because the aberrant left pulmonary artery passes *between* the trachea and the esophagus. Echocardiographic identification is not as reliable as magnetic resonance imaging because the airways cannot be displayed consistently; however, certain anatomical features can be visualized. The origin of the left pulmonary artery is far to the right of the main pulmonary artery–right pulmonary artery junction.[11] Both the subcostal frontal and sagittal sweeps can illustrate this;

however, in a small percentage of cases, the angulation between the main pulmonary artery and the right pulmonary artery may be minimal; this makes it hard to distinguish the start of the right pulmonary artery and thus limits the ability of echocardiography to diagnose this anomaly.

It can coexist with other malformations such as tetralogy of Fallot and truncus arteriosus (Figures 26 and 27).

References

1. Moes CAF, Benson LN, Burrows PE, Freedom RM, Williams W, Duckworth JWA. The subclavian artery as the first branch of the aortic arch. *Pediatr Cardiol* 1991; 12:29–43.

2. Kutsche LM, Van Mierop LHS. Anatomy and pathogenesis of aorticopulmonary septal defect. *Am J Cardiol* 1987; 59:443–447.

3. Murdison KA, Andrews BAA, Chin AJ. Ultrasonographic display of complex vascular rings. *J Am Coll Cardiol* 1990; 15:1645–1653.

4. Rice MJ, Seward JB, Hagler DJ, Mair DD, Tajik AJ. Visualization of aortopulmonary window by two-dimensional echocardiography. *Mayo Clin Proc* 1982; 57:482–487.

5. Alboliras ET, Chin AJ, Barber G, Helton JG, Pigott JD. Detection of aortopulmonary window by pulsed and color Doppler echocardiography. *Am Heart J* 1988; 115:900–902.

6. Ramaciotti C, Chin AJ. Non-invasive diagnosis of coarctation with patent ductus arteriosus in the neonate. *Am Heart J* 1993; 125: 179–185.

7. Wilson DI, Cross IE, Goodship JA, Brown J, Scambler PJ, Bain HH, Taylor JF, et al. A prospective cytogenetic study of 36 cases of DiGeorge syndrome. *Am J Hum Genet* 1992; 51:957–963.

8. Driscoll DA, Budarf ML, Emanuel BS. A genetic etiology for DiGeorge syndrome: consistent deletions and microdeletions of 22q 11. *Am J Hum Genet* 1992; 50:924–933.

9. Lin AE, Chin AJ, Devine W, Park SC, Zackai E. The pattern of cardiovascular malformation in the CHARGE association. *Am J Dis Child* 1987; 141:1010–1013.

10. Smallhorn JF, Anderson RH, Macartney FJ. Cross-sectional echocardiographic recognition of interruption of aortic arch between left carotid and subclavian arteries. *Br Heart J* 1982; 48:229–235.

11. Yeager SB, Chin AJ, Sanders SP. Two-dimensional echocardiographic diagnosis of pulmonary artery sling in infancy. *J Am Coll Cardiol* 1986; 7:625–629.

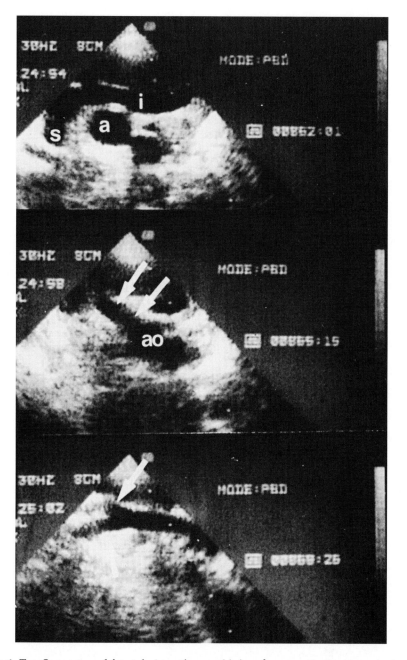

Figure 1: *Top:* Suprasternal frontal view of normal left arch. a = aorta; i = innominate vein; s = right superior vena cava. *Middle:* The first branch (arrows) courses to the patient's right. ao = aorta. *Bottom:* The first branch bifurcates (arrow), strongly suggesting it is an innominate artery. To prove it, one should trace each limb of the bifurcation to make certain that it is a carotid or a subclavian artery.

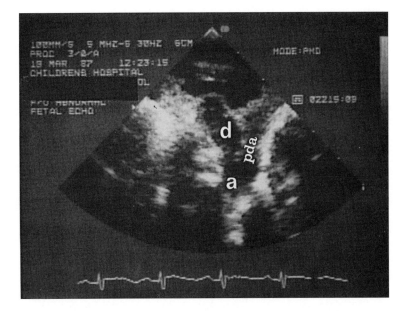

Figure 2: Suprasternal frontal view of the distal (d) portion of a left aortic arch, continuing into a left upper descending aorta (a). A (left-sided) patent ductus arteriosus (pda) is visible.

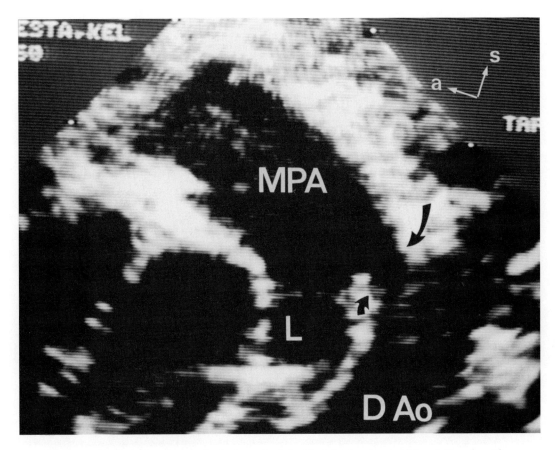

Figure 3: High parasternal sagittal view of a left-sided ductus (arrows) in a left arch with left upper descending aorta (DAo). L = left pulmonary artery; MPA = main pulmonary artery.

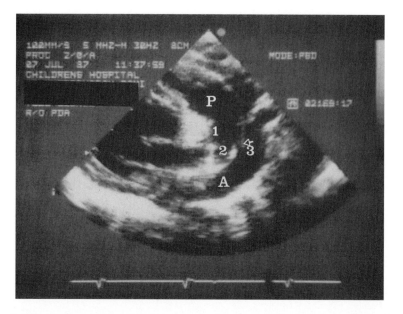

Figure 4: "Three-finger" sign. High parasternal parasagittal view. 1 = right pulmonary origin; 2 = proximal left pulmonary artery; 3 = ductus arteriosus; A = descending aorta; P = main pulmonary artery.

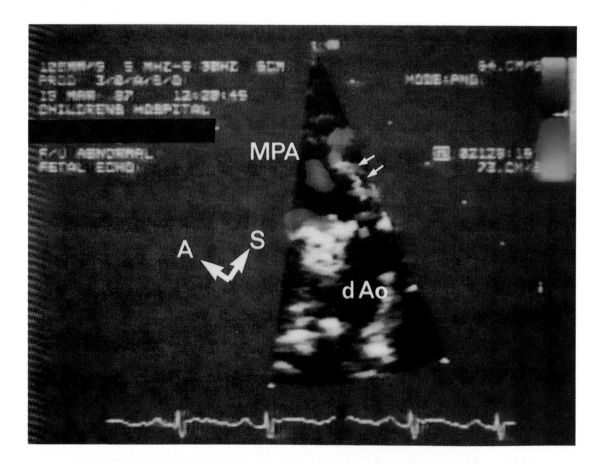

Figure 5: Color flow mapping of restrictive ductus arteriosus with left-to-right flow (arrows), same view as in Figure 4. MPA = main pulmonary artery; dAo = descending aorta.

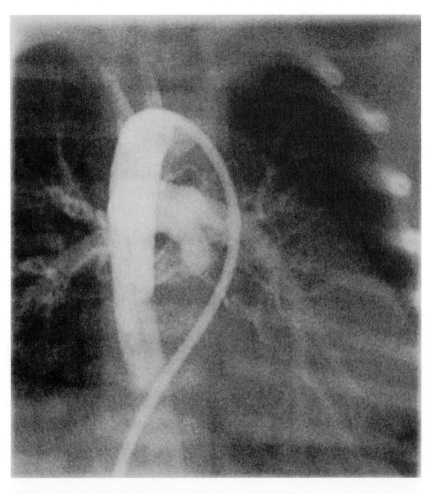

Figure 6: Anteroposterior angiogram of right aortic arch with right upper descending aorta and right-sided ductus arteriosus. The right carotid and right subclavian arteries are seen.

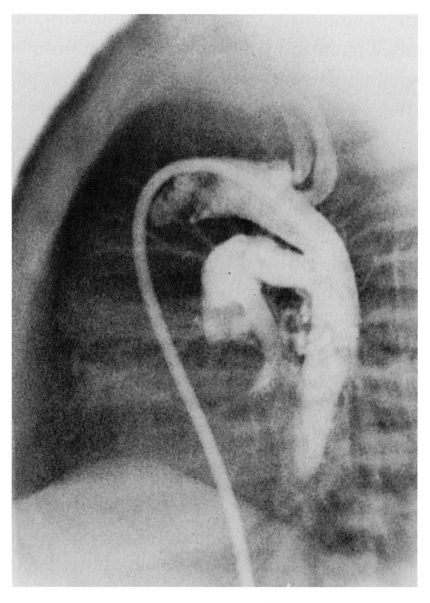

Figure 7: Lateral angiogram of patient shown in Figure 6.

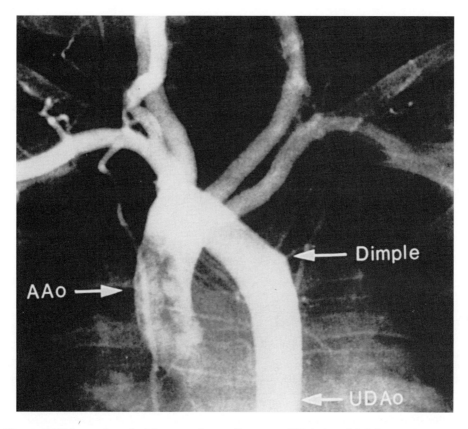

Figure 8: Right aortic arch, *left* upper descending aorta (UDAo), and left ligamentum arteriosum. AAo = ascending aorta. Used with permission of Elsevier Publishing.

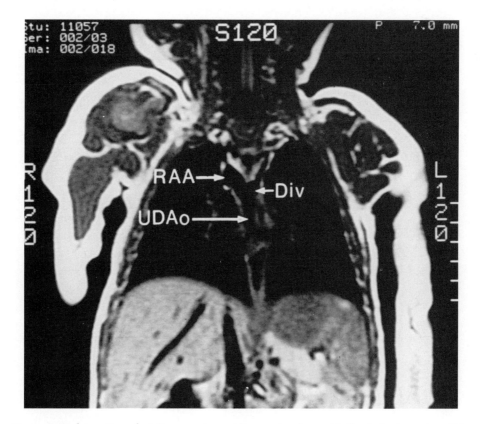

Figure 9: Right aortic arch, left upper descending aorta, aberrant left subclavian artery. Div = diverticulum of Kommerell; RAA = distal part of right aortic arch; UDAo = left upper descending aorta. Used with permission of Elsevier Publishing.

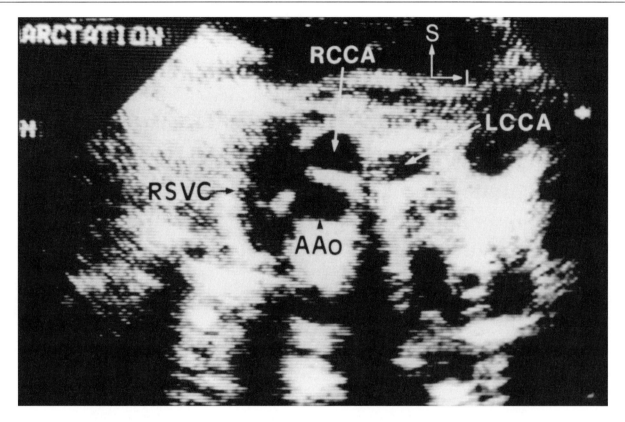

Figure 10: Suprasternal frontal view of double aortic arch. The ascending aorta (AAo) has not yet bifurcated. LCCA = left common carotid artery; RCCA = right common carotid artery; RSVC = right superior vena cava. Used with permission of Elsevier Publishing.

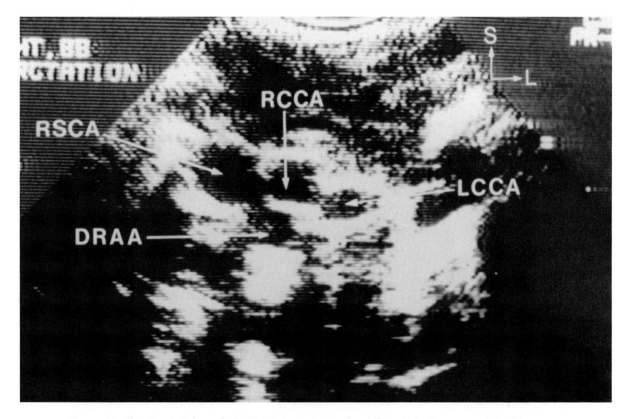

Figure 11: The distal right arch (DRAA) gives rise to the right subclavian artery (RSCA). LCCA = left common carotid artery. Used with permission of Elsevier Publishing.

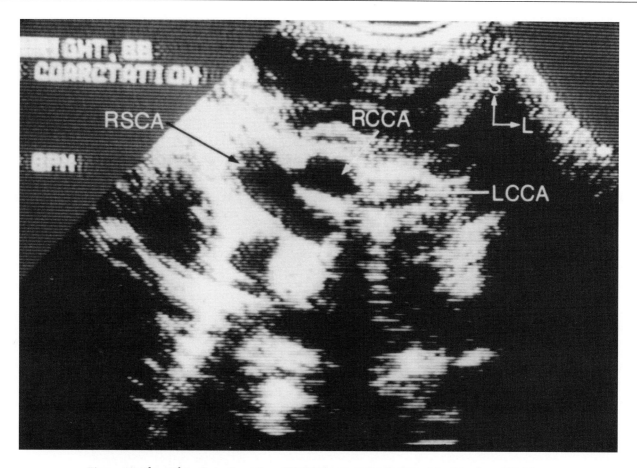

Figure 12: The right subclavian artery (RSCA) is more clearly traced in this plane. RCCA = right common carotid artery; LCCA = left common carotid artery. Used with permission of Elsevier Publishing.

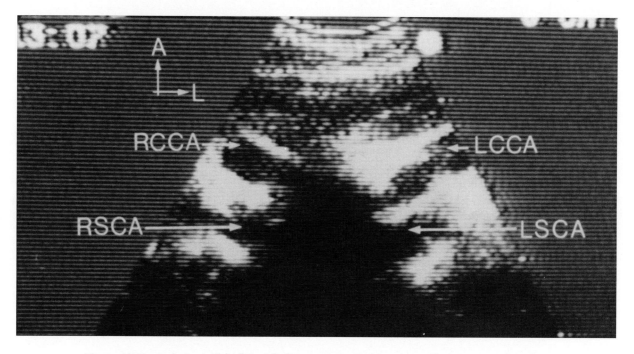

Figure 13: Typical view of brachiocephalic vessels in double aortic arch. RCCA = right common carotid artery; LCCA = left common carotid artery; RSCA = right subclavian artery; LSCA = left subclavian artery. Used with permission of Elsevier Publishing.

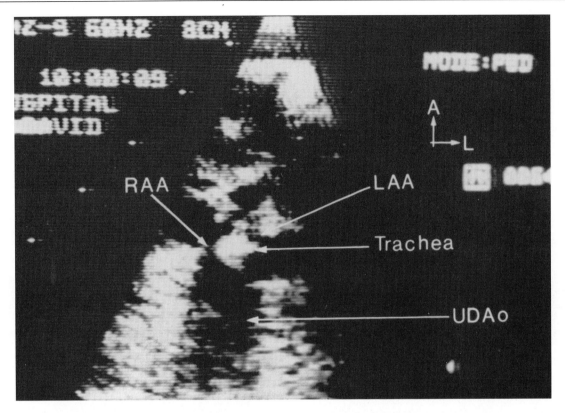

Figure 14: The encirclement of the trachea by a double arch can sometimes be displayed. LAA = left arch; RAA = right arch; UDAo = left upper descending aorta. Used with permission of Elsevier Publishing.

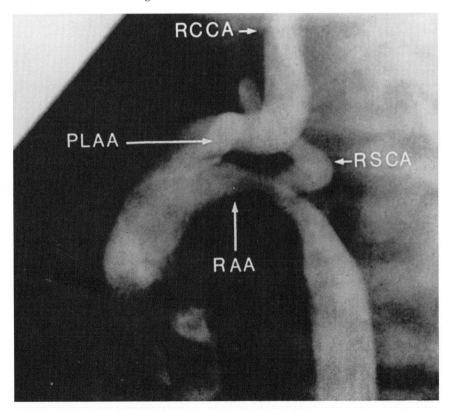

Figure 15: Lateral angiogram of patient shown in Figure 11. This patient had atresia of a segment of the left arch. PLAA = proximal left arch; RCCA = right common carotid artery; RSCA = right subclavian artery; RAA = right arch.

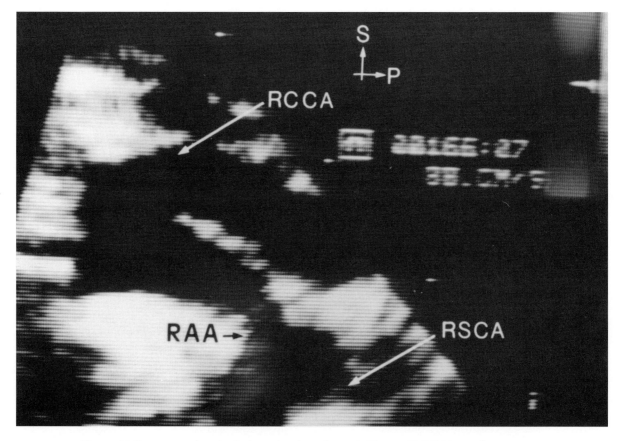

Figure 16: Suprasternal sagittal view of patient shown in Figure 15. RCCA = right common carotid artery; RAA = right arch; RSCA = right subclavian artery.

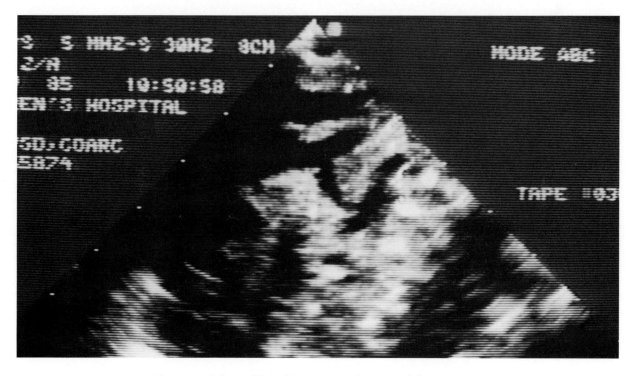

Figure 17: Subcostal left oblique view of aortic arch hypoplasia.

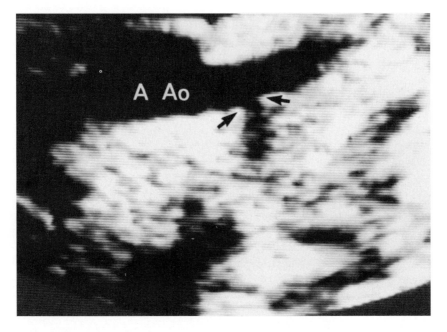

Figure 18: Suprasternal left oblique view of aortic arch hypoplasia. This patient has severe stenosis (arrows) just distal to the left common carotid artery takeoff. AAo = ascending aorta.

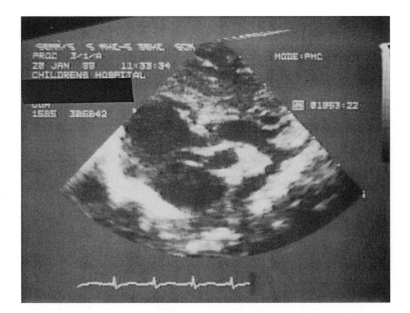

Figure 19: Suprasternal left oblique view of coarctation.

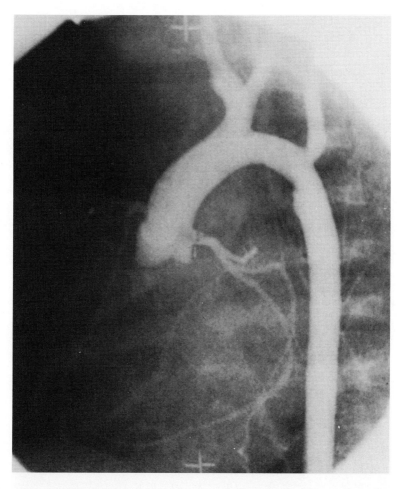

Figure 20: Left oblique angiogram of left aortic arch showing how the second vessel is not always the left carotid artery. In this patient, the left carotid arises from the innominate artery, so the second vessel is the left subclavian artery.

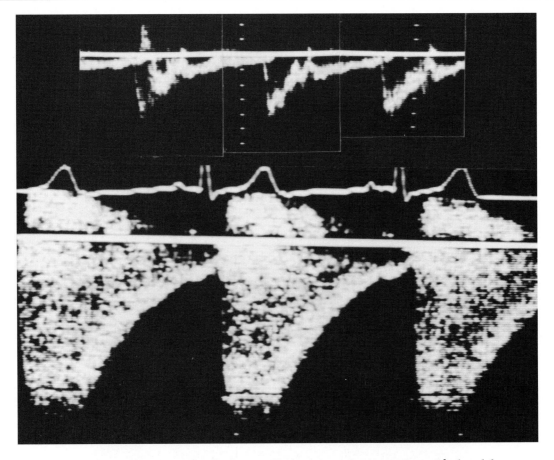

Figure 21: *Top:* Pulsed Doppler display proximal to coarctation in a patient with closed ductus. Flow is continuous and laminar. *Bottom:* Continuous wave Doppler display of maximal velocity distal to coarctation. High-velocity continuous flow is seen.

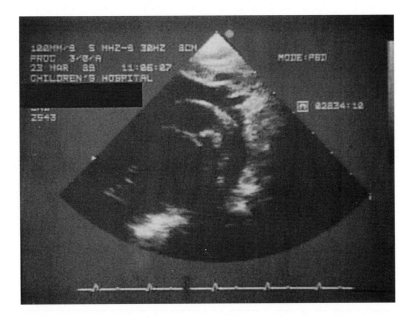

Figure 22: Suprasternal view of transposition of the great arteries, coarctation, and patent ductus arteriosus.

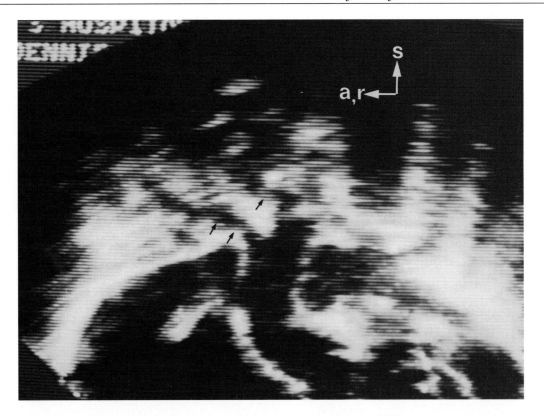

Figure 23: Subcostal left oblique view of first two vessels from the arch (compare with Figure 20).

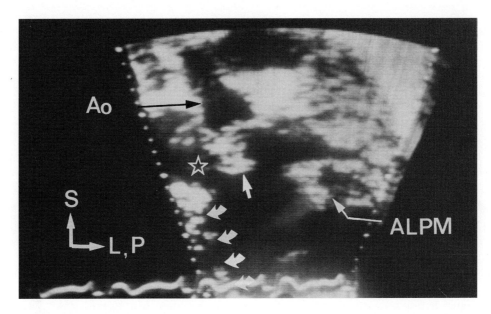

Figure 24: Subcostal left oblique view of subaortic stenosis in interrupted aortic arch. Single white arrow = infundibular septum; star = malalignment-type ventricular septum; curved white arrows = ventricular septum. Ao = aorta; ALPM = anterolateral papillary muscle.

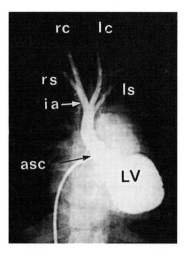

Figure 25: Anteroposterior angiogram of type A interrupted aortic arch. asc = ascending aorta; ia = innominate artery; lc = left carotid artery; ls = left subclavian artery; rc = right carotid artery; rs = right subclavian artery.

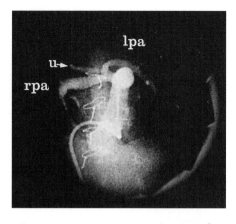

Figure 27: Postoperative angiogram of patient shown in Figure 26. The sling was not recognized intraoperatively; thus, the sling can still be seen on the postoperative study. lpa = left pulmonary artery; u = right upper pulmonary artery; rpa = right pulmonary artery.

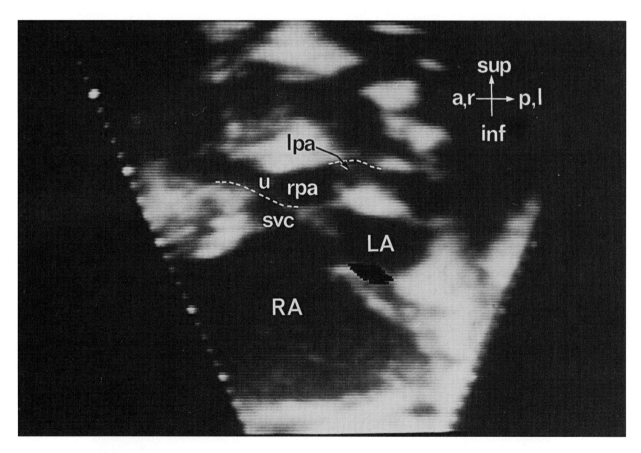

Figure 26: Subcostal left oblique view of pulmonary artery sling in truncus arteriosus. This is far to the right of the usual plane in which the left pulmonary artery is seen. The left pulmonary artery arises from the right pulmonary artery at a point where the right pulmonary artery bifurcates. lpa = left pulmonary artery; rpa = right pulmonary artery; svc = right superior vena cava; u = right upper pulmonary artery; LA = left atrium; RA = right atrium.

Chapter 19

Coronary Arteries, Aortic Sinuses of Valsalva

A. Anomalous Origin of Left Coronary Artery from the Pulmonary Artery

The embryologic mechanism[1] for this anomaly is still unclear.

Although it was hoped that the introduction of 7.5 MHz transducers would make this anomaly easier to detect, it was the advent of Doppler color flow imaging that actually had a greater impact. As with other malformations in which two structures are separated by a thin wall (see Chapter 18, section A, and Chapter 6, section G), the difficulty an echocardiographer encounters is attempting to tell when false dropout occurs. The parasternal short axis view of the aortic root is the easiest way to identify coronary arterial ostia; however, in this anomaly the left coronary artery ostium actually lies in the left pulmonary sinus of Valsalva or slightly more cephalad. It courses to its usual juxta-aortic tract and then travels normally to its bifurcation. The apposition of the coronary artery wall and the aortic wall can result in the false perception of continuity, even when a 7.5 MHz transducer is employed. Only occasionally is the course of the anomalous left coronary artery sufficiently different that two-dimensional imaging alone can convincingly demonstrate pulmonary artery origin (Figure 1).

Doppler color flow imaging, just as it does for aortopulmonary window and unroofed coronary sinus, displays blood flow moving *across* the area of echo dropout verifying that it is true rather than false dropout. The etiology of the color flow (from coronary artery to pulmonary root) is collateral circulation from the right coronary arterial bed. While the previously suggested two-dimensional technique of sizing the right coronary artery depends on the same physiology, Doppler color flow imaging[2] can detect *small* left-to-right shunts (i.e., those that would not result in noticeable dilation of the right coronary artery).

The two-dimensional display of wall motion in this anomaly often reveals global rather than the expected regional diminution in shortening and in wall thickening. Magnetic resonance imaging techniques may eventually explain this observation.

Doppler color flow imaging can also identify the mitral regurgitation which seems to be secondary to ischemic myocardium.

This anomaly can, on rare occasions, coexist with other heart malformations such as tetralogy of Fallot.

B. Coronary Arterio-Cameral Fistulae

The two most common varieties[3] are right coronary artery-to-right ventricle and left coronary artery-to-right ventricle; however, many other types have been reported. (When they occur in the setting of suprasystemic ventricular pressure, they have been termed *ventriculo-coronary connections*. See Chapter 17, section B.)

The affected coronary artery is dilated up to the point of the fistula. The most difficult aspect of their display is to ascertain whether there is more than one drainage destination.

In cases of ventriculo-coronary connections, it is necessary to do cardiac catheterization to identify coronary segments of stenosis or atresia.

C. Aortico-Left Ventricular Tunnel

This rare anomaly[4-6] is an abnormal connection between the ascending aorta and the left ventricle that typically runs through the infundibular septum.

D. Aortic Sinus of Valsalva Aneurysm

Although most commonly involving the right sinus of Valsalva, any sinus can be involved. Drainage sites in cases of rupture depend on the sinus involved; right sinus of Valsalva aneurysms usually rupture into the right ventricle. Noncoronary sinus of Valsalva aneurysms[7] rupture into the right atrium (Figure 2). Left sinus of Valsalva aneurysms are the least common and can rupture into the left atrium (Figure 3).

References

1. Hutchins GM, Kessler-Hanna A, Moore GW. Development of coronary arteries in the embryonic human heart. *Circulation* 1988; 77:1250–1257.
2. Karr SS, Parness IA, Spevak PJ, van der Velde ME, Colan SD, Sanders SP. Diagnosis of anomalous left coronary artery by Doppler color flow mapping: distinction from other causes of dilated cardiomyopathy. *J Am Coll Cardiol* 1992; 19:1271–1275.
3. Sanders SP, Parness IA, Colan SD. Recognition of abnormal connections of coronary arteries with the use of Doppler color flow mapping. *J Am Coll Cardiol* 1989; 13:922–926.
4. Humes RA, Hagler DJ, Julsrud PR, Levy JM, Feldt RH, Schaff HV. Aortico-left ventricular tunnel: diagnosis based on two-dimensional echocardiography, color flow Doppler imaging, and magnetic resonance imaging. *Mayo Clin Proc* 1986; 61:901–907.
5. Wu JR, Huang TY, Chen YF, Lin YT, Roan HR. Aortico-left ventricular tunnel: two-dimensional echocardiographic and angiocardiographic features. *Am Heart J* 1989; 117:697–699.
6. Sreeram N, Franks R, Walsh K. Aortic-ventricular tunnel in a neonate: diagnosis and management based on cross sectional and colour Doppler ultrasonography. *Br Heart J* 1991; 65:161–162.
7. Gleason MM, Hardy C, Chin AJ, Pigott JD. Ruptured sinus of Valsalva aneurysm in childhood. *Am Heart J* 1987; 114:1235–1238.

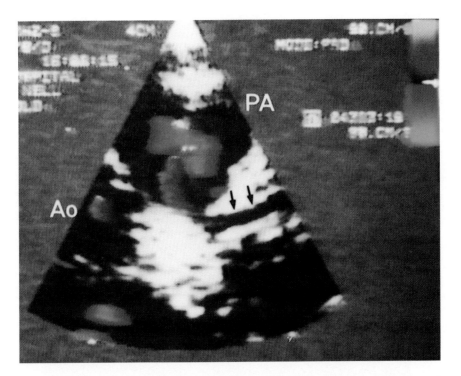

Figure 1: Parasternal view. Doppler color flow imaging showing flow from the anomalous left coronary artery (arrows) to the pulmonary root.

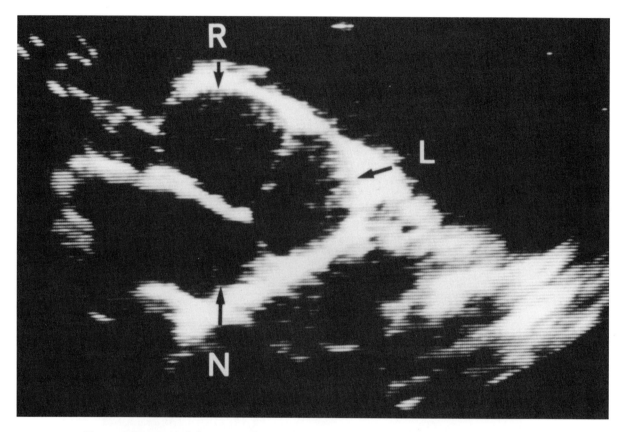

Figure 2: Parasternal short axis of sinus of Valsalva aneurysm. The noncoronary (N) sinus is involved. Note that the tricuspid annulus abuts the right coronary-noncoronary commissure. Thus, the site of rupture of this aneurysm was into the right atrium.

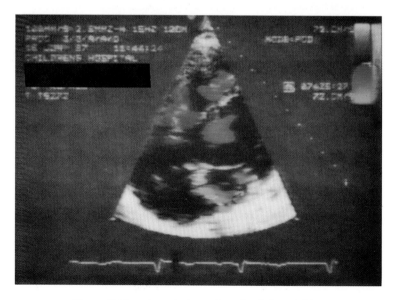

Figure 3: Parasternal view of aortico-left atrial jet.

Chapter 20

Preoperative Magnetic Resonance Imaging:

Form and Function

Mark Alan Fogel, MD

Magnetic resonance imaging (MRI) has been shown to be an effective means of demonstrating a wide variety of congenital cardiovascular lesions.[1–4] Since the advent of ECG gating and other compensatory techniques that allow the display of moving structures, imaging fidelity has been high enough to define cardiovascular anatomy as well as physiology.

MRI has many advantages as an imaging modality. It is completely noninvasive and avoids ionizing radiation. There is no limitation of windows, and any imaging plane is possible. The images are obtained and stored in digital form, making off-line analysis easy to perform. This is especially useful since contiguous parallel slices are obtained and allow for accurate oblique sectioning of the volume set. Since routine MRI constructs images typically over 384 heartbeats (128 phase encoded lines multiplied by 3 excitations), *averaged* motion and blood flow are obtained. This has the advantage of capturing pictures that better show the long-term functioning of the ventricle or blood flow. Newer technologies enable MRI to magnetically tag the myocardium and blood,[5–7] and to phase-encode velocity in blood vessels.[8,9] Finally, MRI is cost-competitive with other technologies.

There are, of course, tradeoffs. MRI can be time-consuming, and claustrophobia may be a problem in the older patient. It requires holding still for long periods of time (up to 90 minutes in long studies); sedation is necessary in young children. The magnetism *itself* may be a problem, because ferromagnetic materials may hinder imaging structures near to it, and pacemakers cannot be allowed near the magnet for risk of failure. Both imaging artifacts as well as problems with ECG gating may also at times preclude image acquisition.

There are numerous types of pulse sequences in use. T1 weighted spin-echo MRI allows for high-resolution imaging, with clearly defined endocardial and epicardial borders (blood-filled spaces contain no signal) at the cost of imaging time. Multiple static images through the thorax are easily obtained; however, multiphase images require an enormous amount of time to acquire if motion display is desired. Cine (gradient echo) MRI can acquire multiphase, single-slice (motion in a single slice), or multislice, single-phase images (identifying flowing blood in many slices) in a much shorter time period, however, at the cost of resolution. Flowing blood gives off a high-intensity signal, myocardium and blood vessels produce a lower intensity signal, and turbulent flow (Reynolds number >2000) gives off no signal. T2 weighted and proton density images allow distinction of various tissue types and are used mainly for cardiac tumor recognition.

SPAMM (*SPA*tial Modulation Magnetization)[6,7] and other magnetic resonance tagging techniques[5] enable MRI to specifically tag various portions of the myocardium and/or blood to allow for calculation of regional strain and wall motion or velocity profiles in a blood vessel. Other software can "phase-encode" velocity in a given blood vessel, and flow may be calculated.[8,9] Future advances have promised real-time imaging (echo planar MRI).

Anatomy, physiology, and function may therefore all be displayed with current technology although the physics of image generation and processing are beyond the scope of this chapter. This chapter and Chapter 24 will describe a few of the many uses of MRI: large amount of anatomical data acquisition quickly utilizing a wide field of view in preoperative evaluation (useful in heterotaxy cases, for example), three-dimensional reconstruction, and regional strain/wall motion analysis.

In many cases, a pediatric cardiologist needs to obtain as much anatomical information as possible noninvasively prior to cardiac catheterization or surgery. The paradigm of this situation is *heterotaxy syndrome*[10] in which the lateralization of blood vessels and organs is deranged (situs ambiguous); heart defects are common. Common parlance is to group such patients into asplenia (or bilateral rightsidedness) and polysplenia (or bilateral leftsidedness) syndromes, although some investigators disagree with calling these *syndromes.* Defining the position or presence of the various abdominal organs, determining venous and arterial connections as well as bronchial anatomy, and diagnosing the cardiac defect may all be done by MRI.

Figure 1 shows a group of axial (A), coronal (B), and sagittal (C) images of a patient with heterotaxy syndrome and double-outlet right ventricle {S,L,L}, large malalignment and atrioventricular canal types of ventricular septal defects, "ipsilateral" pulmonary veins, interrupted inferior vena cava with azygous continuation to the right superior vena cava, the hepatic veins draining to the right atrium, and a left superior vena cava to coronary sinus. The complex cardiac anatomy is well delineated in the three orthogonal views. The subaortic and subpulmonic regions are seen well on the sagittal images. In addition, the liver is midline on the coronal and axial images, the stomach is on the right, and there are bilateral hyparterial bronchi (coronal images).

Figure 2 also shows a group of axial (A), coronal (B), and sagittal (C) images of a patient with heterotaxy syndrome who has truncus arteriosus type A1 with a large ventricular septal defect, right aortic arch (with mirror-image branching) which descends on the right and crosses over the left at the level of the diaphragm, interrupted left inferior vena cava with left azygous continuation to a left superior vena cava which drains to the left-sided atrium, and a right superior vena cava and hepatic veins draining to the right-sided atrium. Note the morphology of the left-sided atrial appendage appears to be morphologically right and the right-sided atrial appendage appears morphologically left (sagittal views). The liver appears midline as well, and tracheal morphology appears normal (coronal views).

A. Three-Dimensional Reconstruction

All modalities acquire tomographic images in two dimensions and require the observer to build a three-dimensional structure mentally. Initially performed with x-ray computerized tomography[11–14] and successfully applied to MRI,[15–25] a volumetric data set, by virtue of the acquisition of contiguous parallel slices, may be reconstructed into a shaded surface display to appear three-dimensional by off-line computer analysis. This approach, which has only recently been attempted by transthoracic[26] and transesophageal[27–30] echocardiography, allows all observers the same three-dimensional perspective from two-dimensional tomographic data and can therefore facilitate communication of anatomy. Three-dimensional reconstruction is a familiar format that both health care workers and nonmedically oriented people can understand. It enables the imager to assess spatial geometry, especially with the ability to rotate structures about any axis and remove pieces of the structure to obtain a better view of the salient points of the anatomy. One of the unique properties is that these alternative viewing angles are used *after* data acquisition. Finally, three-dimensional reconstruction allows for true volume measurements.

The first step in MRI-based three-dimensional reconstruction is to select a region of interest of each image (Figures 3A and 3B) and segment the image into its component structures (Figure 3C). These segments are then transformed into a binary image (i.e., 1's and 0's, black and white). This is accomplished through a process called "thresholding" (Figure 3D), which basically assigns all pixels under a certain value 0 and over a certain value 1 and allows for isolation of each structure under study. This is done for each component in the image, the computer keeping track of the relative position of each one. The binary images are then edited (Figure 3E), to clean up any artifacts that may have been generated by this process.

Next, each binary image for a given structure is stacked one on top of the other and a linear interpolation is done between the images to refine the borders of the final three-dimensional picture (Figure 3F). Then, a shaded surface display is constructed by surface detection (Figure 3G), surface shading (Figure 3H), and color coding (e.g., aorta–red, pulmonary artery–blue, etc.) each structure and adding it to the final product.

Finally, a single-frame view and movie may be created to display the perspective desired.

The following are three examples of where shaded surface displays are particularly useful:

1. Rings and Slings

These are great vessel malformations where vascular structures completely surround the trachea and esophagus.[31] Patients may be asymptomatic or manifest severe respiratory (stridor and/or wheezing) or esophageal (dysphagia) compromise. Which vessels or parts of vessels make up the various parts of the ring is a function of the lesion. Furthermore, there may be additional embarrassment from a saccular outpouching of the descending aorta (diverticulum of Kommerel) impinging on trachea and the esophagus.[32]

Figure 4 shows axial (upper images) and coronal (lower images) planes of a patient with a *double aortic arch*.[33–35] Both datasets display the ascending aorta dividing into a dominant right and a smaller left branch, encircling the trachea and esophagus, and joining the descending aorta posteriorly. As is common in this lesion, the right aortic arch is larger than the left. Figure 5 shows the three-dimensional reconstruction in a number of different views: anterior (A), posterior (B), transverse (C), and with all structures removed except the aorta (C and D). One can appreciate the ring much better from this prospective.

Figure 6 shows three views [anterior (A), posterior (B), and transverse (C)] of a patient with a *right aortic arch with an aberrant left subclavian artery*[36] arising posteriorly from a diverticulum of Kommerel. The great vessels arising from the aorta from proximal to distal are the left carotid, right carotid, right subclavian and left subclavian. The anterior and right lateral portions of the ring are formed by the aorta, the posterior portion from the diverticulum, and the left lateral portion from the left ligamentum (not shown).

Figure 7 is also a patient with a *right aortic arch with an aberrant left subclavian artery*,[36] but who is status post a Fontan procedure. Both views are laterals and show the compression of the trachea by the ring with the aorta in the image (A) and removed (B) to more clearly see the effect.

Figure 8 displays the reconstruction of a *pulmonary artery sling*[37,38] in which the left pulmonary artery arises from the right pulmonary artery and courses behind the trachea. Both images are transverse views, which clearly display the salient features of this anatomy, with the trachea shown in one picture (A) and removed in the other (B).

2. Complex Cardiac Anatomy

Relationships between the atria and atrioventricular valves, the atrioventricular valves to ventricles, the ventricles to great arteries, and the position of the heart in the chest[39] may be hard to reconstruct in three dimensions in an observer's mind. Lesions such as heterotaxy,[10] supero-inferior ventricles, criss-cross atrioventricular relations,[39] and others may be better comprehended by three-dimensional display rather than tomographic images. Not only does this give the pediatric cardiologist a powerful tool for diagnosis, it gives the cardiothoracic surgeon a feel for the relationships of all cardiovascular structures within the chest.

Figure 9 depicts the three-dimensional reconstruction of a patient with supero-inferior ventricles and criss-cross atrioventricular relationships who is status post a Senning procedure.[40–42] With standard tomographic imaging, the spatial relationship of criss-cross atrioventricular valves and supero-inferior ventricles is not well appreciated. Three-dimensional reconstruction allows these important points of the anatomy to be visualized effortlessly. Figure 9A (anterior) shows the supero-inferior relationship of the ventricles and B (transverse) shows the relationship of the *"neo-right"* and *"neo-left"* atrium (to be discussed in Part II). If various structures are removed (transverse views, Figures 9C and 9D), the viewer can appreciate what is meant by the criss-cross relationship of the atrioventricular valves.

Goldenhar's syndrome is a pattern of facial and vertebral anomalies which have hemifacial microsomia, and facioauriculovertebral abnormalities[43] with approximately 25% having cardiovascular defects.[44] Figure 10 displays one such patient with extreme levocardia and tetralogy of Fallot. The spin-echo image (A) shows a four-chamber view displaying the ventricular septal defect and the extreme malposition of the heart with the apex pointing to the left axilla. Three-dimensional reconstruction with rotation to the left axilla (B) and to the lateral position (C) enables one to view the malformation much more clearly. In B, the overriding aorta and ventricular septal defect (VSD) are seen. The lateral view (C) shows the azygous vein clearly draining to the left superior vena cava and the relative positions of some of the important structures in the chest.

3. Perspective

Three-dimensional reconstruction allows for a broader perspective and appreciation of the relative positions and volumes of structures in the chest. This may be important, for example, in the case of anomalous origin of the innominate artery from the aorta causing tracheal compression.[45–48] Figure 11 shows the three-dimensional reconstruction of the MRI data of just such a patient who is rotated in various positions and with structures removed. The upper left picture is an anteroposterior view with the aorta (orange), trachea (green), esophagus (yellow), and pulmonary artery (red) present. The upper right image is also an anteroposterior view; however, the aorta is removed to display the indentation on the trachea. The lower images show all four structures rotated in the posteroanterior view (lower left) and the lateral view (lower left). These images give the observer a much better sense of the positions of the structures in question.

Figure 12 are images of a patient with Williams syndrome[49,50] who has supravalvar aortic stenosis with tubular hypoplasia of the ascending and transverse aorta. The spin-echo image (A) gives a sense of the tubular hypoplasia, but it is only until the data are reconstructed in three dimensions (B) can one appreciate the volumes involved.

The relationship of the great vessels to each other, the ventricles, and salient intracardiac anatomy (e.g., VSD location) is also very important anatomical infor-

mation preoperatively. Figure 13 displays the anatomy of a patient with double-outlet right ventricle {S,D,D}[51] in both the anterior (A) and the transverse (B) views. The anterior view (A) clearly shows both great vessels over the right ventricle, with the aorta to the right of the pulmonary artery. The transverse view (B) with the right ventricle and pulmonary artery removed clearly show the VSD to lie beneath the aorta.

Finally, no MRI chapter on preoperative evaluation of the patient with congenital heart disease would be complete without an image of a coarctation of the aorta.[52] Figure 14 contains spin-echo (left) and cine (center and right) images of a patient with just such an anomaly. The spin-echo image clearly displays the anatomy of the coarctation. The cine images at end-diastole (center) and at 100 msec into systole (right) display areas of turbulence (arrows) during systole. The patient also had a bicuspid aortic valve that also shows turbulence (two left-most arrows of the right image).

In summary, in vascular rings, aortic anomalies, and complex malformations, MRI has made a contribution to preoperative management. The chapter on postoperative MRI (Chapter 24) will discuss additional concepts.

References

1. Didier D, Higgins CB, Fisher M, Osakai L, Silverman NH, Cheitlin MD. Congenital heart disease: gated magnetic resonance imaging in 72 patients. *Radiology* 1986; 158:227–235.

2. Fletcher BD, Jacobstein MD, Nelson AD, Riemenschneider TA, Alfidi RJ. Gated magnetic resonance imaging of congenital cardiac malformations. *Radiology* 1984; 150:137–140.

3. Higgins CB, Byrd BF, Farmer DW, Osakai L, Silverman N, Cheitlin MD. Magnetic resonance imaging in patients with congenital heart disease. *Circulation* 1984; 70:851–860.

4. Reed JD, Soulen RL. Cardiovascular MRI: current role in patient management. *Radiol Clin North Am* 1988; 26:589–606.

5. Zerhouni EA, Parish DM, Rogers WJ, Yang A, Shapiro EP. Human heart: tagging with MR imaging. A method for non-invasive assessment of myocardial motion. *Radiology* 1988; 169:59–63.

6. Axel L, Dougherty L. MR imaging of motion with spatial modulation of magnetization. *Radiology* 1989; 171:841–845.

7. Axel L, Dougherty L. Heart wall motion: improved method of spatial modulation of magnetization for MR imaging. *Radiology* 1989; 172:349–350.

8. Walker MF, Souza SP, Dumoulin CL. Quantitative flow measurement in phase contrast MR angiography. *J Comput Assist Tomogr* 1988; 12:304–313.

9. Nishimura DG. Time of flight angiography. *Magn Reson Med* 1990; 14:194–201.

10. Gutgesell HP. Cardiac malposition and heterotaxy. In: Garson A, Bricker JT, McNamara DG (eds). *The Science and Practice of Pediatric Cardiology*. Lea & Febiger, Philadelphia/London, 1990, pp 1280–1303.

11. Sinak LJ, Liu YH, Block M, Mair DD, Julsrud PR, Hoffman EA, Hagler DJ, et al. Anatomy and function of the heart and intrathoracic vessels in congenital heart disease: evaluation with the Dynamic Spatial Reconstructor. *J Am Coll Cardiol* 1985; 5:705–765.

12. Sinak LJ, Hoffman EA, Julsrud PR, Mair DD, Seward JB, Hagler DJ, Harris LD, et al. The Dynamic Spatial Reconstructor: investigating congenital heart disease in four dimensions. *Cardiovasc Intervent Radiol* 1984; 7:124–139.

13. Farmer DW, Lipton MJ, Webb WR, Ringertz H, Higgins CB. Computed tomography in congenital heart disease. *J Comput Assist Tomogr* 1984; 8:677–687.

14. Ritman EL, Kinsey JH, Robb RA, Gilbert BK, Harris LD, Wood EH. Three-dimensional imaging of

the heart, lungs, and circulation. *Science* 1980; 210:273–280.

15. Vannier MW, Gutierrez FR, Canter CE, Hildebolt CF, Pilgram TK, McKnight RC, Laschinger J, et al. Evaluation of congenital heart disease by three-dimensional magnetic resonance imaging. *J Digit Imaging* 1991; 4:153–158.

16. Vannier MW, Gutierrez FR, Laschinger JC. Three-dimensional magnetic resonance imaging. *Top Magn Reson Imaging* 1990; 2:61–65.

17. Yoffie RL, Vannier MW, Gutierrez FR, Knapp RH, Canter CE. Three-dimensional magnetic resonance imaging of the heart. *Radiol Technol* 1989; 60:305–309.

18. Vannier MW, Gutierrez FR, Laschinger JC, Gronemeyer S, Canter CE, Knapp RH. Three-dimensional magnetic resonance imaging of congenital heart disease. *Radiographics* 1988; 8:857–871.

19. Laschinger JC, Vannier MW, Gutierrez FR, Gronemeyer S, Weldon CS, Spray TL, Cox JL. Preoperative three-dimensional reconstruction of the heart and great vessels in patients with congenital heart disease: technique and initial results. *J Thorac Cardiovasc Surg* 1988; 96:464–473.

20. Higgins CB, Holt W, Pflugfelder P, Sechtem U. Functional evaluation of the heart with magnetic resonance imaging. *Magn Reson Med* 1988; 6:121–139.

21. Laschinger JC, Vannier MW, Gronemeyer S, Gutierrez F, Rosenbloom M, Cox JL. Non-invasive three-dimensional reconstruction of the heart and great vessels by ECG-gated magnetic resonance imaging: a new diagnostic modality. *Ann Thorac Surg* 1988; 45:505–514.

22. Bittner V, Cranney GB, Lotan CS, Pohost GM. Overview of cardiovascular nuclear magnetic resonance imaging. *Cardiol Clin* 1989; 7:631–649.

23. Cline HE, Lorensen WE, Herfkens RJ, Johnson GA, Glover GH. Vascular morphology by three dimensional magnetic resonance imaging. *Magn Reson Imaging* 1989; 7:45–54.

24. Axel L, Herman GT, Udupa JK, Bottomley PA, Edelstein WA. Three dimensional display of nuclear magnetic resonance (NMR) cardiovascular images. *J Comput Assist Tomogr* 1983; 7:172–174.

25. Baffa JM, Hoffman EA, Axel L, Fellows KE, Weinberg PM. Three dimensional display of airway compression by vascular structures using magnetic resonance imaging. *Circulation* 1990; 82(Suppl III):III-154 (abstract).

26. Fulton D, Pandian N, Wollschlager H, Mumm B, Romero B. Dynamic 3-dimensional echocardiographic imaging of congenital heart defects in in-

fants and children by computer-controlled tomographic parallel slicing using a single integrated ultrasound instrument. *Circulation* 1992; 86(Suppl I):I-498 (abstract).

27. King DL, Gopal AS, Shao MYC. Three-dimensional echocardiography: in vitro validation in fixed hearts of infarct size measurements. *Circulation* 1992; 86(Suppl I):I-269 (abstract).

28. Hibberd AG, Siu SC, Handschumacher MD, Jiang L, Newell JB, Levine RA. Three-dimensional echocardiography: increased accuracy for left ventricular volume compared with angiography. *Circulation* 1992; 86(Suppl I):I-270 (abstract).

29. Gerber TC, Foley DA, Belohlavek M, Greenleaf JF, Seward JB. Comparison of different approaches to 3-dimensional reconstruction of the aorta from transesophageal echocardiography. *Circulation* 1992; 86(Suppl I):I-272 (abstract).

30. Jiang L, Siu SC, Handschumacher MD, Guerrero JL, de Prada JV, King ME, Picard MH, et al. Three-dimensional echocardiography: in vivo validation for right ventricular volume and function. *Circulation* 1992; 86(Suppl I):I-272 (abstract).

31. Morrow WR, Huhta JC. Aortic arch and pulmonary artery anomalies. In: Garson A, Bricker JT, McNamara DG (eds). *The Science and Practice of Pediatric Cardiology*. Lea & Febiger, Philadelphia/ London, 1990, p 1421.

32. Shuford WH, Sybers RG, Hogan GB. *The Aortic Arch and Its Malformations*. Charles C. Thomas, Springfield, MA, 1974, p 20.

33. Edwards JE. Anomalies of the derivatives of the aortic arch system. *Med Clin North Am* 1948; 32:925.

34. Riker WL. Anomalies of the aortic arch and their treatment. *Pediatr Clin North Am* 1954; Feb:181–195.

35. Stewart JR, Kinkaid OW, Edwards JE. *An Atlas of Vascular Rings and Related Malformations of the Aortic Arch System*. Charles C. Thomas, Springfield, MA, 1964, pp 14–37.

36. Shuford WH, Sybers RG, Hogan GB. *The Aortic Arch and Its Malformations*. Charles C. Thomas, Springfield, MA, 1974, pp 41–92.

37. Gumbiner CH, Mullins CE, McNamara DG. Pulmonary artery sling. *Am J Cardiol* 1980; 45:311–315.

38. Campbell CD, Wernly JA, Koltip PC, Vitullo D, Replogle RL. Aberrant left pulmonary artery (pulmonary artery sling): successful repair and 24-year follow-up report. *Am J Cardiol* 1980; 45:316–320.

39. Van Praagh R, Weinberg PM, Smith SD, Foran RB, Van Praagh S. Malpositions of the heart. In: Adams FH, Emmanouilides GC, Riemenschneider TA (eds). *Moss' Heart Disease in Infants, Children and*

Adolescents. Williams & Wilkins, Baltimore, 1989, pp 530–580.

40. Senning A. Surgical correction of transposition of the great vessels. *Surgery* 1959; 45:966.

41. Quaegebeur JM, Rohmer J, Brom AJ, Tinkelenberg J. Revival of the Senning operation in the treatment of transposition of the great arteries. *Thorax* 1977; 32:517–524.

42. Parenzan L, Locatelli G, Alfieri O, Villani M, Invernizzi G. The Senning operation for transposition of the great arteries. *J Thorac Cardiovasc Surg* 1978; 76:305–311.

43. Rollnick BR, Kaye CI. Hemifacial microsomia and variants: pedigree data. *Am J Med Genet* 1983; 15:233–53.

44. Greenwood RD, Rosenthal A, Sommer A, Wolff G, Craenen J. Cardiovascular malformations in oculoauriculovertebral dysplasia (Goldenhar syndrome). *J Pediatr* 1974; 85:816–818.

45. Moes CAF, Izukawa T, Trusler GA. Innominate artery compression of the trachea. *Arch Otolaryngol* 1975; 101:733–738.

46. Macdonald RE, Fearon B. Innominate artery compression syndrome in children. *Ann Otol Rhinol Laryngol* 1971; 80:535–540.

47. Ardito JM, Ossoff RH, Tucker GF, DeLeon SY. Innominate artery compression of the trachea in infants with reflex apnea. *Ann Otol Rhinol Laryngol* 1980; 89:401–405.

48. Gross RE. Arterial malformations which cause compression of the trachea or esophagus. *Circulation* 1955; 11:124.

49. Williams JC, Barratt-Boyes BG, Lowe JB. Supravalvar aortic stenosis. *Circulation* 1961; 24:1311.

50. Jones KL, Smith DW. The Williams elfin facies syndrome: a new perspective. *J Pediatr* 1975; 86:718–723.

51. Silka MJ. Double-outlet ventricles. In: Garson A, Bricker JT, McNamara DG (eds). *The Science and Practice of Pediatric Cardiology.* Lea & Febiger, Philadelphia/London, 1990, pp 1213.

52. Shuford WH, Sybers RG, Hogan GB: *The Aortic Arch and its Malformations.* Charles C. Thomas, Springfield, MA, 1974, pp 215–244.

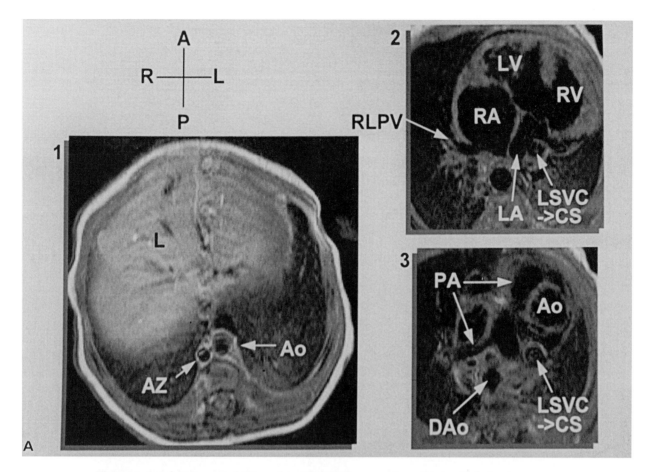

Figure 1: Axial (A), coronal (B), and sagittal (C) images of a patient with heterotaxy syndrome and double-outlet right ventricle {S,L,L}, large malalignment and atrioventricular canal types of ventricular septal defects, "ipsilateral" pulmonary veins, interrupted inferior vena cava with azygous continuation to the right superior vena cava, the hepatic veins draining to the right atrium, and a left superior vena cava to coronary sinus. (A) Images 1–3 are inferior to superior, (B) images 1–5 are posterior to anterior, (C) images 1–5 are right to left. A = anterior; Ao = aorta; AZ = azygous; DAo = descending aorta; HV = hepatic veins; I = inferior, IVC = inferior vena cava; L = left; L (in image) = liver, LA = left atrium; LPA = left pulmonary artery; LSVC → CS = left superior vena cava to coronary sinus; LV = left ventricle; P = posterior; PA = pulmonary artery; R = right; RA = right atrium; RLPV = right lower pulmonary vein; RPA = right pulmonary artery; RV = right ventricle; RVOT-SUB; Ao = right ventricular outflow tract-subaortic; RVOT-SUB PA = right ventricular outflow tract-subpulmonic; S = superior; S (in image) = stomach; T = trachea; VSD = ventricular septal defect.

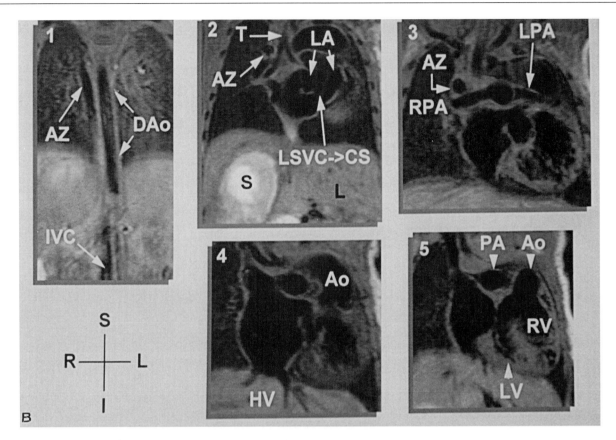

Figure 1B.

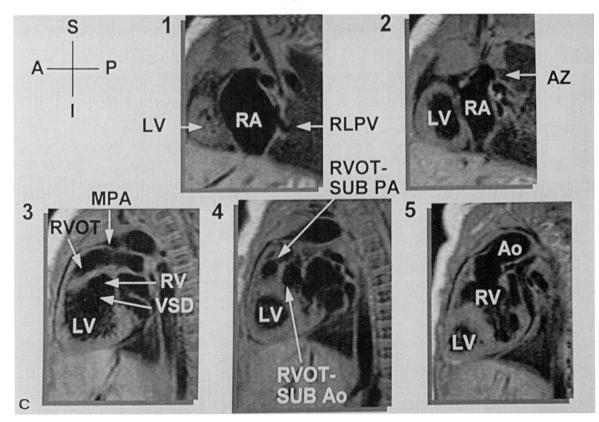

Figure 1C.

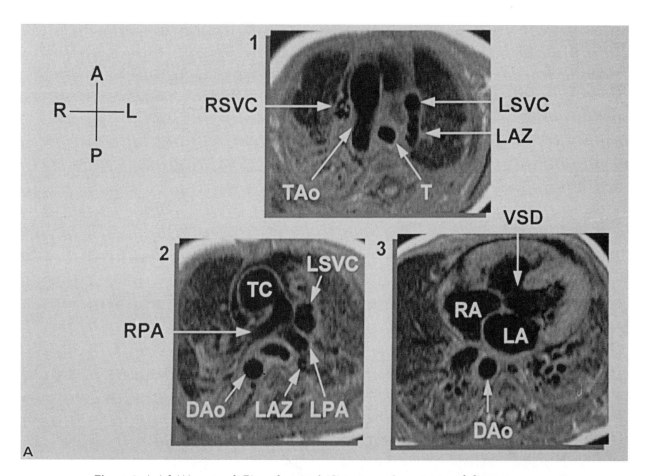

Figure 2: Axial (A), coronal (B), and sagittal (C) images of a patient with heterotaxy syndrome who has truncus arteriosus type A1 with a large ventricular septal defect, right aortic arch which descends on the right and crosses over to the left at the level of the diaphragm, interrupted left inferior vena cava with left azygous continuation to a left superior vena cava with drains to the left-sided atrium, and a right superior vena cava and hepatic veins draining to the right-sided atrium. (A) Images 1–3 are superior to inferior, (B) images 1–5 are posterior to anterior, (C) images 1–5 are left to right. A = anterior; AAo = ascending aorta; Ao = aorta; AZ = azygous; DAo = descending aorta; E = esophagus with esophageal atresia; HV = hepatic veins; I = inferior; In LIVC → LAZ = interrupted left inferior vena cava with continuation to a left azygous; L = left; LA = left-sided atrium; LAA = morphological left atrial appendage; LAZ = left azygous; LInn = left innominate artery; LPA = left pulmonary artery; LSVC = left superior vena cava; LV = left ventricle; MPA = main pulmonary artery; P = posterior; PA = pulmonary artery; R = right; RA = right sided atrium; RPA = right pulmonary artery; RSVC = right superior vena cava; RV = right ventricle; S = superior; SP = spine; T = trachea; TAo = transverse aortic arch; TC = truncus; VSD = ventricular septal defect.

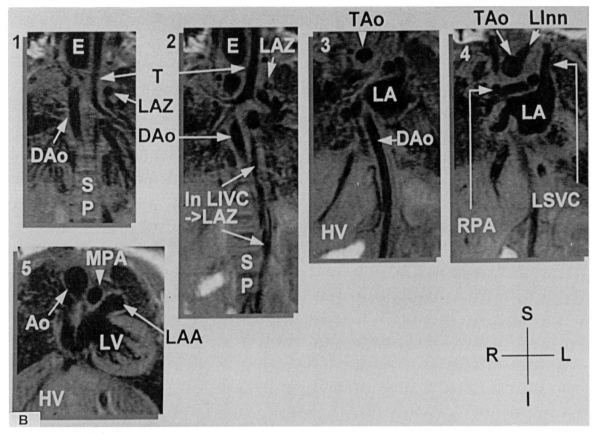

Figure 2B.

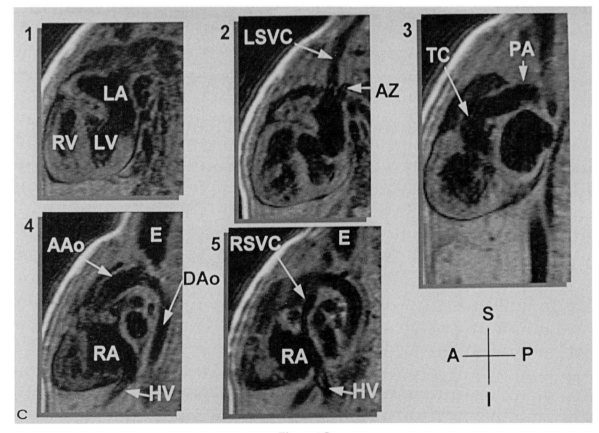

Figure 2C.

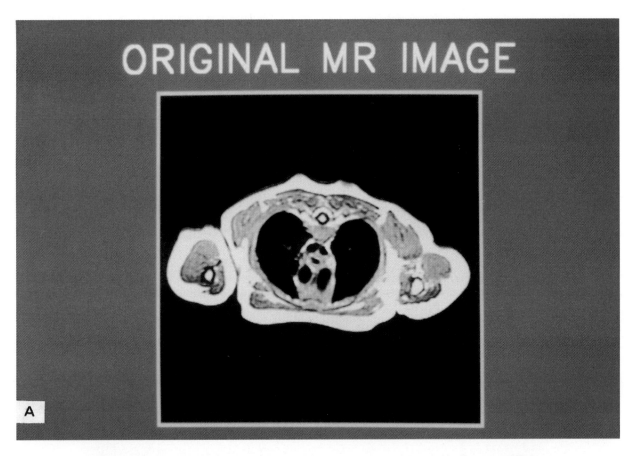

Figure 3: The process of three-dimensional reconstruction. (A) Original transverse MR image superior in the thorax. (B) Selection of a region of interest to construct in three dimensions. (C) Segmenting the image into its component structure, in this case, the aortic arch is isolated while the trachea, lungs, and pulmonary artery are removed. (D) From the gray scale images (left), a binary image is created (right) which displays just the aorta. (E) The binary image is edited to remove any artifacts created by the post processing; the image on the right has an excess structure removed at its lower part in red, see (D). (F) Each binary image for a given structure is stacked one on top of the other and a linear interpolation is done between the images to refine the borders of the final three-dimensional picture. (G) A shaded surface display is constructed by surface detection of the interpolated images to create a three-dimensional picture. (H) Shading is performed to enhance the three-dimensional view. (Photographs courtesy of Paul M. Weinberg, MD.)

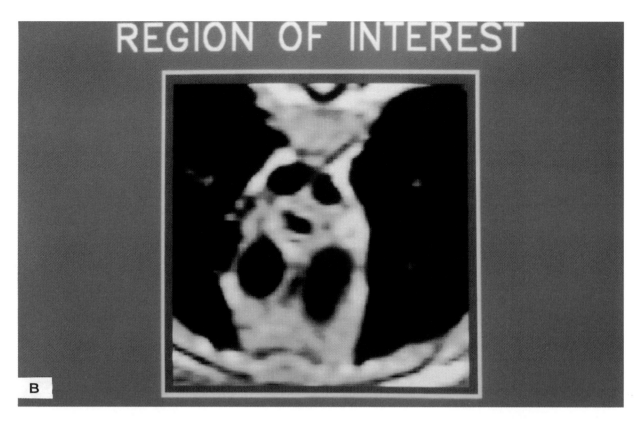

Figure 3B.

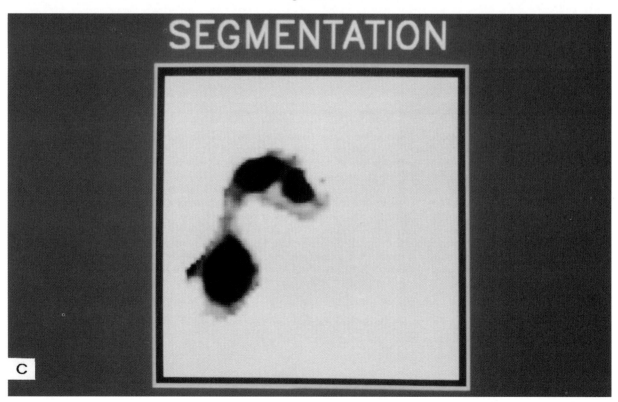

Figure 3C.

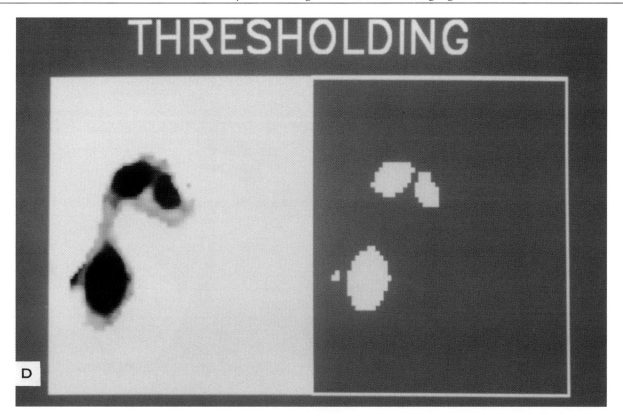

Figure 3D.

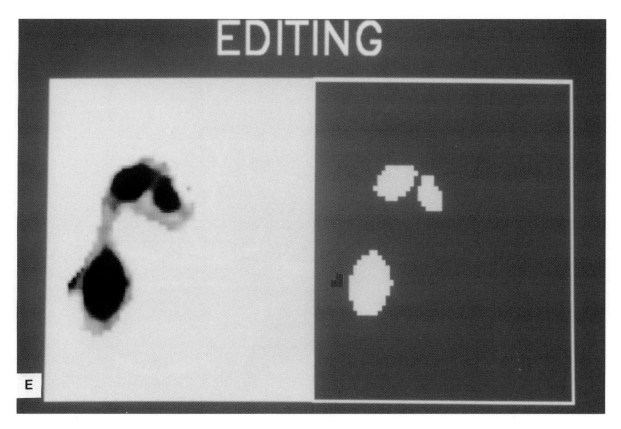

Figure 3E.

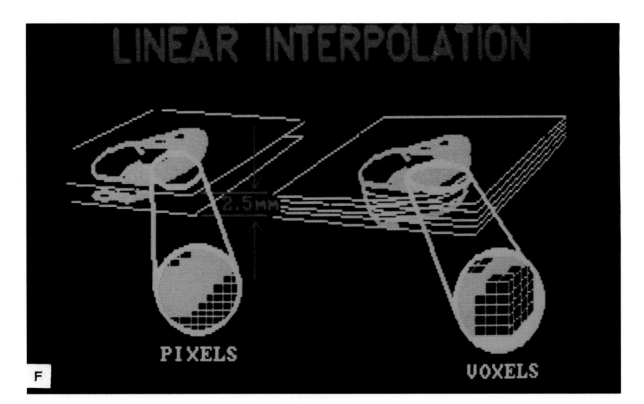

Figure 3F.

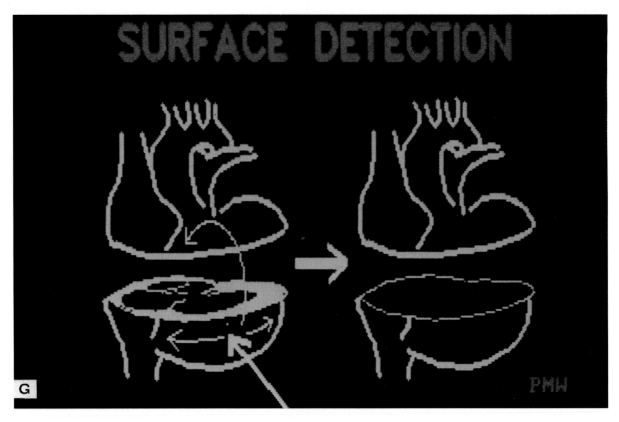

Figure 3G.

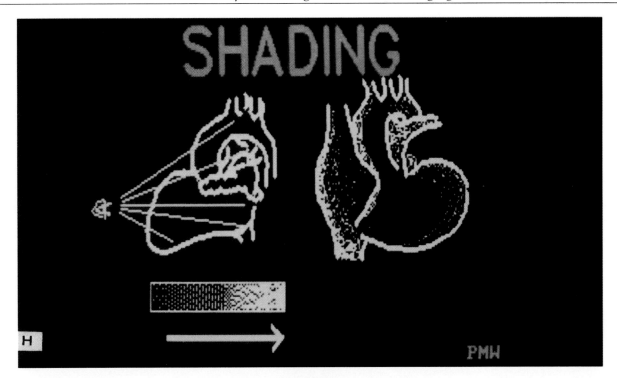

Figure 3H.

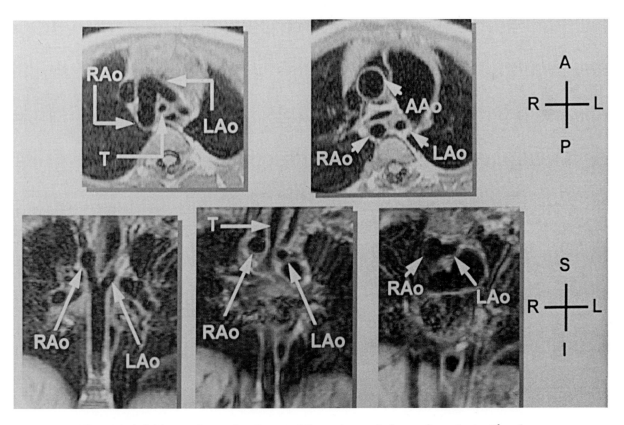

Figure 4: Axial (upper images) and coronal (lower images) planes of a patient with a double aortic arch. The left upper image is superior to the right upper image. The aorta is orange, the trachea is green, and the pulmonary artery is pink. A = anterior; AAo = ascending aorta; I = inferior; L = left; LAo = left aortic arch; P = posterior; R = right; RAo = right aortic arch; S = superior; T = trachea.

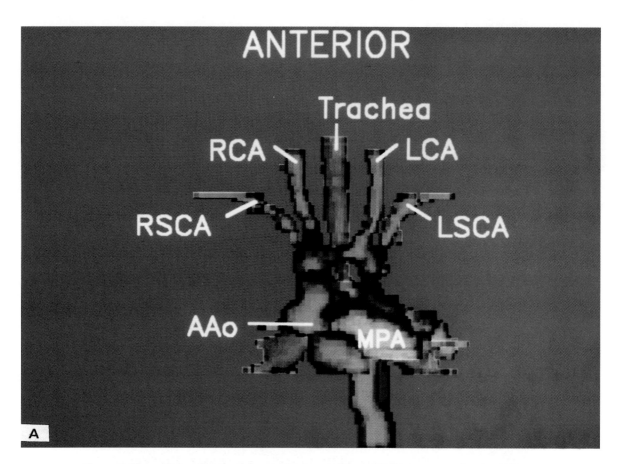

Figure 5: Three-dimensional reconstruction in a number of different ways: anterior (A), posterior (B), transverse (C), and with all structures removed except the aorta (C and D). The aorta is orange, the trachea is green, and the pulmonary artery is pink. AAo = ascending aorta; AoV = aortic valve; DAo = descending aorta; LAoA = left aortic arch; LCA = left carotid artery; LSCA = left subclavian artery; MPA = main pulmonary artery; RAoA = right aortic arch; RCA = right carotid artery; RSCA = right subclavian artery. (Photographs courtesy of Paul M. Weinberg, MD.)

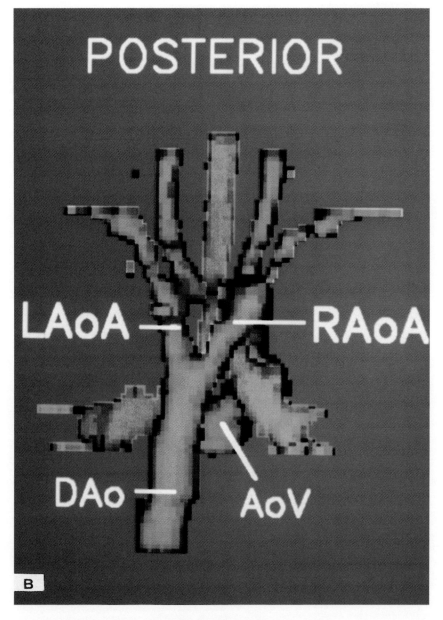

Figure 5B.

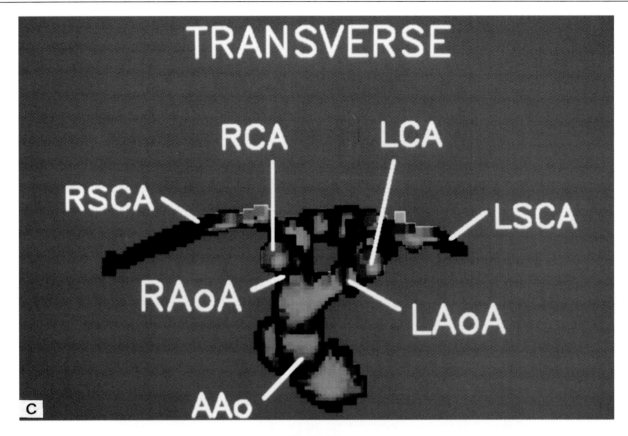

Figure 5C.

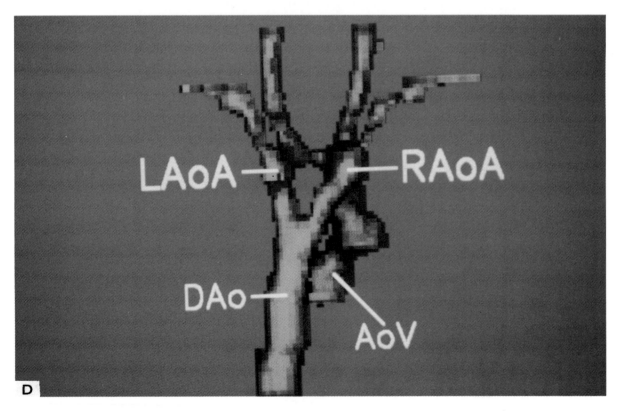

Figure 5D.

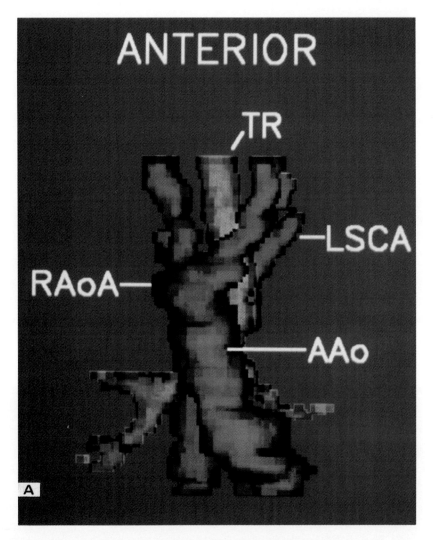

Figure 6: Three views [anterior (A), posterior (B) and transverse (C)] of a patient with a right aortic arch with an aberrant left subclavian artery[36] arising posteriorly from a diverticulum of Kommerel. The lower images progress from posterior to anterior as images go from left to right. The aorta is orange, the trachea is green, and the pulmonary artery is pink. AAo = ascending aorta; DAo = descending aorta; Divertic = diverticulum of Kommerel; Dvrtc = diverticulum of Kommerel; LCA = left carotid artery; LSCA = left subclavian artery; RAoA = right aorta arch; RCA = right carotid artery; RSCA = right subclavian artery; Tr = trachea. (Photographs courtesy of Paul M. Weinberg, MD.)

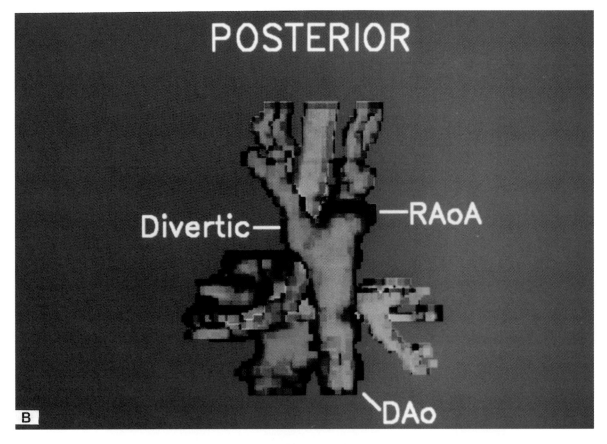

Figure 6B.

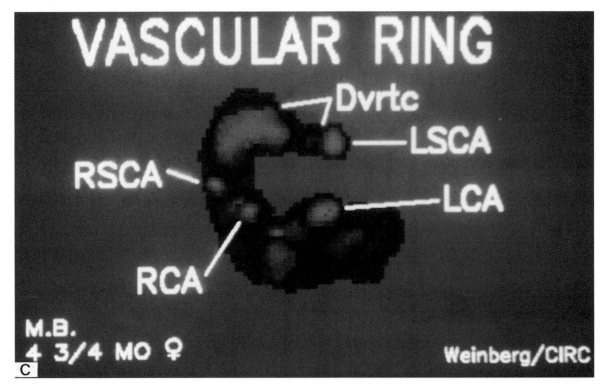

Figure 6C.

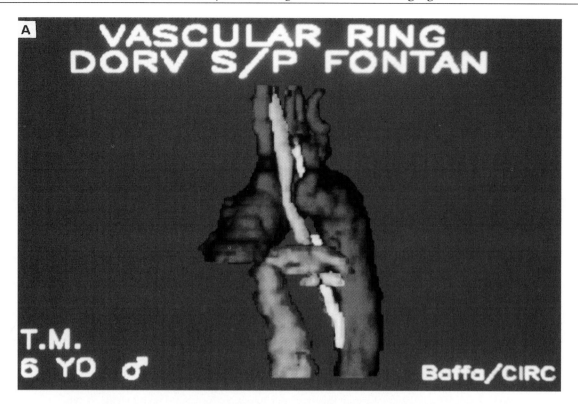

Figure 7: A patient with a right aortic arch with an aberrant left subclavian artery, who is status post a Fontan procedure. Both views are laterals and show the compression of the trachea by the ring with the aorta in the image (A) and removed (B). The aorta is orange, the trachea is green, the esophagus is yellow, and the pulmonary artery is pink. (Photographs courtesy of Paul M. Weinberg, MD.)

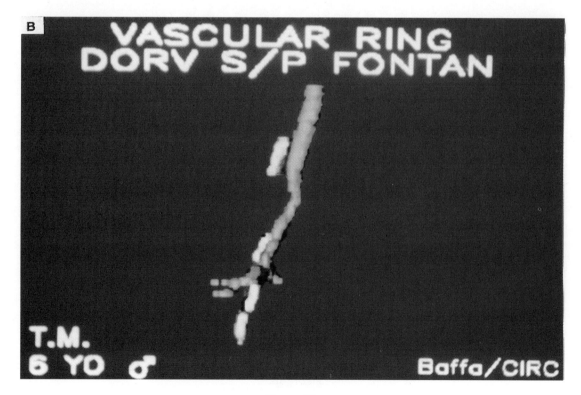

Figure 7B.

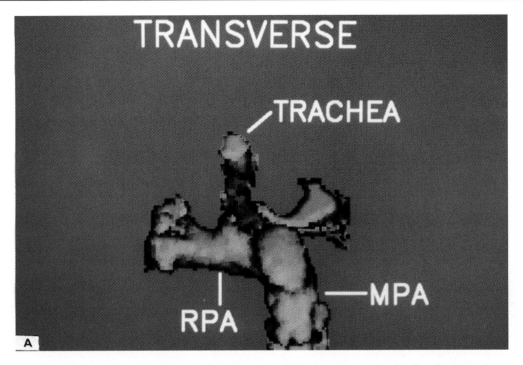

Figure 8: Three-dimensional reconstruction of a pulmonary artery sling that has the left pulmonary artery and coursing behind the trachea. Both images are transverse views, which clearly display the salient features of this anatomy, in which the trachea is shown in one picture (A) and removed in the other (B). The trachea is green and the pulmonary artery is pink. LPA = left pulmonary artery; MPA = main pulmonary artery; RPA = right pulmonary artery. (Photographs courtesy of Paul M. Weinberg, MD.)

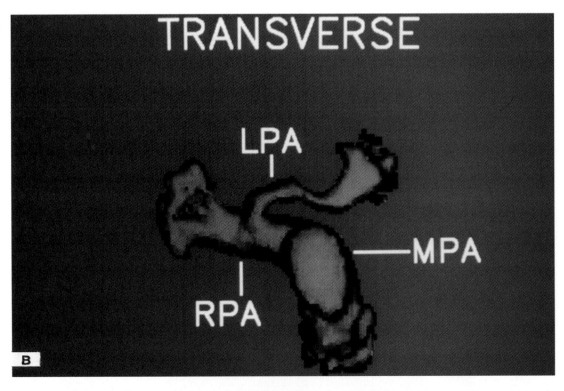

Figure 8B.

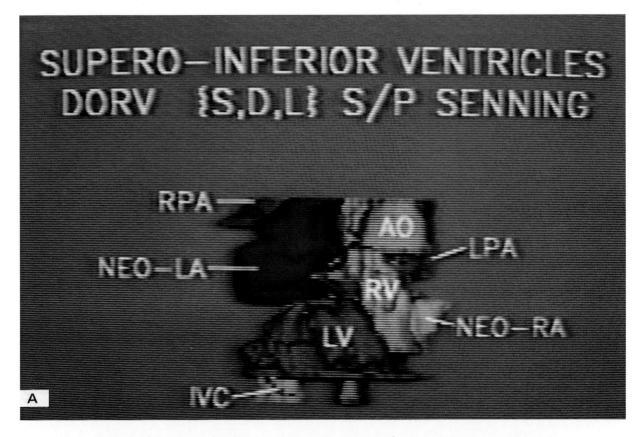

Figure 9: Three-dimensional reconstruction of a patient with supero-inferior ventricles and criss-cross atrioventricular relationships after a Senning procedure. (A) Anterior view shows the supero-inferior relationship of the ventricles and (B) the transverse view shows the relationships of the *"neo-right"* and *"neo-left"* atrium. If various structures are removed in the transverse views (Figures C and D), the viewer can appreciate what is meant by the criss-cross relationship of the atrioventricular valves. AAo = ascending aorta; Ao = aorta; DORV = double outlet right ventricle; IVC = inferior vena cava; LPA = left pulmonary artery; LPV'S = left pulmonary veins; LV = left ventricle; MV = mitral valve; neo-LA = pulmonary venous pathway; neo-RA = systemic venous pathway; RPA = right pulmonary artery; RPV'S = right pulmonary veins; RV = right ventricle; S/P = status post; SVC = superior vena cava; TV = tricuspid valve. (Photographs courtesy of Paul M. Weinberg, MD.)

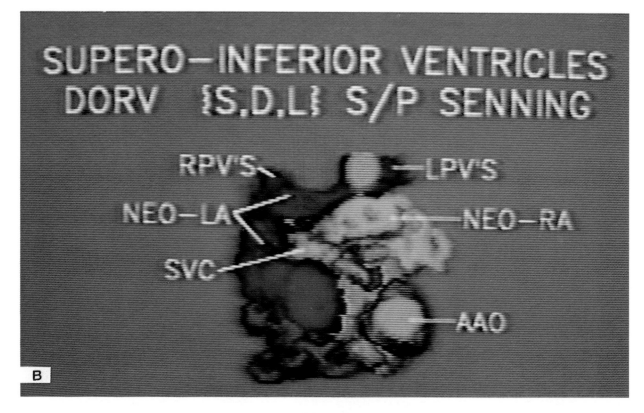

Figure 9B.

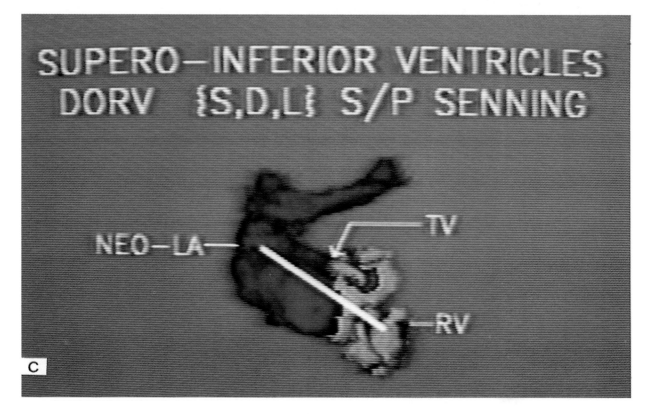

Figure 9C.

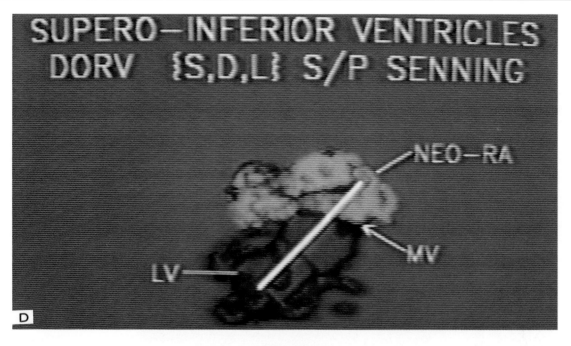

Figure 9D.

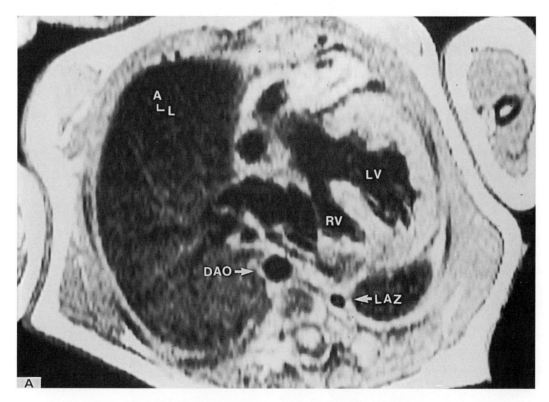

Figure 10: A patient with Goldenhar's syndrome, extreme levocardia, and tetralogy of Fallot. The spin-echo image (A) shows a four-chamber view displaying the ventricular septal defect and the extreme malposition of the heart with the apex pointing to the left axilla. Three-dimensional reconstruction with rotation to the left axilla (B) and to the lateral position (C) enables one to view the malformation much more clearly. In B, the overriding aorta and ventricular septal defect are seen. The lateral view (C) shows the azygous vein clearly draining to the left superior vena cava and the relative positions of some of the important structures in the chest. A = anterior; AAo = ascending aorta; Az = azygous; L = left; LV = left ventricle; RSVC = right superior vena cava; RV = right ventricle; TR = trachea; VSD = ventricular septal defect. (Photographs courtesy of Paul M. Weinberg, MD.)

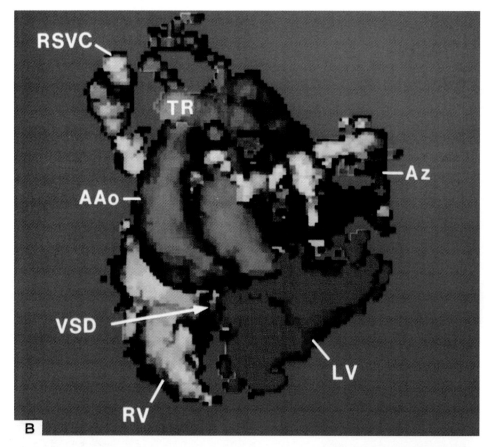

Figure 10B.

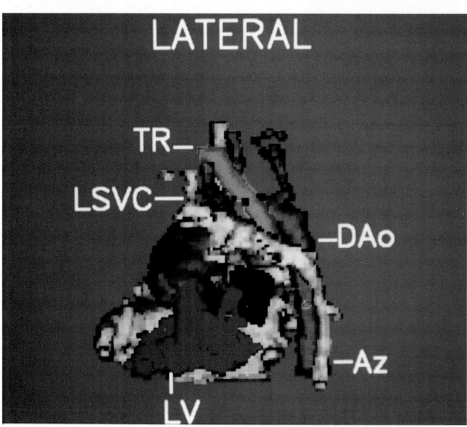

Figure 10C.

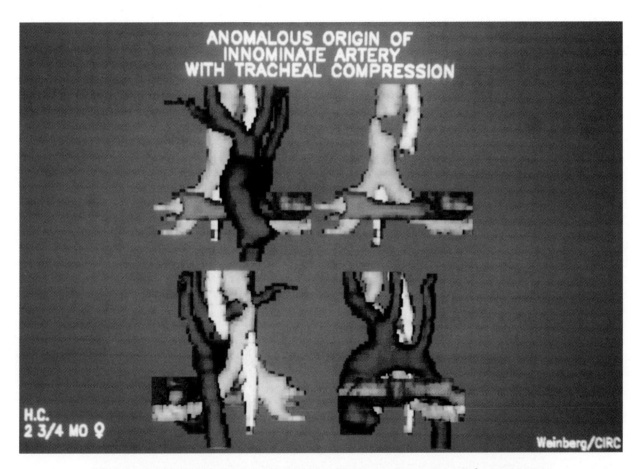

Figure 11: Three-dimensional reconstruction of an anomalous origin of the innominate artery from the aorta causing tracheal compression. The upper left picture is an anteroposterior view with the aorta (orange), trachea (green), esophagus (yellow), and pulmonary artery (red) present. The upper right image is also an anteroposterior view, however, the aorta is removed to display the indentation on the trachea. The lower images show all four structures rotated in the posteroanterior view (lower left) and lateral view (lower left). These images give the observer a much better sense of the positions of the structures in question. (Photographs courtesy of Paul M. Weinberg, MD.)

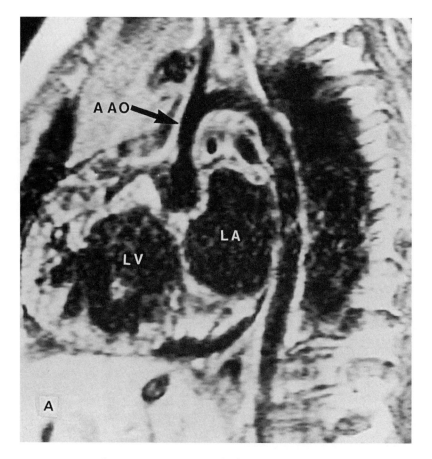

Figure 12: A patient with Williams syndrome who has supravalvar aortic stenosis with tubular hypoplasia of the ascending and transverse aorta. The spin-echo image (A) gives a sense of the tubular hypoplasia, but it is only until the data are reconstructed in three dimensions (B) can one appreciate the volumes involved. AAo = ascending aorta; LAO = left anterior oblique view. (Photographs courtesy of Paul M. Weinberg, MD.)

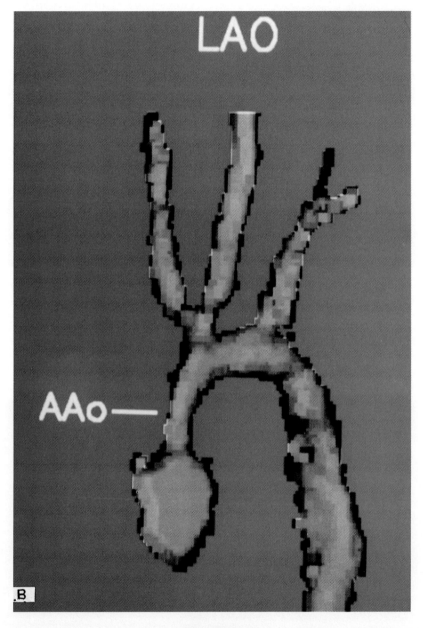

Figure 12B.

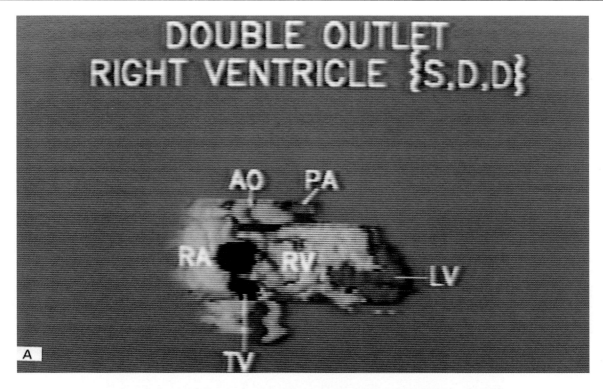

Figure 13: A patient with double-outlet right ventricle {S,D,D} in both the anterior (A) and the transverse (B) views. The anterior view (A) clearly shows both great vessels over the right ventricle, with the aorta to the right of the pulmonary artery. The transverse view (B) with the right ventricle and pulmonary artery removed clearly show the ventricular septal defect to lie beneath the aorta. AO = aorta; LA = left atrium; LV = left ventricle; PA = pulmonary artery; RA = right atrium; RV = right ventricle; TV = tricuspid valve; VSD = ventricular septal defect. (Photographs courtesy of Paul M. Weinberg, MD.)

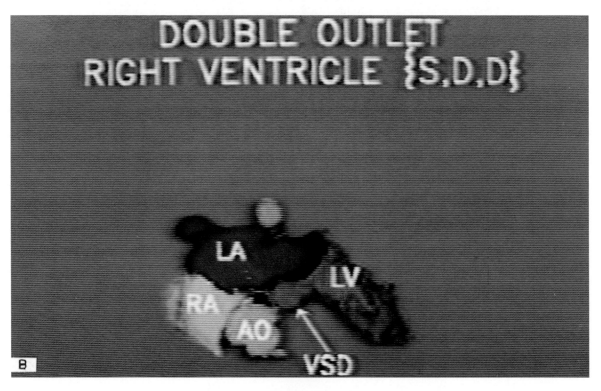

Figure 13B.

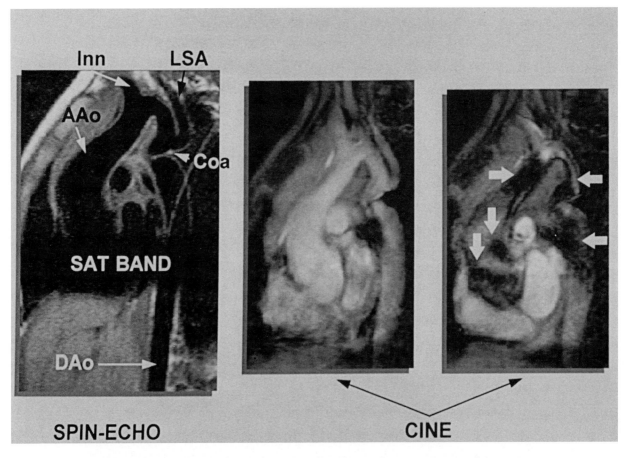

Figure 14: Spin-echo (left) and cine (center and right) images of a patient with coarctation of the aorta. The spin-echo image clearly displays the anatomy of the coarctation. The cine images at end-diastole (center) and at 100 msec into systole (right) display areas of turbulence (arrows) during systole. The patient also had a bicuspid aortic valve which also shows turbulence (two left-most arrows of the right image). AAo = ascending aorta; Coa = coarctation site; DAo = descending aorta; Inn = innominate artery; LSA = left subclavian artery; SAT BAND = saturation band placed to obtain clearer images of the coarctation.

Part II

Imaging of the Postoperative Patient

Chapter 21

Intensive Care Unit Imaging

Over the last decade, there has been a gradual trend toward utilizing more noninvasive techniques in the early postoperative period. In the early 1980s, surgeons and intensivists relied on echocardiography only for identification of gross abnormalities, such as large effusions (Figure 1). Surface imaging has gradually been extended so that even venous stenoses can now be detected (Figure 2). The ability of transthoracic imaging to identify many important anatomical residua is being complemented by growing use of *intra*operative transesophageal imaging. Whether the latter will eventually become the province of dedicated cardiac anesthesiologists is not yet clear; however, in many situations, a rapid examination following the patient's liberation from cardiopulmonary bypass may rule out the presence of significant anatomical residua, thus allowing the team of care-providers to concentrate on ventilatory and intravascular volume management during the first postoperative night. A secondary benefit may be the elimination of many late postoperative catheterizations previously performed to "screen" for residua.

Particular strengths of transthoracic imaging[1] are detection of arch obstruction (Figure 3) and residual shunting at the ventricular level. Particular weaknesses are discerning branch pulmonary artery architecture and displaying the lumen of prosthetic conduits.

The hardest skills to learn are knowing what information is crucial, practicing how to obtain that information in an expeditious manner, and recognizing when the patient's ventilatory status is being compromised by the echocardiographic examination. It is often not feasible to image a patient using surface windows for 60 minutes; thus, exams have to be more focused. If at all possible, a starting 5-minute look from a wide-field-of-view window is still very helpful for orientation, though. Knowing what information is crucial depends on familiarity with the reconstructive surgical techniques employed.

References

1. Chin AJ, Vetter JM, Seliem MA, Jones AA, Andrews BA. Role of early postoperative surface echocardiography in the pediatric cardiac intensive care unit. *Am J Cardiol* (in press).

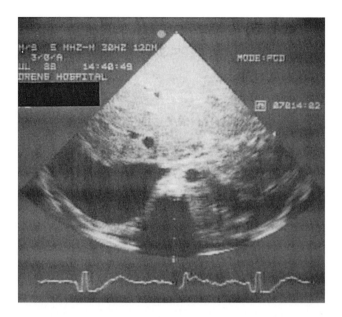

Figure 1: Transverse abdominal view showing right pleural effusion in posterior hemithorax.

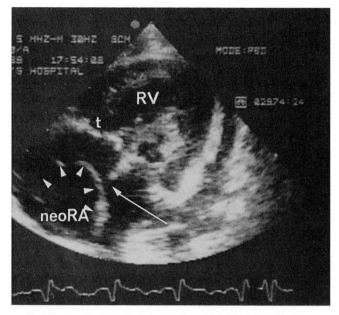

Figure 2: Hypoplastic left heart syndrome after Fontan procedure. Low parasternal view of pulmonary venous pathway obstruction (unlabeled arrow) produced by intra-atrial baffle (arrowheads) protruding into the surgically created atrial septal defect. neo-RA = neo-right atrium; RV = right ventricle; t = tricuspid valve.

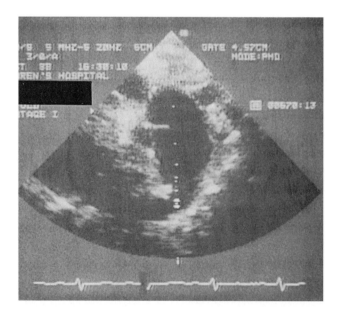

Figure 3: Hypoplastic left heart syndrome after Norwood procedure. Although parasternal windows may be difficult to use early postoperatively, the suprasternal window is usually still accessible. Details of arch anatomy can be displayed, and Doppler interrogation is feasible. The sample volume is just distal to the distal-most portion of the arch gusset.

Chapter 22

Surgery of the Ascending Aorta/Aortic Arch

A. Subclavian Flap Angioplasty

The sequelae of subclavian flap angioplasty are: (1) residual narrowing proximal to the takeoff of the left subclavian artery (when a "reverse" subclavian flap is constructed for arch hypoplasia), (2) narrowing at the repair site, or (3) narrowing immediately distal to the subclavian flap (i.e., insufficient length of the flap). The display of all of these variants is best accomplished from the suprasternal window with left oblique views. In the older child in whom the suprasternal notch is frequently not an effective window, magnetic resonance imaging displays the distal arch well.

B. Patch Augmentation of the Aortic Arch

The two main types of patch repair are: (1) long patch augmentation of the entire aortic arch, and (2) relatively short patch augmentation of the discrete coarctation. The residua of the former procedure are narrowing at either the proximal or the distal end of the patch. The patch repair of discrete coarctation can rarely be followed by aneurysm formation. Again, suprasternal left oblique and sagittal views are most helpful.

C. Interrupted Aortic Arch Repair Without Graft

There are essentially two general methods[1–3] of accomplishing repair of interrupted aortic arch without

the use of a tube graft: (a) an end-to-side anastomosis of the distal arch with the proximal arch, and (b) augmentation of the orifices of the proximal and distal arch portions (by extension onto arterial branches) followed by "side-to-side" anastomosis.

The suprasternal frontal sweep allows the examiner to roughly estimate the degree of obliquity to use in order to display the length of the anastomosis site, e.g., whether a left oblique view or a sagittal view would be preferable. Continuous wave Doppler interrogation is best performed from the parasternal or suprasternal windows, depending on the location of the anastomosis.

The cases of malalignment-type ventricular septal defect with coexistent subaortic stenosis[2] will have undergone a proximal pulmonary artery-to-ascending aorta anastomosis in addition to the interrupted arch repair. Cases with other anomalies occur frequently.[4–6]

Cases with trivial or mild subaortic narrowing may be managed by ventricular septal defect closure alone. The subaortic region must be carefully monitored by serial echocardiographic examinations since the subaortic narrowing can progress.

D. Interrupted Aortic Arch Repair With Graft

Aortic arch grafts[7,8] may or may not be visualized with ultrasound, depending on their orientation. As expected, a suprasternal frontal sweep aids in the identification of both the ascending aortic end and the descending aortic end of the graft. From these two points, the experienced examiner can usually mentally reconstruct the likely course of the graft (conduit) and choose the appropriate sector orientation to display the "long axis" of the graft.

What is more difficult is aligning the continuous wave Doppler cursor with jets across anastomotic sites.

E. Aortic Root Replacement

In pediatrics, this operation is used most often for Marfan syndrome patients and typically includes prosthetic aortic valve replacement. There are other syndromes that have dilatation of the ascending aorta (Ehler-Danlos, Fragile X, and Takayasu's disease). Because the orientation of the aortic root and ascending aorta is quite variable, it is impossible to predict which sector orientation will yield the optimal images. A sequela of aortic root replacement is aneurysm formation immediately proximal or immediately distal to the prosthetic root. Transesophageal imaging or magnetic resonance scanning may be superior to surface echocardiography.

F. Repair of Sinus of Valsalva Aneurysm

The two most common sequelae[9,10] are aortic valve regurgitation and residual left-to-right shunt. The eval-

uation of the former is covered in Chapter 2; the assessment of the latter is best accomplished with foreknowledge of where the original drainage site was located. Parasternal short axis views of the aortic sinuses are a reasonable way to start.

Aortico-left ventricular tunnel[11,12] may be treated in a similar manner.

G. Repair of Supravalvar Aortic Stenosis

As the vast majority of such patients are older than 4 years, the supravalvar aortic region is often difficult to display from subcostal and parasternal windows. Even the suprasternal window is difficult to employ as the patients approach adolescence, and MRI is probably more suitable for serial long-term follow-up (see Chapter 20).

H. Repair of Double Aortic Arch

It is unusual to have cardiovascular sequelae from repair of double aortic arch inasmuch as repair actually consists of ligation and division of a segment of the ring. The most common sequela is persistent stridor; tracheal or bronchial malformation can coexist with double aortic arch. Symptoms may not immediately change following release of the ring.

References

1. Moerman P, Dumoulin M, Lauweryns J, van der Hauwaert LG. Interrupted right aortic arch in DiGeorge syndrome. *Br Heart J* 1987; 58:274–278.

2. Yasui H, Kado H, Nakano E, Yonenaga K, Mitani A, Tomita Y, Iwao H, et al. Primary repair of interrupted aortic arch and severe aortic stenosis in neonates. *J Thorac Cardiovasc Surg* 1987; 93:539–545.

3. Moulton AL, Bowman FO. Primary definitive repair of type B interrupted aortic arch, ventricular septal defect, and patent ductus arteriosus. *J Thorac Cardiovasc Surg* 1981; 82:501–510.

4. Moes CAF, Freedom RM. Aortic arch interruption with truncus arteriosus or aorticopulmonary septal defect. *AJR* 1980; 135:1011–1016.

5. Braunlin E, Peoples WM, Freedom RM, Fyler DC, Goldblatt A, Edwards JE. Interruption of the aortic arch with aorticopulmonary septal defect. *Pediatr Cardiol* 1982; 3:329–335.

6. Berry TE, Bharati S, Muster AJ, Idriss FS, Santucci B, Lev M, Paul MH. Distal aortopulmonary septal defect, aortic origin of the right pulmonary artery, intact ventricular septum, patent ductus arteriosus and hypoplasia of the aortic isthmus: a newly recognized syndrome. *Am J Cardiol* 1982; 49:108–116.

7. Norwood WI, Lang P, Castaneda AR, Hougen TJ. Reparative operations for interrupted aortic arch with ventricular septal defect. *J Thorac Cardiovasc Surg* 1983; 86:832–837.

8. DeLeon SY, Idriss FS, Ilbawi MN, Tin N, Berry T. Transmediastinal repair of complex coarctation and interrupted aortic arch. *J Thorac Cardiovasc Surg* 1981; 82:98–102.

9. Burakovsky VI, Podsolkov VP, Sabirow BN, Nasedkina MA, Alekian BG, Dvinyaninova NB. Ruptured congenital aneurysm of the sinus of Valsalva. *J Thorac Cardiovasc Surg* 1988; 95:836–841.

10. Eliot RS, Woodburn RL, Edwards JE. Conditions of the ascending aorta simulating aortic valvular incompetence. *Am J Cardiol* 1964; 14:679–694.

11. Bash SE, Huhta JC, Nihill MR, Vargo TA, Hallman GL. Aortico-left ventricular tunnel with ventricular septal defect: two-dimensional/Doppler echocardiographic diagnosis. *J Am Coll Cardiol* 1985; 5:757–760.

12. Grant P, Abrams LD, DeGiovanni JV, Shah KJ, Silove ED. Aortico-left ventricular tunnel arising from the left aortic sinus. *Am J Cardiol* 1985; 55:1657–1658.

<h1>Chapter 23</h1>

<h1>Coronary Artery Surgery</h1>

A. Intrapulmonary Artery Tunnel from Aorta to Left Coronary Artery

Among the types of surgical repairs[1] for anomalous left coronary artery arising from the pulmonary artery (PA) (Figure 1) is one reported by Takeuchi.[2,3] An aorticopulmonary window is created, and a hemi-cylindrical patch is used to create a pathway for blood from the aorta to reach the PA origin of the coronary artery, regardless of where it is.[4]

As in another intra-PA baffle procedure, the Aubert procedure (see Chapter 24, section B3), the PA lumen is usually augmented anteriorly with a second patch in order to prevent "supravalvar" pulmonary artery obstruction; however, late-onset obstruction is still occasionally observed. Residual leaks around the baffle suture line are the next most frequently observed sequela; these result in left-to-right shunts. Narrowing of the aorticopulmonary window is a theoretical concern, also.

Subcostal sagittal and right oblique views can display the baffle in the infant. Parasternal views may allow visualization of the entire baffle (Figure 2) and the relationship of the baffle to the anterior aspect of the main pulmonary artery and to the origin of the right pulmonary artery (Figure 3); they are usually necessary for Doppler interrogation.

B. Closure of Coronary Arterio-Cameral Fistula

Because of the great variety of fistulae,[5,6] it is important to know the preoperative diagnosis prior to attempting a postoperative examination. (The minimum information needed is which coronary artery was involved. This will at least allow deduction of *potential* drainage sites.) Since multiple drainage sites can exist in a given patient, the examiner should not only display the site recognized preoperatively but also other potential sites. For example, for a right coronary artery-to-right ventricle fistula, it is prudent to examine not only the right ventricular orifice which was identified by the surgeon but also the right atrium near the right atrioventricular groove.

Since color Doppler echocardiography is the mainstay of noninvasive identification, use of the parasternal window is preferred.

References

1. Bunton R, Jonas RA, Lang P, Rein AJJT, Castaneda AR. Anomalous origin of left coronary artery from pulmonary artery. *J Thorac Cardiovasc Surg* 1987; 93:103–108.

2. Chin AJ, Larsen RL, Seliem MA, Andrews BA, Jones A, Vetter J, Lieb D. Non-invasive imaging of intra-arterial baffles in infants and children. *J Am Soc Echo* 1993; 6:45–50.

3. Takeuchi S, Imamura H, Katsumoko K, Hayashi I, Katohgi I, Yozu R, Ohkura M, et al. New surgical method for repair of anomalous left coronary artery from pulmonary artery. *J Thorac Cardiovasc Surg* 1979; 78:7–11.

4. Steussy HF, Caldwell RL, Wills ER, Waller BF. High takeoff of the left main coronary artery from the pulmonary trunk: potentially fatal combination with pulmonary trunk banding. *Am Heart J* 1984; 108:619–21.

5. Liberthson RR, Sagar K, Berkoben JP, Weintraub RM, Levine FH. Congenital coronary arteriovenous fistula. *Circulation* 1979; 59:849–853.

6. Urruti CO, Falaschi G, Ott DA, Cooley DA. Surgical management of 56 patients with congenital coronary artery fistula. *Ann Thorac Surg* 1983; 35:300–307.

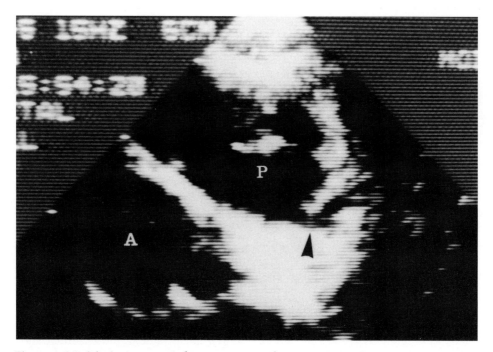

Figure 1: Modified parasternal short axis view. The anomalous left coronary artery (arrowhead) arises from the pulmonary (P) root. A = aorta. Used by permission of American Society of Echocardiography.

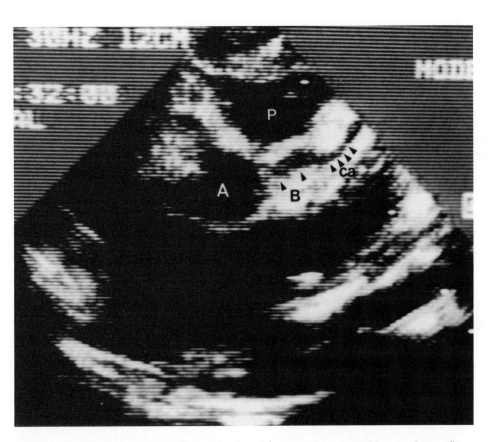

Figure 2: Modified parasternal short axis view. The tunnel is created by a polytetrafluo-rethylene baffle (B) which directs flow from the surgically created aortico-pulmonary window to the coronary artery (ca). P = pulmonary root; A = aorta. Used by permission of American Society of Echocardiography.

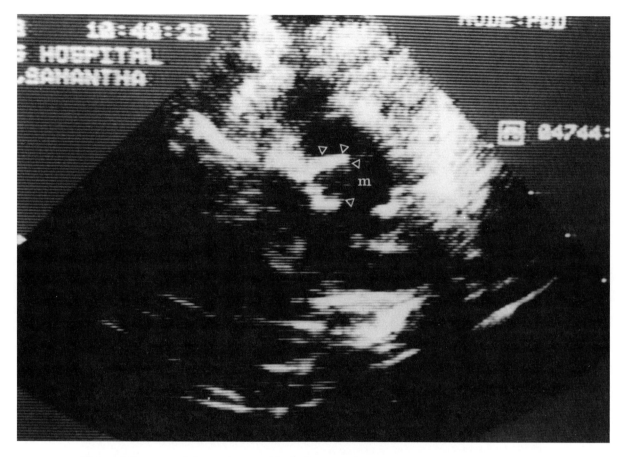

Figure 3: Parasternal short axis view. The baffle (arrowheads) is seen in cross-section; it protrudes into the lumen of the main (m) pulmonary artery.

Chapter 24

Aorto-Pulmonary Artery Surgery

A. Shunts

1. Waterston Shunt (Ascending Aorta-to-Right Pulmonary Artery)

The Waterston shunt typically lies on the right posterolateral aspect of the ascending aorta. Deformity of the proximal right pulmonary artery can occur such that the distal right pulmonary artery receives most of the shunt flow. (The variant in which the left pulmonary artery receives most of the shunt flow is much less common.)

This type of shunt is no longer routinely employed; modified or classic Blalock-Taussig shunts are less likely to deform the branch pulmonary arteries and are easily ligated later on. Thus, the population of Waterston cases presenting for noninvasive assessment consists mostly of adolescents and young adults. Display of subtle deformities of the branch pulmonary arteries is rarely feasible from the subcostal window in this size of patient. Occasionally a high parasternal or suprasternal window can afford adequate visualization (frontal view for the right pulmonary artery and left oblique view for the left pulmonary artery); however, magnetic resonance scanning and transesophageal imaging may be more suitable techniques.

2. Classic Blalock-Taussig Anastomosis

The classic Blalock-Taussig anastomosis is constructed on the side opposite the aortic arch. The suprasternal frontal view typically provides the best display of the shunt (Figure 1). The entire shunt can usually be traced using a sweep from posterior to anterior (Figure 2). The most common site of stenosis is at the pulmonary artery insertion site. Color Doppler has helped tremendously with the tracing of shunts.

Continuous wave Doppler (with or without 2-D image or color Doppler guidance) and the simplified Bernoulli formula have been utilized by Marx et al.[1] to estimate the trans-shunt maximal instantaneous gradient; however, their work has yet to be reproduced by other laboratories. A theoretical limitation to the clinical application of their methodology arises from the fact that many individuals initially treated by shunt procedures do not have two normal-size ventricles; thus, definitive surgical treatment consists of a modified Fontan procedure, candidacy for which relies on precise hemodynamic characterization of the pulmonary vascular bed. Marx has not reported whether the accuracy of their method is sufficient to guide surgical management decisions in the Fontan candidate.

Other limitations to the use of the modified Bernoulli equation in this setting stem from the fact that a classic Blalock-Taussig shunt is a nondiscrete obstruction and that it results, if properly constructed, in essentially a right-angle trajectory of flow at its distal end. The validity of maximal instantaneous gradient estimations in this geometry has not been established in the in-vivo environment. Flow in the shunt (proximal to the anastomotic site) is low velocity, continuous, and laminar (Figure 3).

3. Classic Glenn Shunt (Right Superior Vena Cava-to-Right Pulmonary Artery)

The classic (uni-lung) Glenn shunt comprises a right superior vena cava-to-right pulmonary artery anastomosis combined with separation of the right pulmonary artery from the remainder of the pulmonary arterial circulation. The suprasternal or high right parasternal windows can occasionally display this shunt, although magnetic resonance imaging is a superior technique.

Contrast injection in an upper extremity vein may give a clue to the presence of arteriovenous fistulae late postoperatively.[2]

The modification currently employed is discussed in Chapter 31, section E.

4. Modified Blalock-Taussig Shunt

In 1993, by far the most frequently employed shunt is the interposition of a tube of prosthetic material (e.g., polytetrafluorethylene) between the innominate artery and the ipsilateral pulmonary artery. The morphological evaluation of such a shunt rests on demonstration that the lumen is uniform in caliber throughout its length. The most frequent sequelae are a kinking of the anastomosis at the innominate artery end and the development of a narrowing (secondary to fibrous tissue or rarely clot) at the pulmonary artery end. As with the classic Blalock-Taussig shunt, a suprasternal frontal sweep from posterior to anterior usually displays the entirety of the shunt (Figure 4). Because the diameter of the shunt resembles that of the right superior vena cava, and because the direction of flow in both structures is cephalad-to-caudad, great care must be taken to distinguish these structures during color Doppler examination. The use of image-directed pulsed Doppler prevents mis-identification; the flow in a modified Blalock-Taussig shunt is essentially independent of respiratory cycle.

5. Conversion to Hemi-Fontan (see Chapter 31, section E)

Recently, interest has revived in staging the Fontan (see Chapter 31, section F). This can be accomplished in several ways. One, adopted by Norwood[3] in 1989, is a superior vena cava-right atrial junction side-to-side anastomosis with the right pulmonary artery. A dam is inserted between this anastomosis and the atrium proper to prevent superior vena caval blood flow reaching the pulmonary venous compartment. When a "cavopulmonary" shunt is performed in a heterotaxy patient with interrupted inferior vena cava with azygos continuation,[4] it diverts all the systemic venous return except the hepatic veins (and coronary veins) to the pulmonary circulation.

Suprasternal frontal imaging is best for displaying the anastomosis. In the infant, the anastomosis can usually be seen from the subcostal window.

B. Other Aorto-Pulmonary Artery Procedures

1. Arterial Switch Procedure with Lecompte Maneuver

After the widespread adoption in the mid-1980s of the arterial switch procedure (Figure 5) as the repair of choice in transposition[5] attention initially became focused on assessment of left ventricular performance and function.[6-9] The most common sequela, however, of the arterial switch has been the development of obstruction to right ventricular outflow. Although the anastomotic site was initially incriminated, subsequent larger studies[10-16] have identified other sites of stenosis occurrence [subvalvar region (Figure 6), the reconstructed sinuses of Valsalva (Figure 7), and the branch pulmonary artery regions]. The mechanism of stenosis development may be different for each site. In the case of branch pulmonary artery stenosis, the most likely etiology is tension on the proximal segment of the left pulmonary artery after the Lecompte maneuver (Figure 8).[17] For the area proximal to the anastomosis, the geometry of the patches used to close the defects created by coronary button excision[18,19] may play an additional role. Subvalvar narrowing may be due to progression of preoperative narrowing of the region underneath the native aortic valve. Narrowing of the neo-aortic anastomosis itself is rare (Figure 9).[19,20] Preoperative dynamic left ventricular outflow tract obstruction disappears postoperatively.[21]

The Lecompte maneuver places the neo-pulmonary valve and the subvalvar region immediately under the sternum, thereby making standard parasternal imaging problematic in many infants. The use of the subcostal and suprasternal windows usually allows visualization of the relevant structures.[20] The subcostal right oblique view (Figure 10) is especially useful for the right ventricular outflow tract, neo-pulmonary valve cusps, sinuses of Valsalva (Figure 11), and right pulmonary artery origin. Suprasternal (or high parasternal) imaging using modified short axis views is the best way to display the branch pulmonary artery origins (Figure 12); often the origins cannot be displayed simultaneously.

Because of the multiple potential levels of stenosis, pulsed Doppler evaluation of each arterial tract must be performed from several windows (Figure 13). The sample volume must be placed sequentially in the outflow tract (Figure 14), above the valve leaflets (Figure 15), and above the anastomotic site. In the case of the neopulmonary artery, the branches should be interrogated (Figure 16), although the right pulmonary artery (Figure 17) is usually at a large (>20°) angle to the ultrasound beam regardless of which window is used. (Likewise, the use of continuous wave Doppler to quantitate right pulmonary artery origin narrowing is probably of less value than consideration of the morphology.) The subcostal (Figure 18) and apical (Figure 19) windows should not be used to interrogate the proximal left pulmonary artery because the angle of incidence can cause false dispersion (Figure 20). To "cross-check" the right-sided outflow tract gradient, right ventricular peak systolic pressure estimate by application of the Bernoulli equation to tricuspid regurgitation jets should be performed. Color Doppler has not added significantly to the conventional Doppler assessment of obstruction except to facilitate the alignment of the continuous wave Doppler beam in the estimation of right ventricular systolic pressure. It must be remembered that color Doppler display is angle-dependent so that multiple windows must be explored (just as with the use of non-image-directed continuous wave Doppler) to ensure that the highest maximal instantaneous gradient is measured. For the evaluation of arterial valve regurgitation,[22,23] color Doppler has great advantages since it allows rapid detection; quantitation of jet widths at the leaflet level allows accurate assessment of regurgitation severity.

Success with the switch has been spectacular recently,[24] and it may have wide uses.[25]

2. Arterial Switch Procedure Without Lecompte Maneuver

The arterial repair of transposition of the great arteries with *side-by-side* great arteries or the Taussig-Bing type of double-outlet right ventricle[26] is more easily managed without the Lecompte maneuver. The orifice of the native distal main pulmonary artery can be extended to the patient's right by incision of the proximal right pulmonary artery. Suture closure of the leftward aspect of the enlarged orifice effectively *transposes* "the pulmonary bifurcation" rightward, allowing the anastomosis with the native proximal aortic root to be made without tension.

The neo-pulmonary artery can usually be seen easily with the subcostal frontal sweep. The entire tract should be surveyed with the Doppler techniques previously mentioned (see the previous section, B1).

3. Aubert Procedure

There are at least three coronary arterial variations that may make translocation as part of an arterial

switch procedure more difficult. First, single coronary artery ostium accompanied by a branch passing *between* the arterial roots necessitates the creation of a flap on the native proximal pulmonary artery in order to minimize the rotation of the button. Second, two closely spaced ostia, arising either from separate sinuses of Valsalva (on either side of a commissure) or arising from the same sinus, make the creation of separate buttons of sufficient aortic tissue more difficult. Third, the oblique intramural course of a coronary artery (e.g., a left coronary arising from the right sinus and passing through the aortic wall for a considerable length to emerge above the left sinus) makes creation of a button problematic; the standard technique of button excision would transect the coronary vessel.

Aubert[27] introduced the idea of creating an aortopulmonary "window" just cephalad to the ostium (or ostia) and insertion of a baffle of polytetrafluorethlene inside the native aortic root (neo-pulmonary root) to supply the coronary circulation (Figure 21). Thus, coronary ostia transplantation is avoided. This technique bears some similarity to the creation of an aortopulmonary window and placement of intrapulmonary artery tunnel (see Chapter 23, section A) in the repair of anomalous origin of the left coronary artery from the pulmonary artery (Figure 22). As with the latter procedure, potential residua include: (a) reduction in aortopulmonary orifice size, (b) a dehiscence in the suture line of the baffle, or most commonly, (c) narrowing of the artery in which the baffle is inserted (neopulmonary artery in the case of transposition of the great arteries). This last complication can be avoided by placement of an augmentation patch on the anterior aspect of the neo-pulmonary artery (Figure 23).

The surgically created aortopulmonary orifice can be displayed in the subcostal sagittal view. A high parasternal approach also works. Intra-arterial narrowing caused by the baffle is best seen in subcostal sagittal or right oblique views or parasternal views.

4. Damus-Kaye-Stansel Procedure

Prior to the widespread utilization of the arterial switch procedure involving coronary artery translocation, several investigators[28–30] proposed another approach to making the morphological left ventricle the systemic pumping chamber. In those cases of transposition which did not have subvalvar or valvar pulmonary stenosis, the main pulmonary artery was transected. The proximal end was anastomosed end-to-side to the ascending aorta while the distal end was connected to the right ventricle by the interposition of a conduit.

The need for a conduit dampened the popularity

of this approach for repair of transposition of the great arteries (TGA) with two ventricles of at least normal size; however, its central theme of using the pulmonary outflow and valve as a passageway to the ascending aorta has been adopted for the multitude of conotruncal malformations which have both malalignment of the infundibular septum (causing subaortic narrowing) and a malalignment-type ventricular septal defect (VSD). Examples with functionally single ventricle include: (a) TGA {S,L,L} and restrictive bulboventricular foramen (outlet foramen),[31] (b) TGA {S,D,D} and right atrioventricular valve atresia (absent right atrioventricular connection). Examples with two ventricles (of at least normal size) include: (a) interrupted aortic arch, malalignment-type VSD, and subaortic stenosis, (b) Taussig-Bing variant of double-outlet right ventricle (i.e., DORV {S,D,D} with bilateral infundibula and no subpulmonary stenosis, but without straddling mitral valve[32]).

The potential residua of proximal pulmonary artery-to-ascending aorta anastomosis are: (a) narrowing of the anastomotic orifice, and (b) native pulmonary valve insufficiency. In the infant, the suprasternal approach is the easiest method of displaying the anastomosis; in older children, magnetic resonance imaging is a major aid. Pulmonary valve regurgitation in this setting is rarely more than mild (as judged by jet width at the leaflet level) but may develop late postoperatively.[33]

The use by Norwood of a different pulmonary artery-to-ascending aorta anastomosis in palliative reconstruction of hypoplastic left heart syndrome will be discussed in the next section.

5. Norwood Procedure

The components of the Norwood[3] procedure (as performed in 1993) include: (1) transection of the proximal main pulmonary artery, (2) homograft patch closure of the distal main pulmonary artery, (3) excision of the ductus arteriosus and contraductal intimal ridge, (4) homograft augmentation (Figure 24) of the aorta (incised from 1 cm caudad to the ductal origin to the ascending aorta at the level of the proximal main pulmonary artery), (5) proximal pulmonary artery-to-ascending aorta-to-augmented arch (three-way) anas-

tomosis (Figure 25), (6) interposition of a 4-mm diameter polytetrafluorethylene shunt between the innominate artery and the right pulmonary artery, and (7) atrial septectomy. Sequelae include obstruction at the most distal portion of the aortic arch augmentation, pulmonary arterial confluence distortion, obstruction at the proximal three-way anastomosis (Figure 26), and residual obstruction at the atrial septal defect level (see Chapter 8).

The principal challenge in imaging this reconstruction is the extensive presence of prosthetic material: (a) homograft constituting the majority of the anterior aspect of the arch, and a large portion of the distal main pulmonary artery (pulmonary arterial confluence), (b) polytetrafluorethylene in the aortopulmonary shunt. Suprasternal imaging is far preferable to subcostal imaging. Left oblique and parasagittal planes are usually the best for the distal arch (Figure 27). High parasternal "transverse" views are best for the display of the proximal aortic reconstruction (Figure 28) as suggested by Weinberg[34] and are mandatory for visualizing the pulmonary arterial confluence (Figure 29). When distal arch narrowing is suggested, it must be confirmed by *pullback* of the sample volume in pulsed Doppler mode (Figure 30) and quantitated by standard or image-directed continuous wave Doppler. The velocity proximal to the distal part of the arch gusset is often >2.0 m/sec; thus, it cannot be neglected. The velocity distal to the distal part of the arch gusset can be as high as 2.8 m/sec without being associated with a peak-to-peak systolic gradient at catheterization. The correlation of Doppler peak instantaneous gradient and peak-to-peak catheter gradients is not high, perhaps because of the coexistent aortic runoff. Shunt stenosis is rare but[35,36] can be quantitatively assessed by evaluating color Doppler jet width (Figure 31) and by quantitating the ratio of diastolic retrograde velocity-time integral to antegrade systolic velocity-time integral.

Finally, the morphological right ventricle occasionally dilates markedly in response to the volume overload. Because of the complex geometry of the right ventricle, rapid measurement of its volume is challenging. Seliem[37] has used a bi-plane method that appears to work well for hypoplastic left heart syndrome, but magnetic resonance imaging may ultimately prove efficient and more reproducible.

References

1. Marx GR, Allen HD, Goldberg SJ. Doppler echocardiographic estimation of systolic pulmonary artery pressure in patients with aortic-pulmonary shunts. *J Am Coll Cardiol* 1986; 7:880–885.

2. McFaul RC, Tajik AJ, Mair DD, Danielson GK, Seward JB. Development of pulmonary arteriovenous shunt after superior vena cava–right pulmonary artery (Glenn) anastomosis. *Circulation* 1976; 55:212–216.

3. Norwood WI. Hypoplastic left heart syndrome. *Ann Thorac Surg* 1991; 52:688–695.

4. Kawashima Y, Kitamura S, Matsuda H, Shimazaki Y, Nakano S, Hirose H. Total cavopulmonary shunt operation in complex cardiac anomalies. *J Thorac Cardiovasc Surg* 1984; 87:74–81.

5. Jatene AD, Fontes VF, Souza LCB, Paulista PP, Neto CA, Sousa JEMR. Anatomic correction of transposition of the great arteries. *J Thorac Cardiovasc Surg* 1982; 83:20–26.

6. Borow KM, Arensman FW, Webb C, Radley-Smith R, Yacoub M. Assessment of left ventricular contractile state after anatomic correction of transposition of the great arteries. *Circulation* 1984; 69:106–112.

7. Colan SD, Trowitzsch D, Wernovsky G, Sholler GF, Sanders SP, Castaneda AR. Myocardial performance after arterial switch operation for transposition of the great arteries with intact ventricular septum. *Circulation* 1988; 78:132–141.

8. Sievers HH, Lange PE, Onnasch DGW, Radley-Smith R, Yacoub MH, Heintzen PH, Regensburger D, et al. Influence of the two-stage anatomic correction of simple transposition of the great arteries on left ventricular function. *Am J Cardiol* 1985; 56:514–519.

9. Lange PE, Onnasch DGW, Stephan E, Wessel A, Radley-Smith R, Yacoub MH, Regensburger D, et al. Two-stage anatomic correction of complete transposition of the great arteries: ventricular volumes and muscle mass. *Herz* 1981; 6:336–343.

10. Norwood WI, Gleason MM, Chin AJ, Murphy JD. Arterial repair for complete transposition in the neonate. *Proceedings First World Congress of Pediatric Cardiac Surgery: Perspectives in Pediatric Cardiology* 1989, Vol. 2, part 2, pp 10–13.

11. Quaegebeur JM, Rohmer J, Ottenkamp J, Buis T, Kirklin JW, Blackstone EH, Brom AG. The arterial switch operation. *J Thorac Cardiovasc Surg* 1986; 92:361–384.

12. Idriss FS, Ilbawi MN, DeLeon SY, Duffy CE, Muster AJ, Berry TE, Paul MH. Arterial switch in simple and complex transposition of the great arteries. *J Thorac Cardiovasc Surg* 1988; 95:29–36.

13. DiDonato RM, Wernovsky G, Walsh EP, Colan SD, Lang P, Wessel DL, Jonas RA, et al. Results of the arterial switch operation for transposition of the great arteries with ventricular septal defect. *Circulation* 1989; 80:1689–1705.

14. Lincoln C, Redington AN, Li K, Mattos S, Shinebourne EA, Rigby ML. Anatomical correction for complete transposition and double outlet right ventricle: intermediate assessment of functional results. *Br Heart J* 1986; 56:259–266.

15. Norwood WI, Dobell AR, Freed MD, Kirklin JW, Blackstone EH, for the Congenital Heart Surgeons Society. Intermediate results of the arterial switch repair: a 20-institution study. *J Thorac Cardiovasc Surg* 1988; 96:854–863.

16. Castaneda AR, Trusler GA, Paul MH, Blackstone EH, Kirklin JW. The early results of treatment of simple transposition in the current era. *J Thorac Cardiovasc Surg* 1988; 95:14–28.

17. Lecompte Y, Zannini L, Hazan E, Jarreau MM, Bex JP, Tu TV, Neveux JY. Anatomic correction of transposition of the great arteries. New technique without the use of a prosthetic conduit. *J Thorac Cardiovasc Surg* 1981; 82:629–631.

18. Yacoub MH, Radley-Smith R. Anatomy of the coronary arteries in transposition of the great arteries and methods for their transfer in anatomical correction. *Thorax* 1978; 33:418–424.

19. Arensman FW, Sievers HH, Lange P, Radley-Smith R, Bernhard A, Heintzen P, Yacoub MH. Assessment of coronary and aortic anastomoses after anatomic correction of transposition of the great arteries. *J Thorac Cardiovasc Surg* 1985; 90:597–604.

20. Gleason MM, Chin AJ, Andrews BA, Barber G, Helton JG, Murphy JD, Norwood WI. Two-dimensional and Doppler echocardiographic assessment of neonatal arterial repair for transposition of the great arteries. *J Am Coll Cardiol* 1989; 13:1320–1328.

21. Yacoub MH, Arensman FW, Keck E, Radley-Smith R. Fate of dynamic left ventricular outflow tract obstruction after anatomic correction of transposition of the great arteries. *Circulation* 1983; 68(Suppl II):II-56–II-62.

22. Caguioa ES, Reinmold SC, Velez S, Lee RT. Influence of aortic pressure on effective regurgitant orifice area in aortic regurgitation. *Circulation* 1992; 85:1565–1571.

23. Martin RP, Ettedgui JA, Qureshi SA, Gibbs JL, Baker EJ, Radley-Smith R, Maisey MN, et al. A quantitative evaluation of aortic regurgitation after anatomic correction of transposition of the great arteries. *J Am Coll Cardiol* 1988; 12:1281–1284.

24. Kirklin JW, Blackstone EH, Tchervenkov CI, Castaneda AR and the Congenital Heart Surgeons Society. Clinical outcomes after the arterial switch operation for transposition. *Circulation* 1992; 86:1501–1515.

25. Mee RBB. Severe right ventricular failure after Mustard or Senning operation. Two-stage repair: pulmonary artery banding and switch. *J Thorac Cardiovasc Surg* 1986; 92:385–390.

26. Kanter K, Anderson R, Lincoln C, Firmin R, Rigby M. Anatomic correction of double-outlet right ventricle with subpulmonary ventricular septal defect (the "Taussig-Bing" anomaly). *Ann Thorac Surg* 1986; 41:287–292.

27. Aubert J, Pannetier A, Couvelly JP, Unal D, Rouault F, Delarue A. Transposition of the great arteries: new technique for anatomical correction. *Br Heart J* 1978; 40:204–208.

28. Damus PS. Correspondence. *Ann Thorac Surg* 1975; 20:724–725.

29. Kaye MP. Anatomic correction of transposition of the great arteries. *Mayo Clin Proc* 1975; 50:638–40.

30. Stansel HC. A new operation for d-loop transposition of the great vessels. *Ann Thorac Surg* 1975; 19:565–567.

31. Doty DB, Marvin WJ, Lauer RM. Single ventricle with aortic outflow obstruction. *J Thorac Cardiovasc Surg* 1981; 81:636–640.

32. Ceithaml E, Puga FJ, Danielson GK, McGoon DC, Ritter DG. Results of the Damus-Stansel-Kaye procedure for transposition of the great arteries and for double-outlet right ventricle with subpulmonary ventricular septal defect. *Ann Thorac Surg* 1984; 38:433–437.

33. Chin AJ, Barber G, Helton JG, Alboliras ET, Aglira BA, Pigott JD, Norwood WI. Fate of the pulmonic valve after proximal pulmonary artery-to-ascending aorta anastomosis for aortic outflow obstruction. *Am J Cardiol* 1988; 62:435–438.

34. Weinberg PM, Chin AJ, Murphy JD, Pigott JD, Norwood WI. Postmortem echocardiography and tomographic anatomy of hypoplastic left heart syndrome following palliative surgery. *Am J Cardiol* 1986; 58:1228–1232.

35. Viitanen A, Salmenpera M, Heinonen J, Hynynen M. Pulmonary vascular resistance before and after cardiopulmonary bypass: the effect of $PaCO_2$. *Chest* 1989; 95:773–778.

36. Jobes DR, Nicolson SC, Steven JM, Miller M, Jacobs ML, Norwood WI. Carbon dioxide prevents pulmonary overcirculation in hypoplastic left heart syndrome. *Ann Thorac Surg* 1992; 54:150–151.

37. Seliem MA, Baffa JM, Vetter JM, Chen S-L, Chin AJ, Norwood WI. Changes in right ventricular geometry and heart rate early after Hemi-Fontan procedure. *Ann Thorac Surg* 1993; 55:1508–1512.

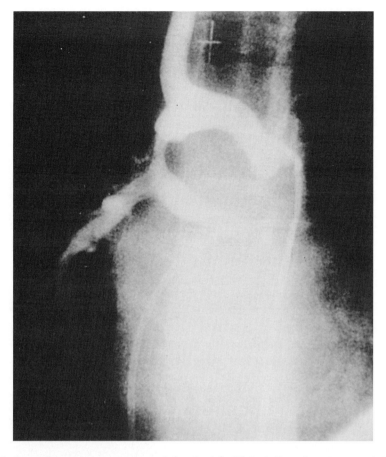

Figure 1: Anteroposterior angiogram of classic right Blalock-Taussig anastomosis in a patient with left aortic arch. Note that the right pulmonary artery has become tented.

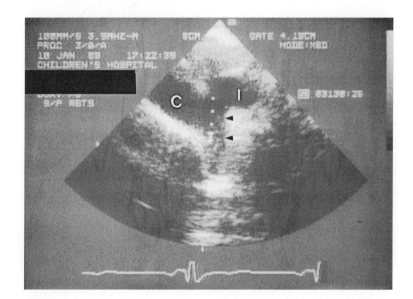

Figure 2: Suprasternal frontal view of a classic right Blalock-Taussig shunt (arrowheads). C = right common carotid artery; I = innominate artery.

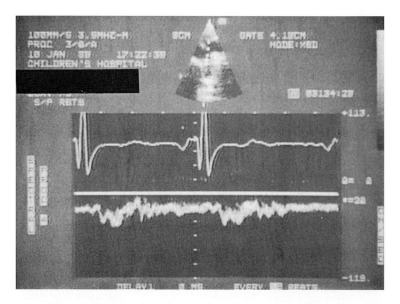

Figure 3: Pulsed Doppler display from the patient in Figure 2. The sample volume is within the proximal portion of the shunt. Note the low-velocity, continuous, laminar flow.

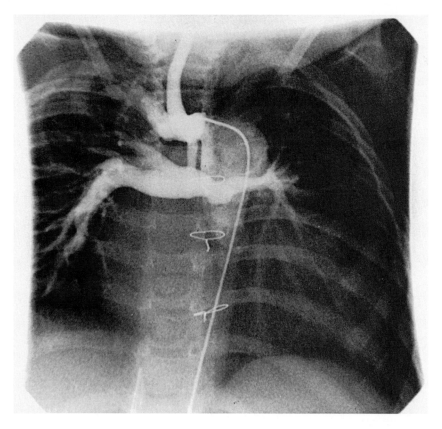

Figure 4: Anteroposterior projection of modified right Blalock-Taussig shunt. In this case, the disparity in size between distal right pulmonary and distal left pulmonary arteries may be due to the size of the reconstructed aortic arch (Norwood procedure for hypoplastic left heart syndrome).

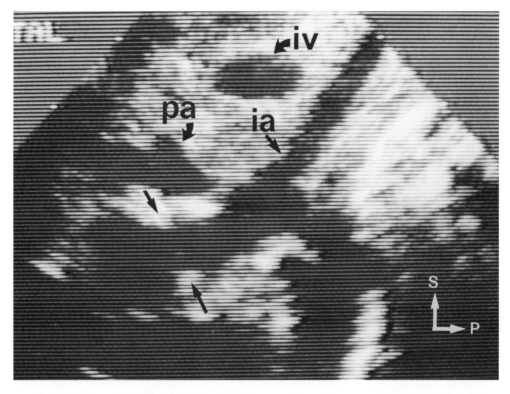

Figure 5: Suprasternal left oblique view of the neo-aorta and the anastomotic site (unlabeled arrows). ia = innominate artery; iv = innominate vein; pa = neo-pulmonary artery.

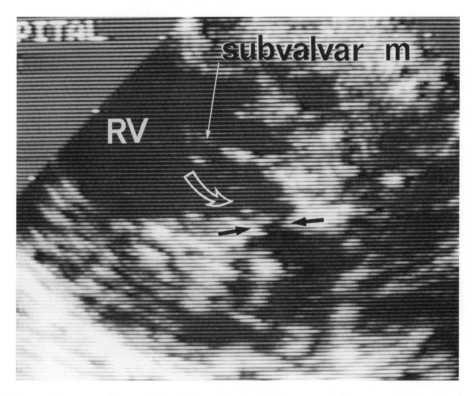

Figure 6: Parasternal view of the right ventricular outflow tract (white arrow) and neo-pulmonary artery. The sinuses of Valsalva (black arrows) appear to be deformed. m = muscle; RV = right ventricle.

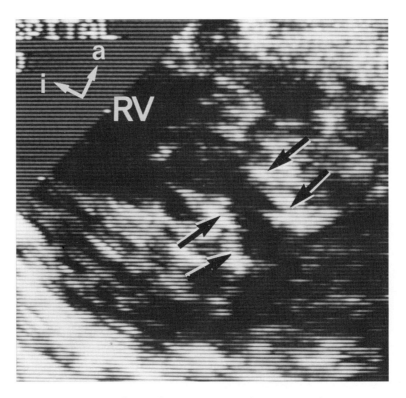

Figure 7: Parasternal view of the patches used to close the defects in the sinuses of Valsalva caused by button excision.

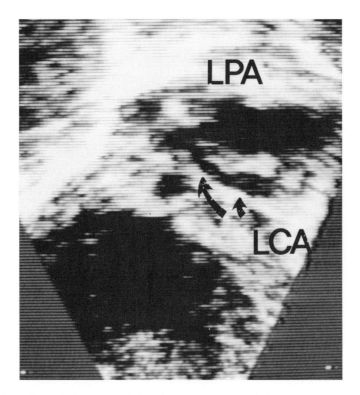

Figure 8: Apical view of proximal left pulmonary artery (LPA) as it courses over the neo-aorta and reimplanted left coronary artery (LCA).

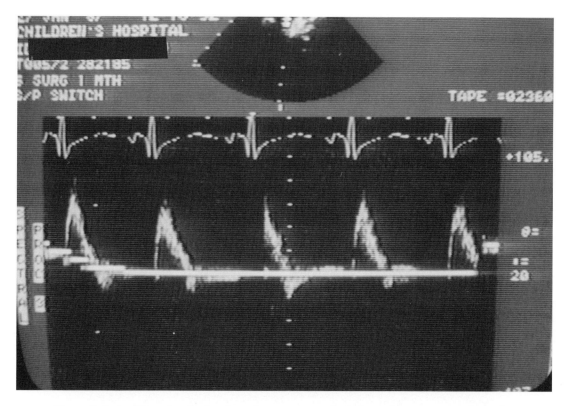

Figure 9: Pulsed Doppler display from the suprasternal window of the neo-aorta above the anastomosis.

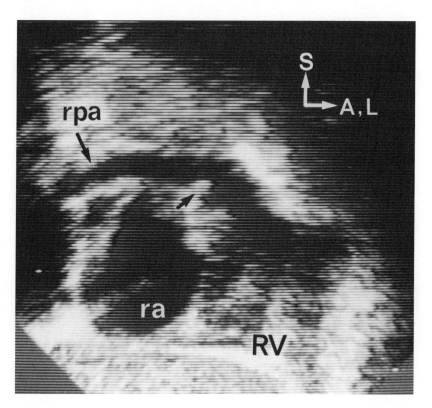

Figure 10: Subcostal right oblique view of neo-pulmonary artery. The anastomosis (unlabeled arrow) and right pulmonary artery (rpa) are displayed. ra = right atrium; RV = right ventricle.

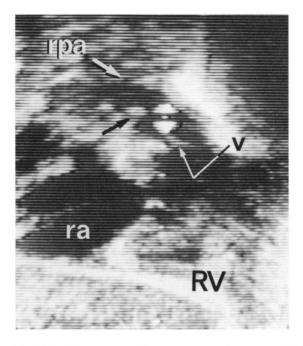

Figure 11: Subcostal right oblique view of the reconstructed sinuses of Valsalva (neo-pulmonary artery). They lie between the anastomosis (unlabeled arrow) and the valve (v) cusps of the neo-pulmonary artery. rpa = right pulmonary artery; ra = right atrium; RV = right ventricle.

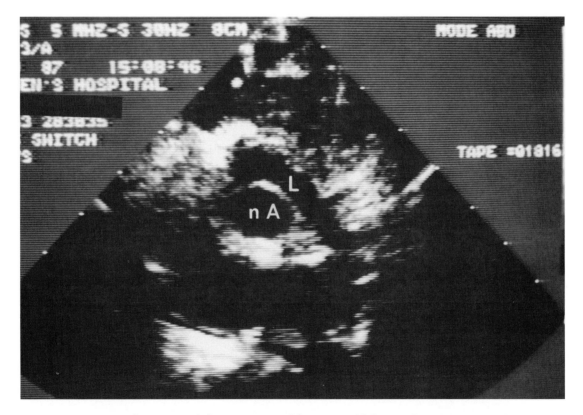

Figure 12: High parasternal short axis view of the proximal left (L) pulmonary artery. nA = neo-aorta.

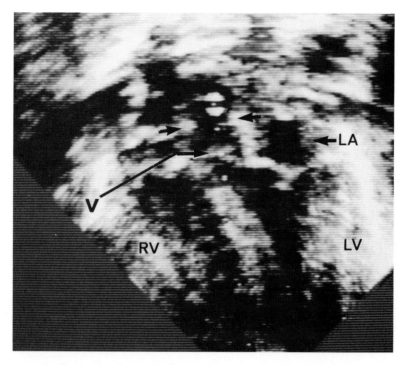

Figure 13: Apical view of neo-aorta. The sample volume is above the anastomosis (unlabeled arrows). LA = left atrium; LV = left ventricle; RV = right ventricle; v = valve cusps.

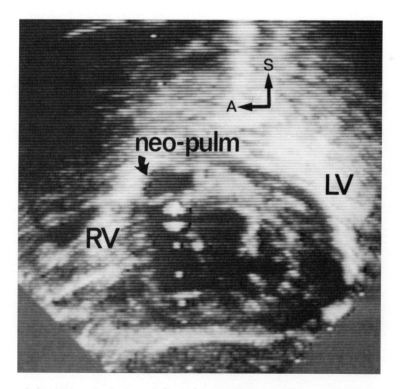

Figure 14: Subcostal sagittal view of the right ventricular outflow tract. neo-pulm = neo-pulmonary root; RV = right ventricle; LV = left ventricle.

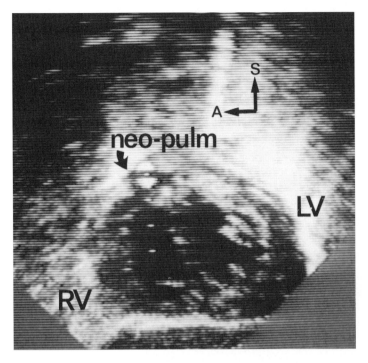

Figure 15: Subcostal sagittal view of patient shown in Figure 14. The sample volume has now been moved above the neo-pulmonary (neo-pulm) cusps. RV = right ventricle; LV = left ventricle.

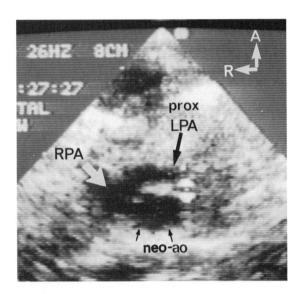

Figure 16: High parasternal view showing pulsed Doppler interrogation of the proximal left pulmonary artery (prox LPA). neo-ao = neo-aorta; RPA = right pulmonary artery.

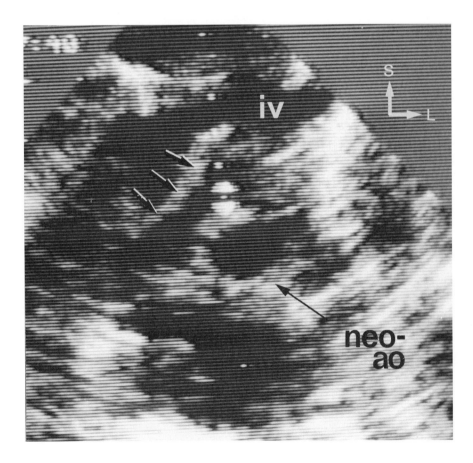

Figure 17: Suprasternal frontal view of the proximal right pulmonary artery (unlabeled arrows). Note how the right pulmonary artery is at a 45° angle to the Doppler cursor.

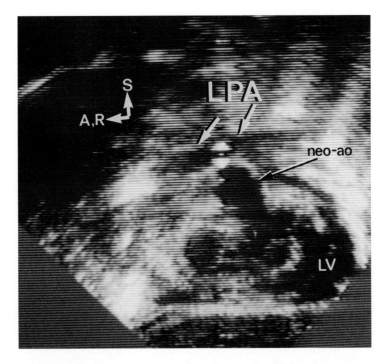

Figure 18: Subcostal left oblique view. Note how the proximal left pulmonary artery (LPA) is almost perpendicular to the Doppler cursor. neo-ao = neo-aorta; LV = left ventricle.

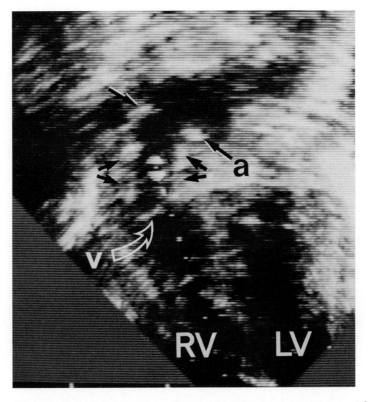

Figure 19: Although the apical view is very helpful for Doppler interrogation of the reconstructed sinuses of Valsalva (unlabeled arrows), the proximal left pulmonary artery is almost perpendicular to the Doppler cursor. a = anastomosis; v = neo-pulmonary valve cusps; LV = left ventricle; RV = right ventricle.

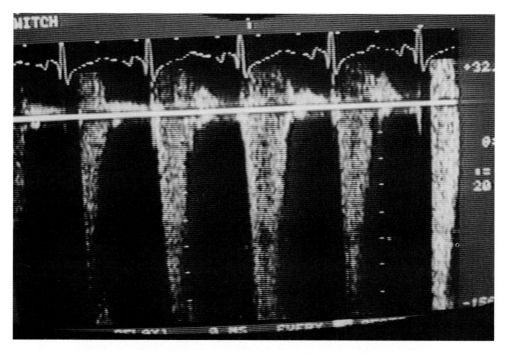

Figure 20: Pulsed Doppler display of left pulmonary artery flow when angle of incidence is >20°.

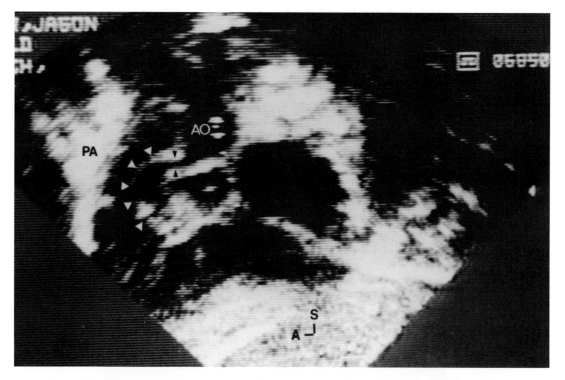

Figure 21: Subcostal sagittal view of Aubert procedure. An aorticopulmonary window (black arrowheads) is surgically created to allow aortic (Ao) blood to be directed by the poly-tetrafluorethylene baffle (white arrowheads) into the coronary circulation. PA = neo-pulmonary artery. Used with permission of American Society of Echocardiography.

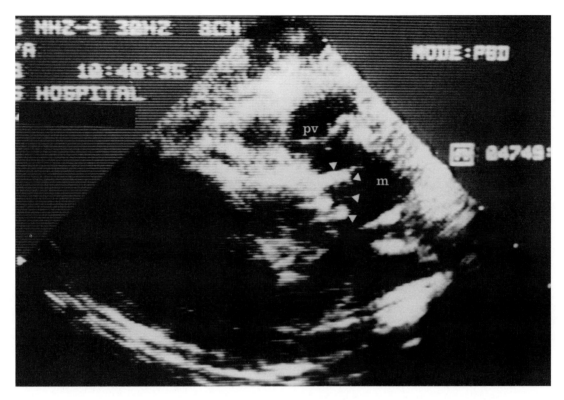

Figure 22: Parasternal view short axis view of the baffle in the Takeuchi procedure. m = main pulmonary artery; pv = pulmonary valve cusps.

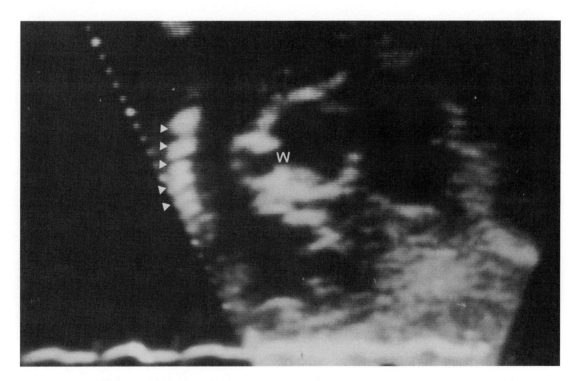

Figure 23: Subcostal sagittal view of the Aubert procedure. Note the augmentation patch (arrowheads) on the anterior aspect of the neopulmonary artery. W = surgically created aorticopulmonary window.

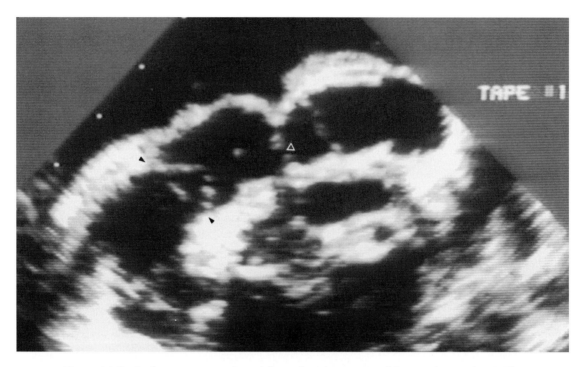

Figure 24: Sagittal postmortem view of the arch augmentation (Norwood procedure). The anterior-most aspect of the suture line (white arrowhead) is visible. This is less than 2 cm cephalad to the native pulmonary annulus (black arrowheads).

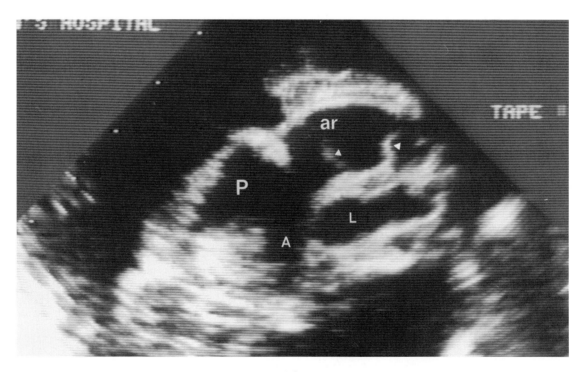

Figure 25: Left oblique postmortem view of the pulmonary artery-to-ascending aorta-to-augmented arch three-way anastomosis (Norwood procedure). The left pulmonary artery-confluence junction (L) lies underneath the arch gusset. When polytetrafluorethylene is used as the gusset material, distortion of the native tissue can occur, producing "wrinkles" or ridges (white arrowheads). This is not seen when homograft is utilized.

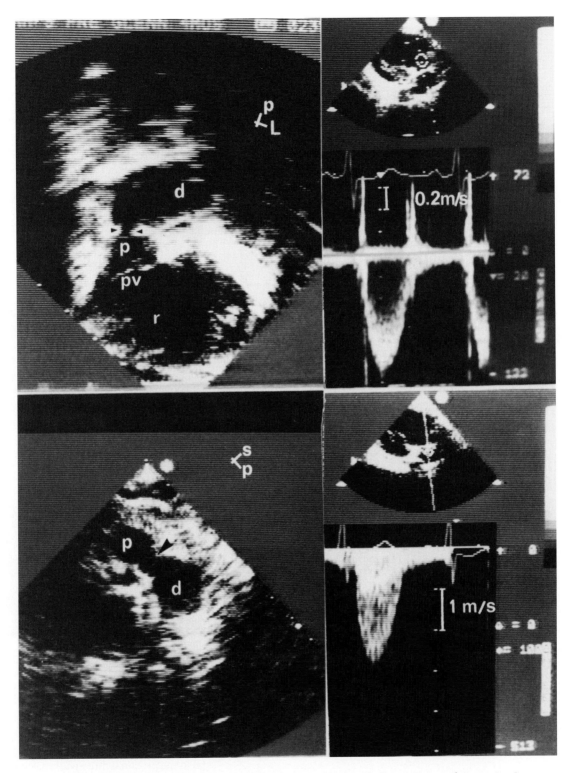

Figure 26: Top left: Low parasternal (nearly apical) view of obstruction at the proximal three-way anastomosis (black arrowheads). **Bottom left:** High parasternal sagittal view of the mild narrowing. **Top right:** Pulsed Doppler trace of the velocity distal to the native pulmonary valve cusps but proximal to the narrowing. **Bottom right:** Continuous wave Doppler interrogation of the narrowing. Used with permission of American College of Chest Physicians.

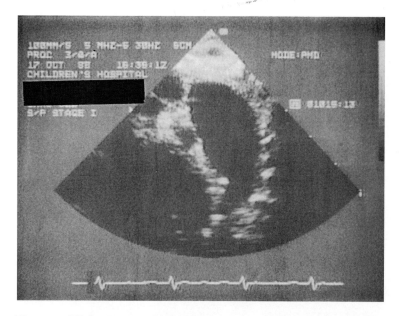

Figure 27: High parasternal left oblique view of the distal arch. Note the abrupt change in caliber as the augmentation patch meets the descending aorta. Obstruction should not be diagnosed by identifying such disparities but rather by measurement of absolute dimensions and by Doppler interrogation.

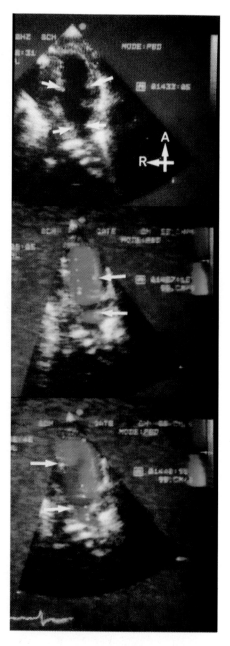

Figure 28: Top: High parasternal transverse views of the arch reconstruction. The arrows show a "normal" result of the Norwood operation. Note that at the distal part of the arch, there is typically an abrupt change in caliber. **Middle:** Same view. Placement of the pulsed Doppler sample volume to assess the velocity distal to the proximal three-way anastomosis. (Arrows denote proximal and distal extent of the augmentation.) **Bottom:** Same view. Placement of the pulsed Doppler sample volume to assess the velocity distal to the distal-most portion of the augmentation patch. The red color denotes the onset of flow reversal in diastole (due to the presence of the aortopulmonary shunt).

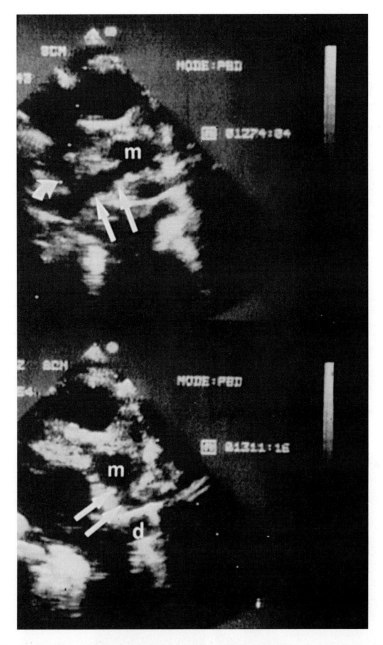

Figure 29: Top: High parasternal transverse view of the right pulmonary artery (long arrows). The pulmonary artery end of the modified right Blalock-Taussig shunt is shown by the short arrow. **Bottom:** High parasternal transverse view of the left pulmonary artery (arrows) before it passes anterior to the descending (d) aorta.

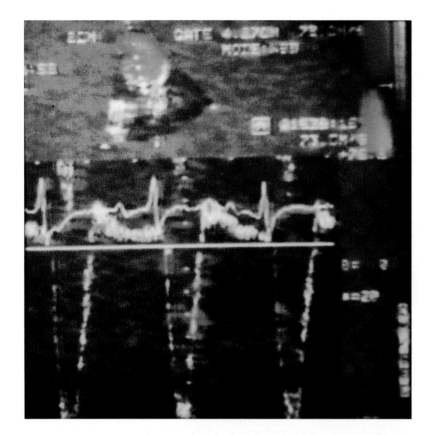

Figure 30: Pulsed Doppler pattern (v_{max} = 2.0 m/sec) distal to distal-most portion of the augmentation patch.

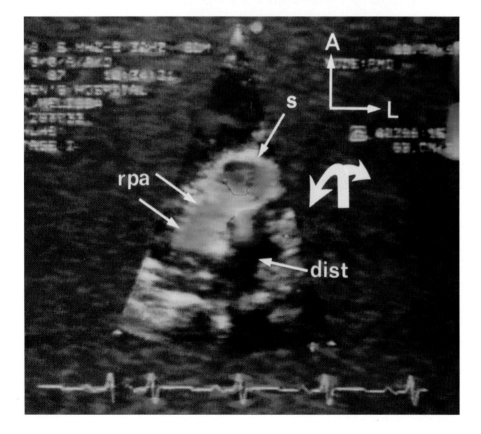

Figure 31: High parasternal transverse view of a patient who had a central (distal arch-to-pulmonary artery confluence) shunt. The width of the shunt can be seen from its aortic end to its pulmonary end by looking at the color jet width. The flow is displayed as red as it traverses the shunt and hits (s) the anterior aspect of the confluence and as blue as it travels down the right pulmonary artery (rpa). The beginning of the left pulmonary artery is also seen.

Chapter 25

Aortic Valve, Truncus, Truncal Valve Surgery

A. Konno Procedure

This procedure,[1] which has as its central feature replacement of the aortic valve, has been used increasingly sparingly. The infundibular septum is incised and augmented by a patch. The free wall of the right ventricular outflow tract is augmented with a patch. Conceived as an annulus-enlarging technique, it is difficult to apply in the infant because of the paucity of acceptable prosthetic valves for this age group. Thus, as reconstructive surgery is extended to younger and younger infants, the Konno procedure is being reserved for older children.

In addition to problems inherent in prosthetic valves, there are the additional potential sequelae of right ventricular outflow tract obstruction and residual ventricular-level shunting.

B. Aortic Valvoplasty

There are several reconstructive techniques[2,3] for aortic regurgitation. The value of transesophageal imaging for quantifying the post-repair regurgitation severity has been demonstrated in adult populations. Relatively little experience has been reported in the pediatric age group.

C. Aortic Valve Replacement (St. Jude Valve)

Potential sequelae are paravalvar leaks, impaired motion of one or both tilting discs to fibrous tissue, or thrombosis causing obstruction[4-6] of any of the three orifices. Transesophageal imaging has markedly facilitated the assessment of mechanical valves.

D. Aortic Valve Replacement (Tissue Valve)

Potential sequelae are paravalvar leaks, stenosis, or regurgitation; degenerative changes are responsible for the latter two. Occasionally, regurgitation occurs acutely due to cuspal rupture. Thus, a patient who has been diligently followed as a stenosis patient can suddenly become a regurgitation patient!

E. Truncus Arteriosus Repair Using Truncal Root Flap

Except for rare variants,[7,8] truncus arteriosus is now straightforward to repair in infancy.

Barbero-Macial[9] introduced a method of repairing truncus without extracardiac conduits. An autologous flap is created and forms a portion of the circumference of the right ventricle-to-pulmonary artery pathway.

Potential sequelae include branch pulmonary artery stenosis and residual aortopulmonary window.

References

1. Konno S, Imai Y, Iida Y, Nakajima M, Tatsuno K. A new method for prosthetic valve replacement in congenital aortic stenosis associated with hypoplasia of the aortic valve ring. *J Thorac Cardiovasc Surg* 1975; 70:909–917.

2. Trusler GA, Moes CAF, Kidd BSL. Repair of ventricular septal defect with aortic insufficiency. *J Thorac Cardiovasc Surg* 1973; 66:394–403.

3. Carpentier A. Cardiac valve surgery: the "French correction." *J Thorac Cardiovasc Surg* 1983; 86:323–337.

4. Baumgartner H, Khan S, DeRobertis M, Czer L, Maurer G. Effect of prosthetic aortic valve design on the Doppler-catheter correlation: an in vitro study of normal St. Jude, Medtronic- Hall, Starr-Edwards, and Hancock valves. *J Am Coll Cardiol* 1992; 19:324–332.

5. Baumgartner H, Khan S, DeRobertis M, Czer L, Maurer G. Discrepancies between Doppler and catheter gradients in aortic prosthetic valves in vitro. *Circulation* 1990; 82:1467–1475.

6. Burstow DJ, Nishimura RA, Bailey KR, Reeder GS, Holmes DR, Seward JB, Tajik AJ. Continuous wave Doppler echocardiographic measurement of prosthetic valve gradients. *Circulation* 1989; 80:504–514.

7. Alves JC, Ferrar AH. Common arterial trunk arising exclusively from the right ventricle with hypoplastic left ventricle and intact ventricular septum. *Int J Cardiol* 1987; 16:99–102.

8. Areias JC, Lopes JM. Common arterial trunk associated with absence of one atrioventricular connexion. *Int J Cardiol* 1987; 17:329–332.

9. Barbero-Macial M, Riso A, Atik E, Jatene A. A technique for correction of truncus arteriosus types I and II without extracardiac conduits. *J Thorac Cardiovasc Surg* 1990; 99:364–369.

Chapter 26

Pulmonary Artery/
Pulmonary Outflow Tract
Surgery

A. Banding

Pulmonary artery banding has been applied less and less as reparative surgery has increasingly become a primary procedure. For patients with functional single ventricle, a way to apply Fontan's operation in the newborn period has not yet been developed; thus, pulmonary artery banding may retain some usefulness as a palliative procedure to prevent pulmonary overcirculation. For the group with single left ventricle and outlet chamber,[1] pulmonary artery banding reduces the size of the outlet foramen (bulboventricular foramen). The mechanism is the change in ventricular geometry following acute volume load reduction. [In this malformation (with either D or L ventricular loop), transection of the main pulmonary artery and end-to-side anastomosis of the proximal pulmonary artery and the ascending aorta combined with creation of a systemic artery-to-pulmonary artery shunt may prove to yield better early and long- term survival.]

Sequelae of pulmonary artery banding include: (1) deformity of the branch pulmonary artery origins by the band migrating distally, (2) "ineffective" protection of the pulmonary vascular bed, and (3) erosion (Figure 1) of the pulmonary artery band into the lumen (Figure 2) of the main pulmonary artery.[2–5]

Deformity of the right pulmonary artery origin can usually be displayed well with the subcostal right oblique view (Figure 3). The left pulmonary artery origin can often be well displayed in the subcostal left oblique view. The parasternal short axis cut is usually helpful as well.

Doppler interrogation of the pulmonary artery distal to the band is not analogous to the interrogation distal to a valvar stenosis for two reasons: (1) pulmonary artery bands constructed with Silastic result in a nondiscrete (long-segment) narrowing, and (2) the distal main pulmonary bifurcates into branches at a point at most a few millimeters from the distal end of the band. Although continuous wave Doppler correlated well with simultaneous, unblinded catheterization-measured instantaneous gradients in a population of larger children, this technique has not been prospectively tested in infants.

B. Repair of Pulmonary Artery Sling

Although initial diagnosis of the anomaly can be accomplished from either the subcostal or the parasternal window in the infant, the display of the left pulmonary artery origin after repair is more easily obtained from the parasternal window. Repair of this anomaly involves transection of the proximal left pulmonary artery, mobilization so that its course is no longer posterior to the trachea, and reanastomosis to the main pulmonary artery. Although morbidity and mortality after this procedure is dependent on the presence and severity of coexistent tracheal abnormalities, patency of the anastomotic site must also be assessed if the long-term growth of the left lung vasculature is to be restored.

C. Transannular Patch Augmentation

Transannular patch augmentation of the pulmonary outflow tract is most commonly utilized in repair of tetralogy of Fallot. Although many surgeons have advocated extensive resection of the infundibular septum as well as free wall muscle, Castaneda introduced the concept of augmentation of the pulmonary outflow by inserting a patch on the infundibular free wall that crossed the annulus and extended distally onto the main pulmonary artery. Resection of infundibular septal muscle was thus unnecessary. (Advocating repair in early infancy, he reasoned that secondary hypertrophic changes would be less marked at that age, necessitating a smaller ventriculotomy.) This type of outflow tract reconstruction is best displayed by the subcostal long axial oblique equivalent view and the subcostal right oblique view.

Pulmonary atresia[6,7] without right ventricular hypoplasia can be repaired without closing the foramen ovale (Figures 4–7).

The other malformation frequently repaired with a transannular patch is transposition of the great arteries, malalignment-type ventricular septal defect, coarctation (or other arch anomaly), and subaortic stenosis. After arterial switch, the native subaortic region becomes the new subpulmonary area. The malalignment of the infundibular septum anteriorly (and to the right) causes subvalvar stenosis. Just as for tetralogy of Fallot, the subpulmonary region can be augmented by a transannular patch, provided that the supply to the anterior descending or circumflex coronary arteries does not traverse the external surface of the right ventricular outflow tract.

D. Resection of Right Ventricular Anomalous Muscle Bundle

Anomalous right ventricular muscle bundle can be of several types (see Chapter 17, section D). Following surgery, the only complication commonly observed is incompletely resected muscle. The subcostal right oblique view is the best way of displaying the morphological features. The continuous wave Doppler assessment is also most consistently achieved from the subcostal window. In those patients with tricuspid regurgitation, estimation of peak systolic right ventricular pressure is helpful as a "cross-check."

References

1. Freedom RM, Benson LN, Smallhorn JF, Williams WG, Trusler GA, Rowe RD. Subaortic stenosis, the univentricular heart, and banding of the pulmonary artery: an analysis of the courses of 43 patients with univentricular heart palliated by pulmonary artery banding. *Circulation* 1986; 73:758–764.

2. Berry CL. Changes in the wall of the pulmonary artery after banding. *J Pathol* 1969; 99:29–32.

3. Cordell AR, Suh SH. The pulmonary artery lesion after banding: influence of different materials. *Ann Surg* 1974; 179:805–812.

4. Mahle S, Nicoloff DM, Knight L, Moller JH. Pulmonary artery banding: long-term results in 63 patients. *Ann Thorac Surg* 1978; 27:216–224.

5. Stark J, Berry CL, Silove ED. The evaluation of materials used for pulmonary artery banding. *Ann Thorac Surg* 1972; 13:163–169.

6. deLeval M, Bull C, Hopkins R, Rees P, Deanfield J, Taylor JFN, Gersony W, et al. Decision making in the definitive repair of the heart with a small right ventricle. *Circulation* 1985; 72(Suppl II):II52–II60.

7. Coles JG, Freedom RM, Lightfoot NE, Dasmahapatra HK, Williams WG, Trusler GA, Burrows PE. Long-term results in neonates with pulmonary atresia and intact ventricular septum. *Ann Thorac Surg* 1989; 47:213–217.

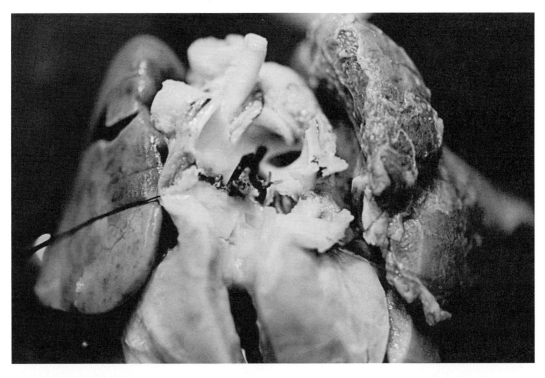

Figure 1: Postmortem frontal view of a full-thickness erosion. From the external surface, no band was seen; however, once the main pulmonary artery was opened, it became obvious that the band had gradually eroded through the wall, with scar tissue being laid down over the outside. Nearly the entire circumference of the band had eroded through.

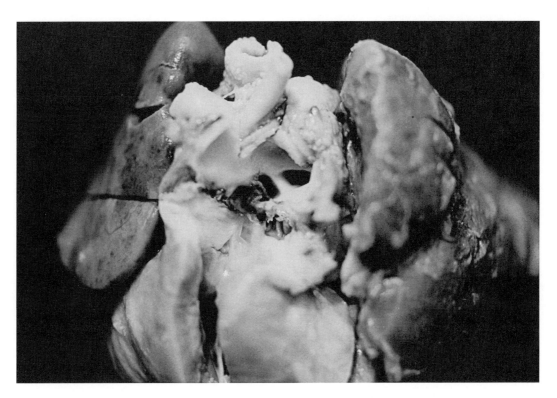

Figure 2: The band is clearly quite proximal; the "ostia" of the right and left pulmonary arteries can be seen clearly.

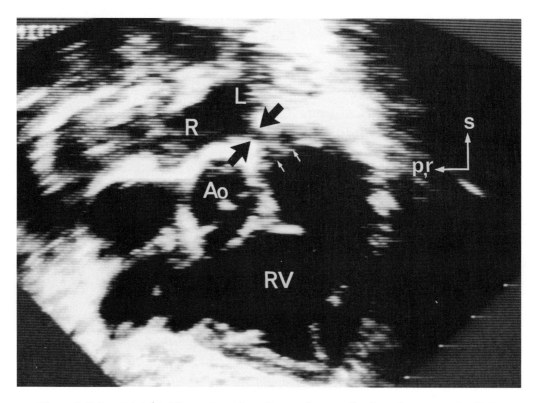

Figure 3: Subcostal right oblique view of a patient with normally aligned great arteries. Pulmonary valve cusps are shown by small unlabeled white arrows. The band (black arrows) is proximal and does not obstruct the right (R) or left (L) pulmonary artery origins. Ao = aorta; RV = right ventricle.

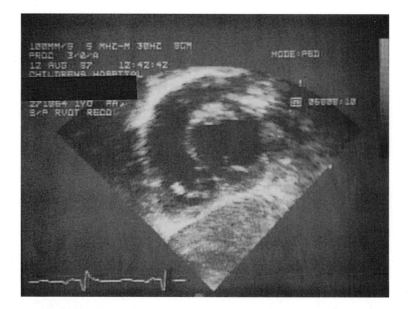

Figure 4: Subcostal sagittal view of transannular patch repair of pulmonary atresia. There is at most mild right ventricular hypoplasia (inflow portion).

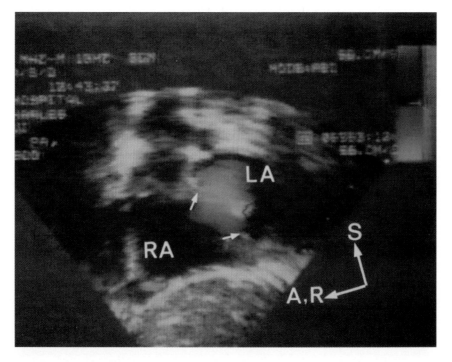

Figure 5: Subcostal left oblique view of patient shown in Figure 4. There is diastolic right-to-left flow across a widely patent foramen ovale (arrows).

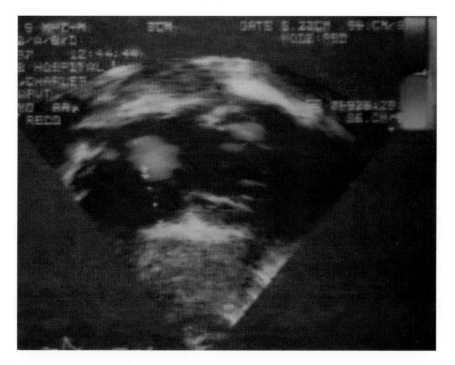

Figure 6: Subcostal frontal view of patient shown in Figure 4. The pulsed Doppler sample volume is positioned in the center of the foramen ovale.

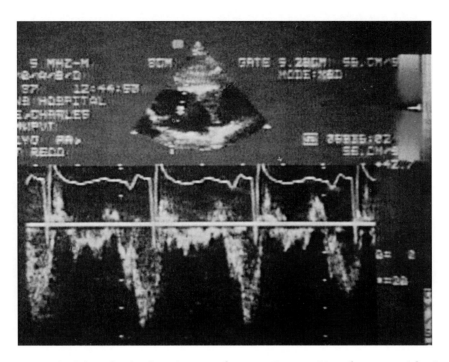

Figure 7: Pulsed Doppler display of patient shown in Figure 6. Note that most of the flow occurs in atrial systole.

Chapter 27

Internal Ventricle-to-Great Artery Tunnels (Baffles)

A. Left Ventricle-to-Aorta Baffle in Transposition, Double-Outlet Right Ventricle, and Other Ventriculo-Arterial Alignments

Unlike the situation in truncus arteriosus or tetralogy of Fallot, the development of narrowing in this pathway following reparative surgery is not rare in double-outlet right ventricle or transposition (Figure 1). The sites of occurrence are either at the original ventricular septal defect[1] or, less commonly, at the midportion of the intraventricular baffle. The mechanism is geometric change following volume load removal. It is important to identify patients who are poor candidates for left ventricle-to-aorta baffles;[2] cases with extensive atrioventricular valve tissue near the ventricular septal defect (Figure 2) or large infundibular septal structures (Figures 3 and 4) are difficult to repair with the Rastelli procedure.[3,4]

Similar to the difficulty encountered in trying to visualize distal arch narrowing in the aortic atresia patient following Norwood reconstruction, the prosthetic material used for the intraventricular baffle can obscure the target area when the subcostal window is employed. This can lead to the erroneous diagnosis of a widely patent left ventricular-to-aorta pathway. The solution is to utilize either the parasternal or the apical window.

Visualization of the left ventricular-to-aorta pathway can be especially challenging in the patient with TGA {S,D,L} or DORV {S,D,L} after Rastelli procedure.

B. Left Ventricle-to-(Native) Pulmonary Artery Intraventricular Baffle in Aortic Outflow Tract Obstruction Associated with Malalignment-type Ventricular Septal Defect

Although aortic atresia and normal-sized mitral valve and left ventricle is relatively uncommon, the malformations of interruption or coarctation with malalignment-type ventricular septal defect and subaortic stenosis are more frequently seen. Successful palliation of these latter malformations depends on addressing the aortic outflow obstruction. Although resection of the infundibular septum[5] has been attempted, in many patients the infundibular septum is hypoplastic. The etiology for aortic outflow obstruction is an unbalanced septation of the arterial outflow portion of the heart. Even in those with a thick infundibular septum, simple resection alone still leaves an aortic valve annulus that is too small. (This is analogous to treating tetralogy of Fallot by excising subpulmonary muscle without addressing the pulmonary valve annulus).

The method of Damus, Kaye, and Stansel[6-8] (see Chapter 24, section B, 4) can be applied to those malformations. Because of the position of the aortic valve and its relationship to coronary arteries, direct transannular enlargement of the left ventricular outflow is cumbersome in the infant. Bypassing the aortic area by redirecting left ventricular blood to the pulmonary valve and creating a supravalvar anastomosis between the great arteries can be a solution in some cases[9,10]; however, the malalignment-type ventricular septal

313

defect in this group of malformations is not as large as it is in tetralogy of Fallot. Furthermore, it can reduce in size when the volume load on the left ventricle is re-moved.[1] Thus, the left ventricle-to-native pulmonary root pathway can become obstructed.

References

1. Rychik J, Jacobs ML, Norwood WI, Chin AJ. Changes in ventricular geometry and ventricular septal defect size following Rastelli operation. *Circulation* 1994 (in press).

2. Moulton AL, deLeval MR, Macartney FJ, Taylor JFN, Stark J. Rastelli procedure for transposition of the great arteries, ventricular septal defect, and left ventricular outflow tract obstruction. *Br Heart J* 1981; 45:20–28.

3. Borromee L, Lecompte Y, Batisse A, Lemoine G, Vouhe P, Sakata R, Leca F, et al. Anatomic repair of anomalies of ventriculo arterial connection associated with ventricular septal defect. II. Clinical results in 50 patients with pulmonary outflow tract obstruction. *J Thorac Cardiovasc Surg* 1988; 95:96–102.

4. Smolinsky A, Castaneda AR, Van Praagh R. Infundibular septal resection: surgical anatomy of the superior approach. *J Thorac Cardiovasc Surg* 1988; 95:486–494.

5. Bove EL, Minich LL, Pridjian AK, Lupinetti FM, Snider AR, Dick M, Beekman RH. The management of severe subaortic stenosis, ventricular septal defect, and aortic arch obstruction in the neonate. *J Thorac Cardiovasc Surg* 1993; 105:289–295.

6. Damus P. Correspondence. *Ann Thorac Surg* 1975; 20:724–725.

7. Kaye MP. Anatomic correction of transposition of the great arteries. *Mayo Clin Proc* 1975; 50:638–640.

8. Stansel HC. A new operation for d-loop transposition of the great vessels. *Ann Thorac Surg* 1975; 19:565–567.

9. Rychik J, Murdison KA, Norwood WI, Chin AJ. Surgical management of severe aortic outflow obstruction in lesions other than hypoplastic left heart syndrome: use of a pulmonary artery-to-aorta anastomosis. *J Am Coll Cardiol* 1991; 18:809–816.

10. Damus PS, Thomson NB, McLoughlin TG. Arterial repair without coronary relocation for complete transposition of the great vessels with ventricular septal defect. *J Thorac Cardiovasc Surg* 1982; 83:316–318.

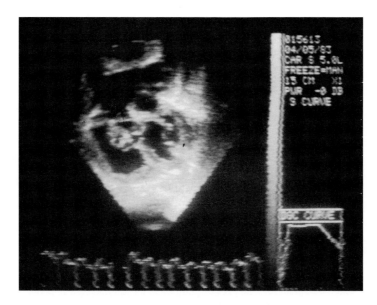

Figure 1: Subcostal sagittal view of transposition of the great arteries {S,D,D} with mal-alignment-type ventricular septal defect. Not only is the infundibular septum bulky but there is accessory tissue in the ventricular septal defect.

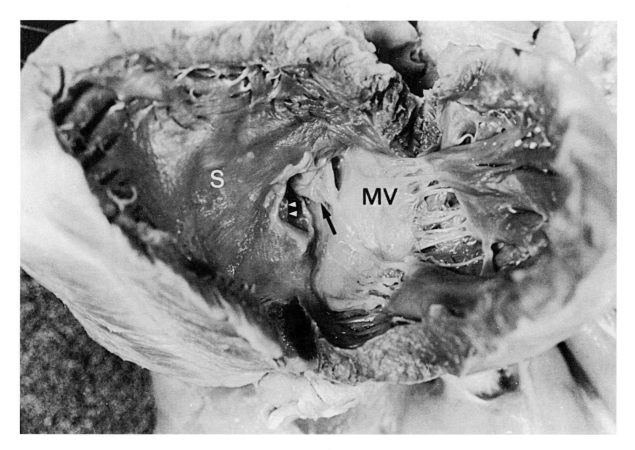

Figure 2: Postmortem view of the left ventricle of the same patient shown in Figure 1. The accessory tissue in the ventricular septal defect (black arrow) is confirmed. MV = mitral valve; S = left septal surface.

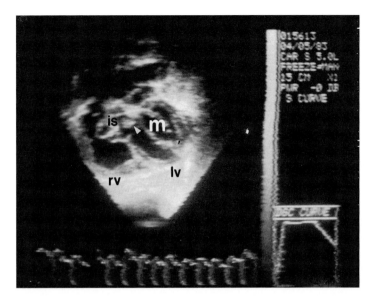

Figure 3: Subcostal sagittal view slightly to the right of the plane shown in Figure 1. The dense attachments of the tricuspid valve to the bulky infundibular septum (is) are seen. lv = left ventricle; m = mitral valve; rv = right ventricle.

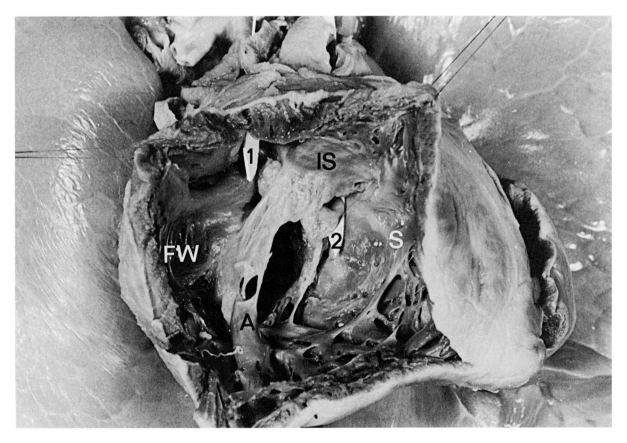

Figure 4: Postmortem view of the right ventricle of the patient shown in Figure 3. 1 = aortic outflow; 2 = pulmonary outflow. A = anterior papillary muscle; FW = free wall; S = right septal surface; IS = infundibular septum. Used with permission of American Journal of Cardiology.

Chapter 28

External Ventricle-to-Great Artery Conduits

A. Right Ventricle-to-Pulmonary Artery Pathways

The most common uses of the right ventricle-to-pulmonary artery conduit are the Rastelli procedure (and its variations), repair of tetralogy of Fallot with pulmonary atresia, and repair of truncus arteriosus (van Praagh types AI, AII, and AIII). The initial use of the valved conduit gave way to the nonvalved synthetic tube and more recently to partial autologous pathways (see Chapter 25). The rationale for the last[1] is that some growth potential may exist, minimizing the need for later "conduit change" operations. A variety of these have been devised, e.g., in truncus arteriosus, suturing a flap of truncal root to the exterior of the left atrial appendage (to form the bottom of the right ventricle-to-pulmonary artery pathway) and then roofing this over with a piece of homograft or polytetrafluoroethylene.

The ultrasonographic display of these pathways remains challenging. Although subcostal imaging is feasible in most infants and young children, it is usually difficult to visualize the distal portion of the right ventricle-to-pulmonary artery path. With those repairs involving autologous tissue, the distal portion of the right ventricle-to-pulmonary artery path together with the branch pulmonary artery origins are the most frequent sites of narrowing.

Multiple parasternal views are often necessary to display the full course. The use of image-directed (and color Doppler-directed) continuous wave Doppler has greatly enhanced the sensitivity and specificity of ultrasonographic assessment of tube conduits. Although the fact that many conduit stenoses are not discrete theoretically limits the use of the simple Bernoulli formula, most conduit patients do have at least trivial tricuspid regurgitation. Interrogation of the latter jet provides an excellent estimate of right ventricular systolic pressure.

B. Left Ventricular Apex-to-Descending Aorta Conduit

Employed most commonly to bypass nondiscrete subaortic stenosis, the apico-aortic conduit[2-4] can often be visualized in infants. (The mid-portion becomes more difficult to see as the patient gets larger.) Transverse views of the body are probably the best way to visualize the mid-portion. The most common sequela is regurgitation of the valve within the conduit.

Obstruction at the ventricular end of the conduit (just distal to the connector) can be seen in rare cases. Obstruction at the level of the valve can develop just as it can occur in right-sided conduits.

Magnetic resonance imaging (see Chapter 34, Figures 4 and 5) is helpful in displaying the course of these conduits.

C. Left Ventricle-to-Pulmonary Artery Conduit

This is commonly utilized for TGA {S,L,L}, VSD, PS[5-7]; for DORV {S,L,L}, VSD, PS; and for TGA {S,D,D}, muscular VSD, PS.[8-10] In TGA {S,L,L} and DORV {S,L,L} patients with levocardia, the conduit is usually best seen in the subcostal frontal view. In cases of dextro-

317

cardia (Figure 1), the conduit can be difficult to visualize from any window because of its extremely posterior site.

A rare complication is the development of an aneurysm near the ventricular (Figures 1 and 2) end of the conduit.

References

1. Barbero-Macial M, Riso A, Atik E, Jatene A. A technique for correction of truncus arteriosus types I and II without extracardiac conduits. *J Thorac Cardiovasc Surg* 1990; 99:364–369.

2. Brown JW, Girod DA, Hurwitz RA, Caldwell RL, Rocchini AP, Behrendt DM, Kirsh MM. Apicoaortic valved conduits for complex left ventricular outflow obstruction: technical considerations and current status. *Ann Thorac Surg* 1984; 38:162–168.

3. Norwood WI, Lang P, Castaneda AR, Murphy JD. Management of infants with left ventricular outflow obstruction by conduit interposition between the ventricular apex and thoracic aorta. *J Thorac Cardiovasc Surg* 1983; 86:771–776.

4. DiDonato RM, Danielson GK, McGoon DC, Driscoll DJ, Julsrud PR, Edwards WD. Left ventricle-aortic conduits in pediatric patients. *J Thorac Cardiovasc Surg* 1984; 88:82–91.

5. Gerlis LM, Wilson N, Dickinson DF. Abnormalities of the mitral valve in congenitally corrected transposition (discordant atrioventricular and ventriculoarterial connections). *Br Heart J* 1986; 55:475–479.

6. Westerman GR, Lang P, Castaneda AR, Norwood WI. Corrected transposition and repair of associated intracardiac defects. *Circulation* 1982; 66(Suppl II):I197–I202.

7. McGrath LB, Kirklin JW, Blackstone EH, Pacifico AD, Kirklin JK, Bargeron LM. Death and other events after cardiac repair in discordant atrioventricular connection. *J Thorac Cardiovasc Surg* 1985; 90:711–728.

8. Crupi G, Pillai R, Parenzan L, Lincoln C. Surgical treatment of subpulmonary obstruction in transposition of the great arteries by means of a left ventricular-pulmonary arterial conduit. *J Thorac Cardiovasc Surg* 1985; 85:907–913.

9. Idriss FS, DeLeon SY, Nikaidoh H, Muster AJ, Paul MH, Newfeld EA, Albers W. Resection of left ventricular outflow tract obstruction in d-transposition of the great arteries. *J Thorac Cardiovasc Surg* 1977; 74:343–351.

10. Wilcox BR, Henry GW, Anderson RH. The transmitral approach to left ventricular outflow tract obstruction. *Ann Thorac Surg* 1983; 35:288–293.

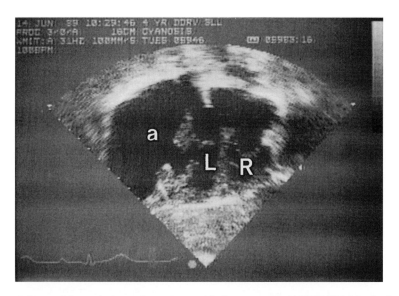

Figure 1: Subcostal frontal view of a patient with dextrocardia, DORV {S,L,L} who had undergone ventricular septal defect closure and placement of a left ventricle-to-pulmonary artery conduit. A fluid-density mass (a) developed in the right hemi-thorax, and by two-dimensional echocardiography it appeared to originate near the ventricular end of the conduit. L = morphological left ventricle; R = morphological right ventricle.

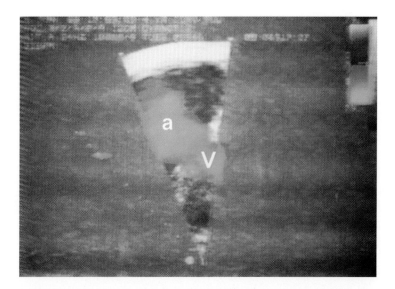

Figure 2: Subcostal frontal view of same patient shown in Figure 1. Color flow imaging confirms that the mass (a) is an aneurysm in direct communication with the morphological left ventricle (v).

Chapter 29

Surgery of the Ventricular Septum

A. Closure of the Malalignment-type Ventricular Septal Defect

The most common sequela is residual ventricular septal defect (VSD); in tetralogy of Fallot, this is typically at the tricuspid valve aspect of the patch. This is best seen in the parasternal short axis view (Figure 1). Incorrect patch placement (e.g., attaching part of the patch to a muscle bundle) is rare. The rare variant with restrictive VSD[1,2] can also be repaired.

In other ventriculo-arterial alignments with malalignment-type VSD, the residual jets are in variable sites. One of the problems that is less frequent in 1993 is incorrect patch placement (Figure 2). Malalignment of the infundibular septum may be more easily appreciated on echocardiography than on angiography (Figure 3). If malalignment is not recognized, the patch may be seated so as to close the left ventricle-to-pulmonary artery path (Figure 4).

B. Closure of the Perimembranous Ventricular Septal Defect

The most common sequela is residual VSD typically at the tricuspid valve aspect of the patch (Figure 5). This is best seen in the parasternal short axis view. Occasionally, a residual "VSD" occurs when a portion of the tricuspid valve becomes situated in the caudal portion of the original defect; this phenomenon results in a left ventricular-to-right atrial jet. The combination of a residual VSD and tricuspid regurgitation should be distinguished from a left ventricle-to-right atrial jet. In the former, interrogating the right atrium will yield an estimate of right ventricular pressure; in the latter, analogous interrogation will yield *left ventricular* pressure (Figure 6).

C. Closure of the Muscular Ventricular Septal Defect

From the right side, it may be difficult for the surgeon to seat the patch so that all jets of a mid-muscular VSD are obliterated. Thus, it is usual to see one or more tiny residual sites of shunting. From an apical left ventriculotomy, the patch is seated more flush with the septal surface.

D. Closure of the Atrioventricular Canal-Type Ventricular Septal Defect

Small residual jets on color flow mapping are frequently seen, presumably because tricuspid valve tensor apparatus can make seating the patch difficult (Figure 7).

References

1. Musewe NN, Smallhorn JF, Moes CAF, Freedom RM, Trusler GA. Echocardiographic evaluation of obstructive mechanism of tetralogy of Fallot with restrictive ventricular septal defect. *Am J Cardiol* 1988; 61:664–667.

2. Flanagan MF, Foran RB, Van Praagh R, Jonas R, Sanders SP. Tetralogy of Fallot with obstruction of the ventricular septal defect: spectrum of echocardiographic findings. *J Am Coll Cardiol* 1988; 11:386–395.

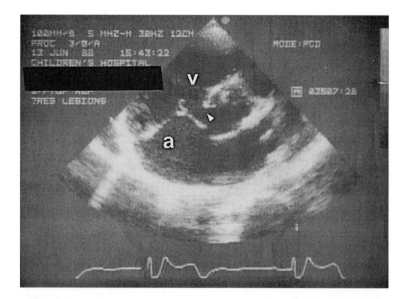

Figure 1: Parasternal short axis view following repair of tetralogy of Fallot. The large residual ventricular septal defect (arrowhead) is at the tricuspid valve aspect of the patch. a = right atrium; v = right ventricle.

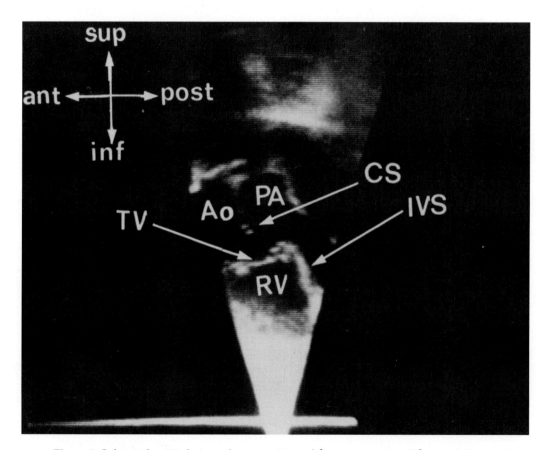

Figure 2: Subcostal sagittal view of transposition of the great arteries. When malalignment of the infundibular septum (cs) coexists, it is important to communicate this clearly to the cardiac surgeon so he can avoid incorrect patch orientation. Ao = aorta; IVS = interventricular septum; TV = tricuspid valve; PA = pulmonary root; RV = right ventricle.

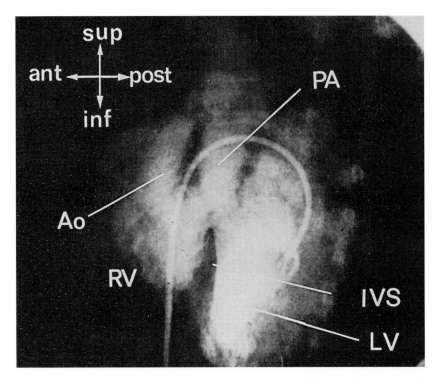

Figure 3: Lateral angiogram of patient in shown in Figure 2. Mild malalignment of the infundibular septum is suggested. PA = pulmonary root; Ao = aorta; RV = right ventricle; LV = left ventricle; IVS = interventricular septum.

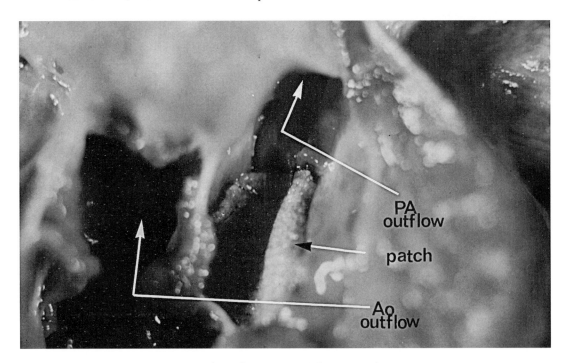

Figure 4: Postmortem view of the right ventricle of the patient shown in Figure 2. Incorrect patch placement has closed off the left ventricle-to-pulmonary artery path.

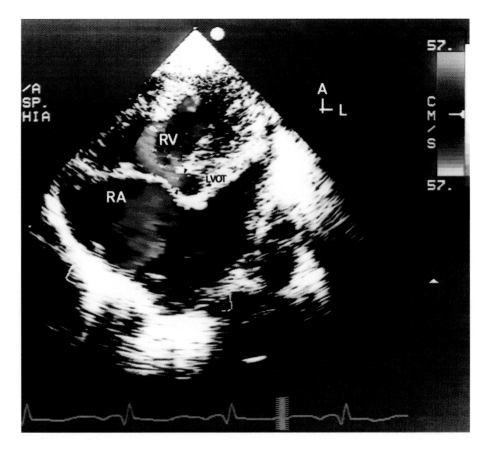

Figure 5: Modified parasternal short axis view of residual ventricular septal defect (unlabeled arrowheads). LVOT = left ventricular outflow tract; RA = right atrium; RV = right ventricle. Used with permission of American College of Chest Physicians.

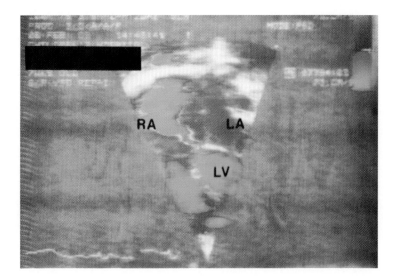

Figure 6: Apical view of a patient whose original defect was a large perimembranous ventricular septal defect. Following patch closure of this defect, the patient was left with a 3-mm left ventricle (LV)-to-right atrial (RA) jet. LA = left atrium.

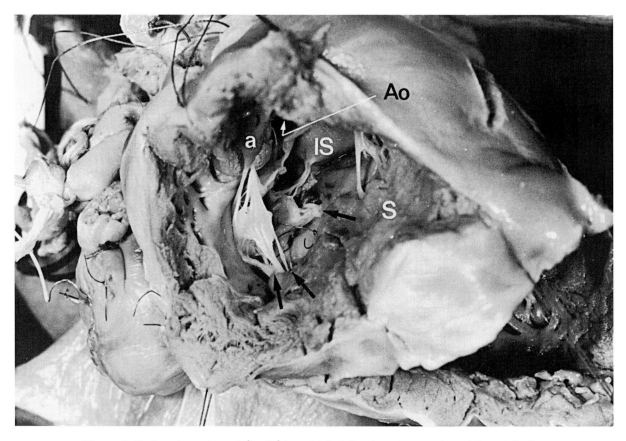

Figure 7: Postmortem view of the right ventricle following closure of an atrioventricular canal-type ventricular septal defect. (The patient who had transposition of the great arteries.) Note the numerous tricuspid valve attachments around the rim of the ventricular septal defect (black arrows). a = anterior papillary muscle; Ao = aortic outflow; IS = infundibular septum; S = right septal surface. Used with permission of American Journal of Cardiology.

Chapter 30

Atrioventricular Valves

A. Repair of Common Atrioventricular Canal

The sequelae of repair of the complete form of common atrioventricular canal are: mitral regurgitation, residual ventricular septal defect, residual left ventricle-to-right atrium shunt, residual left ventricular outflow tract obstruction, and mitral stenosis.

Mitral regurgitation can be due to unsuccessful valvoplasty (Figure 1) or to sudden dehiscence[1] (of either the valvoplasty itself or its suspension from the septal patch). Although theoretically the degree of preoperative regurgitation might be thought to correctly predict the degree of postoperative regurgitation, we have not found this to be the case (except in the rare situation in which true deficiency of valve tissue exists). Thus, whatever malcoaptation of leaflets exists preoperatively, artful valvoplasty can create a reasonably competent valve.

As for sudden dehiscence, the most important contribution of echocardiography is to provide evidence of a *change* in both valve morphology (Figure 2) and function (Figure 3); therefore, it seems advisable to perform an echocardiography/Doppler examination prior to hospital discharge in patients following repair of the complete form of common atrioventricular canal.

Mitral stenosis is rare and may be limited to patients with solitary left ventricular papillary muscle (Figure 4). Extensively suturing[2] the mitral "cleft" (septal commissure) can narrow the effective orifice (Figure 5).

B. Tricuspid Valvoplasty or Annuloplasty

In lesions such as hypoplastic left heart syndrome and transposition following Mustard (or Senning), tricuspid valve regurgitation can occasionally progress and become a significant hemodynamic problem. Two reconstructive approaches exist: reducing annular size (annuloplasty) and directly adjusting leaflet coaptation (valvoplasty). Annuloplasty appears to be more frequently successful, although numbers are small. Tricuspid valve replacement (Figures 6 and 7) is a last resort, largely because it does not appear to return the morphological right ventricle to a favorable geometry.

A variety of approaches also exist for the reconstruction of the tricuspid valve in Ebstein's anomaly.[3]

C. Mitral Valvoplasty or Annuloplasty

Excluding cases of common atrioventricular canal, need for mitral valve reconstruction[4] is relatively uncommon in childhood. As with the tricuspid valve, two basic approaches exist: annuloplasty or valvoplasty. For cases of isolated cleft mitral valve, valvoplasty is usually the chosen method. For regurgitation in the setting of ventricular dysfunction, annuloplasty is preferred.

D. Mitral Valve Replacement (St. Jude Valve)

"Malfunctions" of St. Jude valves consist of paravalvar leaks, impaired motion of one or both tilting discs due to fibrous tissue, or thrombosis causing obstruction of any of the three prosthesis orifices. Although the apical window (Figure 8) is helpful for stenosis detection, the shadow produced by closed disks (Figure 9) prevents the identification of regurgitation. Parasternal views (Figure 10) may help. Transesophageal imaging has markedly facilitated the assessment of artificial mitral valves.

E. Mitral Valve Replacement (Tissue Valve)

The use of porcine valves in infants and children has plummeted since the early 1980s. Frequently, valve regurgitation can be appreciated from transthoracic imaging, although transesophageal echocardiography has been very successful as well.

References

1. Chin AJ, Keane JF, Norwood WI, Castaneda AR. Complete common atrioventricular canal repair in infancy. *J Thorac Cardiovasc Surg* 1982; 84:437–445.

2. David I, Castaneda AR, Van Praagh R. Potentially parachute mitral valve in common atrioventricular canal: pathological anatomy and surgical importance. *J Thorac Cardiovasc Surg* 1982; 84:178–186.

3. Quaegebeur JM, Sreeram N, Fraser AG, Bogers AJJC, Stumper OFW, Hess J, Bos E, Sutherland GR. Surgery for Ebstein's anomaly: the clinical and echocardiographic evaluation of a new technique. *J Am Coll Cardiol* 1991; 17:722–728.

4. Stellin G, Bortolotti U, Mazzucco A, Faggian G, Guerra F, Daliento L, Livi U, Gallucci V. Repair of congenitally malformed mitral valve in children. *J Thorac Cardiovasc Surg* 1988; 95:480–485.

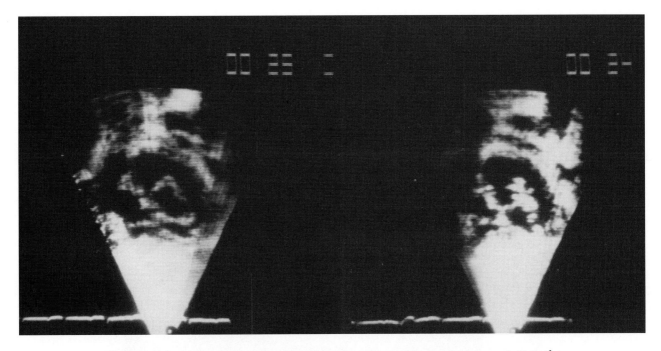

Figure 1: Subcostal sagittal view of transitional common atrioventricular canal. Note the triangular orifice in diastole (left panel) and the T-shaped coaptation line in systole (right panel).

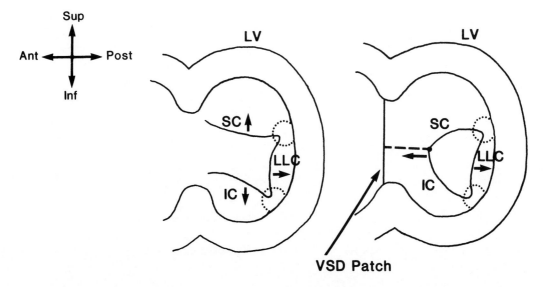

Figure 2: Schematic of repair that includes suturing the cleft (septal commissure), denoted by dashed line. **A:** preoperative arrangement. **B:** postoperative arrangement. IC = inferior leaflet; LLC = left lateral leaflet; SC = superior leaflet. Used with permission of American Journal of Cardiology.

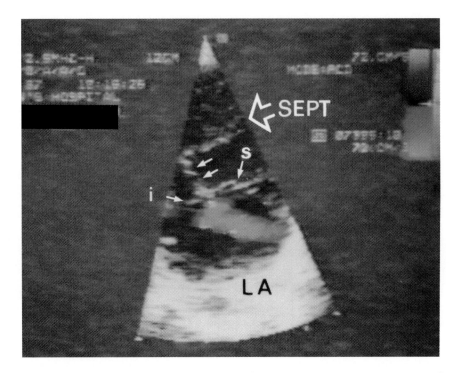

Figure 3: Modified parasternal short axis view of the sutured cleft (unlabeled arrows). There is mild mitral regurgitation. Compare with Figure 2B. i = inferior leaflet free edge; s = superior leaflet free edge; SEPT = interventricular septum.

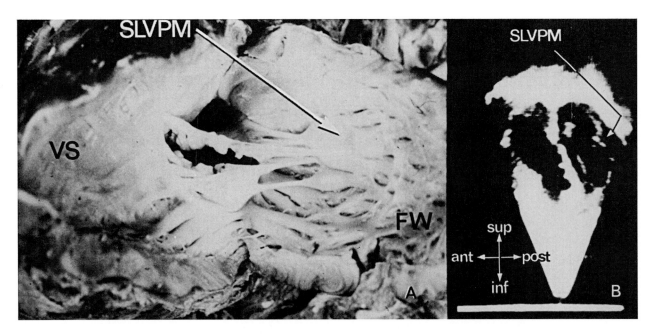

Figure 4: A: postmortem view of the left ventricle. A solitary papillary muscle (SLVPM) group is seen. FW = free wall; VS = ventricular septum. **B:** antemortem subcostal sagittal view of SLVPM.

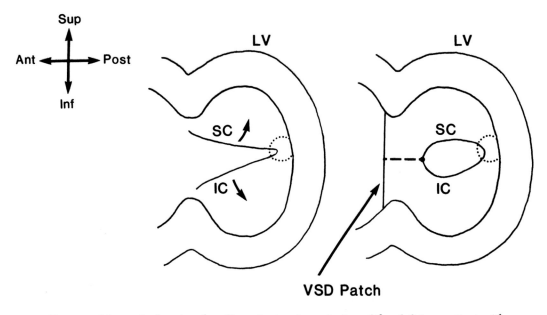

Figure 5: Schematic showing the effect of extensive suturing of the cleft in a patient with solitary left ventricular papillary muscle. Used with permission of the American Journal of Cardiology.

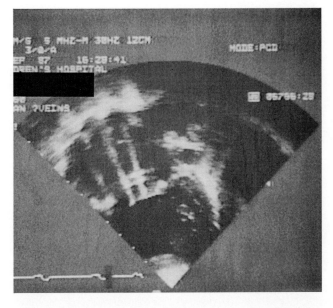

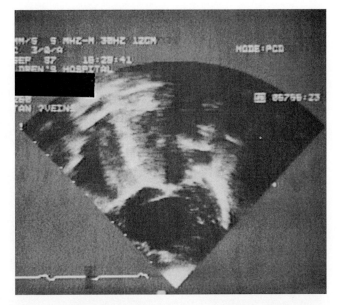

Figure 6: Apical view of prosthetic tricuspid valve (St. Jude) in the open position. This patient had previously undergone staged repair of hypoplastic left heart syndrome.

Figure 7: Apical view of the patient shown in Figure 6. In the closed position, the prosthesis "shadows" the right atrium, making the assessment of paravalvar regurgitation from this window impossible.

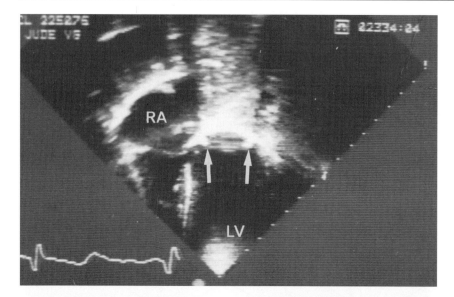

Figure 8: Apical view of St. Jude mitral prosthesis. Although the disks are difficult to resolve, the sewing ring (arrows) can be identified. LV = left ventricle; RA = right atrium.

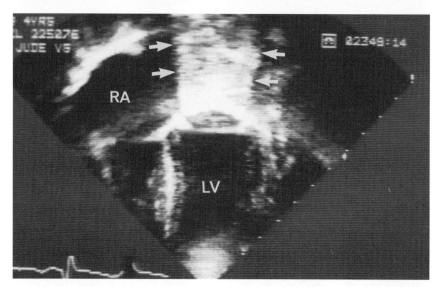

Figure 9: Apical view of patient shown in Figure 8. Shadowing by closed disks is recognized by the sharp "edges" (arrows); thus, it is easily distinguished from left atrial thrombus. LV = left ventricle; RA = right ventricle.

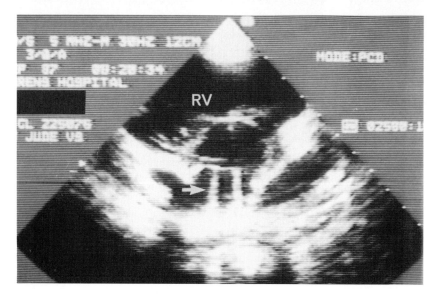

Figure 10: Parasternal short axis view of St. Jude disks in open position. RV = right ventricle.

Chapter 31

Atrial/Vena Caval/Pulmonary Venous Operations

A. Repair of Total Anomalous Pulmonary Venous Connection to Coronary Sinus

As suggested by Van Praagh,[1] the simplest method to repair this lesion is to unroof the coronary sinus (i.e., create a coronary sinus septal defect) and then patch-close the ostium (mouth) of the coronary sinus (Figure 1). This assumes that there is no obstruction *within* the coronary sinus itself. In cases where obstruction has been identified preoperatively, the unroofing must be extended (Figure 2) to include the site of the narrowing.

Subcostal imaging (frontal and left oblique views) can identify a residual shunt.

B. Repair of Partial Anomalous Pulmonary Venous Connection to the Right Superior Vena Cava

The redirection of an anomalous right pulmonary vein[2] can be accomplished by constructing an intra-caval baffle that encloses both the ostium of the right pulmonary vein and the high atrial septal defect. (In the rare case of anomalous right upper pulmonary vein and *intact* atrial septum, the surgeon first creates the atrial septal defect.) In order to avoid subsequent superior caval obstruction, a patch is utilized to augment the cava.

The potential sequelae of this repair are: obstruction of the right upper pulmonary vein, residual atrial-

level shunting through a peri-baffle leak, and obstruction of the right superior vena cava. In general, the greater the distance between the anomalous pulmonary vein and the left atrium, the more frequent are post-repair sequelae.

Suprasternal imaging is best to identify obstruction. In the infant, subcostal imaging may be successful, too.

C. Mustard Procedure

The most frequent hemodynamically important complications of the Mustard operation[3-5] are: (1) obstruction within the superior caval pathway,[6] and (2) obstruction within the pulmonary venous pathway.[7,8] Obstruction within the inferior caval pathway seems to be quite rare.

Aziz[9] reported a two-dimensional echocardiographic technique for displaying these venous pathways. It becomes harder to image the baffle from surface windows in the older child; transesophageal imaging facilitates display in these cases.

D. Senning Procedure

Obstruction of either the pulmonary or systemic venous pathway[10,11] is the most common hemodynamic complication of the Senning procedure.[12] The atrial compartments resemble two interlocking hemitori.[13,14] The pulmonary venous path can be displayed by the subcostal frontal (Figure 3) and sagittal (Figure

333

4) views. The superior and inferior caval paths can best be displayed by the left oblique (Figure 5) and right oblique (Figure 6) views, respectively. Ideally, at least two views (Figure 7) should be obtained of each structure. Pulmonary venous obstruction appears as a waist in the "outside" hemi-torus (Figure 8). Narrowing in the superior vena cava pathway occurs at the superior caval-(neo) right atrial junction.

Although diagnosis relied initially on dimension measurements, the advent of color Doppler-directed (Figure 9) pulsed Doppler interrogation has facilitated the recognition of pulmonary (Figure 10) and systemic venous pathway stenosis in infants. (Moreover, spin-echo and cine magnetic resonance imaging have allowed the identification of such residua in older children and in young adults.) As with most venous stenoses, the temporal pattern of flow[8] is more important than the absolute velocity. Mild obstruction is associated with mild elevation of maximal instantaneous velocity from 1 m/sec to 2 m/sec, with relative preservation of the phasic pattern distal to the narrowing. With severe obstruction, the phasic pattern is lost, and the dispersion of velocities is conspicuous with an often ill-defined envelope. The velocity waveform *proximal* to the narrowing remains laminar but decreases in amplitude and, with severe obstruction, becomes continuous.

Two-dimensional echocardiography is a noninvasive way of answering such questions as whether growth of the atrial compartments is affected by the age at repair. Over a 3-year period, 22 unselected early survivors of a Senning procedure for transposition of the great arteries or double-outlet right ventricle were assessed prospectively with the same scanning techniques as were employed in an earlier (retrospective) study.[13] Group I consisted of seven patients repaired as *neonates* (ages at operation 4 to 23 days, median 10 days), and group II consisted of 15 patients repaired after the first month of life (ages at operation 1.6 to 25 months, median 4.7 months). In group I, the oldest patient underwent augmentation of the neo-left atrium (pulmonary venous atrium) with in situ pericardium at the time of primary repair.[15] Theoretically, this type of pericardial flap should grow since its blood supply is not interrupted, remaining hinged on the right pulmonary hilum. In group II, five patients underwent neo-left atrium augmentation at the time of primary repair, four with a pericardial patch and one with in situ pericardium. Patients were followed for a median interval of 11 months.

In group I, superior and inferior vena cava dimension products remained in the normal range throughout the study period. In four out of seven (Figure 11), the pulmonary venous pathway dimension product remained above 200 but below 600 mm^2/m$^{4/3}$.

Two of these four underwent cardiac catheterization, confirming the absence of pulmonary venous obstruction; the other two have no clinical or roentgenographic evidence of pulmonary venous obstruction.

One group I patient (patient A, Figure 11) had an atypically small pulmonary venous pathway dimension product on the third postoperative day but was not tachypneic. Five and a half months later, his pulmonary venous dimension product was still small, but he now manifested marked tachypnea. Cardiac catheterization showed a 20 mm Hg mean gradient; after reoperation, his pulmonary venous dimension product returned to the normal range. Another group I patient (patient B, Figure 11) had a normal pulmonary venous pathway dimension product in the early postoperative period, cardiac catheterization (performed to rule out a residual right-to-left atrial-level shunt), confirming the absence of pulmonary venous obstruction. Four months later, the pulmonary venous dimension product had fallen to 80 mm^2/m$^{4/3}$. Because of low output syndrome, reoperation was undertaken emergently; the narrowest portion of the pulmonary venous pathway was "pinhole-sized." Following surgery, the pulmonary venous pathway dimension product returned to normal. Finally, the remaining group I patient (patient G, Figure 11) had a progressive increase in pulmonary venous pathway size, late postoperative catheterization proving the presence of moderate tricuspid regurgitation.

In group II, the superior and inferior vena cava dimension products remained above the lower limits of normal in all 15 patients, with cardiac catheterization data (available in 14) confirming the absence of gradients.

Of six with typical appearance of the neo-left atrium and normal pulmonary venous pathway dimension products throughout the study interval, five had confirmatory catheterization data, and the other has no clinical or roentgenographic evidence of pulmonary venous obstruction. Nine group II patients had pulmonary venous pathways outside the normal range or atypical appearance of the neo-left atrium and illustrated the entire spectrum of etiologies!

One patient (patient C, Figure 11) had a small pulmonary venous dimension product on the third postoperative day. After catheterization showed a 12 mm Hg gradient, reoperation was performed prior to hospital discharge.

Another patient (patient F, Figure 11) had a small pulmonary venous dimension product at both 19.9 and 32.0 months postoperatively; a 7 mm Hg mean gradient was measured at catheterizations following each echocardiogram.

Of four patients with a dimension product of >600 mm^2/m$^{4/3}$ at the time of their *first* postoperative echocardiogram, two had poor right ventricular shortening,[16,17] while the other two had severe tricuspid regurgitation at catheterization and have since undergone valve replacement.

Two patients were initially normal but developed large pulmonary venous pathways later. Patient H has a moderate-size residual ventricular septal defect, while patient D (Figure 11) developed severe bradycardia from sick sinus syndrome in the interval.

Finally, patient E (Figure 11) had a normal pulmonary venous dimension product; however, marked systolic pulsation of the supratricuspid portion of the neo-left atrium was observed. The portion of the neo-left atrium closest to the pulmonary vein orifices did not exhibit the systolic expansion. At catheterization, severe tricuspid regurgitation and an 11 mm Hg gradient between the proximal and distal portions of the neo-left atrium was noted. Thus, the *combination* of severe tricuspid regurgitation and moderate pulmonary venous pathway obstruction can be associated with a normal dimension product measurement.

Two-dimensional echocardiography illustrates that true *late-onset* pulmonary venous obstruction (patient B, Figure 11) can occur following the Senning procedure; prospective diagnosis of both early (i.e., residual) and late-onset pulmonary venous obstruction has been successful using two-dimensional imaging alone, except in the case (patient E, Figure 11) of *combined* tricuspid regurgitation and pulmonary venous obstruction. Since the incidence of late pulmonary venous obstruction in group I (1/7) and group II (2/15) were similar, early age at repair does not appear to predispose to poor atrial compartment growth.[18] Interestingly, the three patients with late pulmonary venous obstruction had all had augmentation of the neo-left atrium at the time of primary repair, suggesting that such a technique does not guarantee the avoidance of late-onset obstruction.

Rare sequelae of the Senning procedure include residual peri-baffle leak (Figure 12) and late dehiscence (Figure 13), both of which may be more easily seen with color flow mapping.

E. Bi-Directional Glenn Anastomosis; Hemi-Fontan

Modifications of the Glenn shunt (see Chapter 24, section A, 5) have had a resurgence in popularity for single ventricle malformations. Since the successful application of Fontan's principle depends on the presence of normal (systolic *and* diastolic) performance of the systemic ventricle and normal pulmonary vascular impedance, attention has focused on minimizing the mag-

nitude and duration of the volume overload imposed by the placement of a systemic artery-to-pulmonary artery shunt. As the pulmonary vascular impedance falls over the first 2 months of life, the Qp/Qs ratio rises to 2.0 or greater, depending on the caliber and length of the shunt. The volume load on the single ventricle thus becomes three times normal. In the adult, volume loads of this magnitude seen in chronic mitral or aortic regurgitation are often well tolerated for many years; however, this may not be the case in the infant, and efforts are under way to determine whether in fact the morphological *right* ventricle behaves differently from the morphological *left* ventricle. Removal of the volume overload (Figure 14) can certainly be accomplished after 4 months of age by takedown of the systemic artery-to-pulmonary artery shunt and construction of a bi-directional superior vena cava-to-pulmonary artery shunt.

Instead of the classic Glenn anastomosis, a side-to-side anastomosis of the superior vena cava and proximal right pulmonary artery can be constructed ("hemi-Fontan"), with the superior vena cava-to-right atrial junction being closed by a flap. The right and left pulmonary arteries thus remain in continuity with one another and, in fact, can be augmented at this time by patch plasty if the prior systemic-to-pulmonary artery shunt caused any distortions.

The evaluation of the patency of this type of Glenn can be done easily from the subcostal window (sagittal plane) or suprasternal window. Residual superior vena cava-to-right atrial leakage can be detected by color Doppler examination.

F. Modified Fontan Procedures

The Fontan procedure has undergone multiple changes in the last 10 years. Atrioventricular anastomoses have given way to atriopulmonary anastomoses (Figures 15 and 16); moreover, the latter have evolved from including a pulmonary venous baffle (Figure 17) to instead including a systemic venous baffle. Among the reasons why many surgeons abandoned the pulmonary venous baffle were frequent dilation of the right atrium, right atrial thrombi, and baffle-related pulmonary venous pathway obstruction (Figure 18 and section G, below). At present, many surgeons are experimenting with fenestrated variants. In 1989, Norwood additionally proposed that radical ventricular geometry changes (Figure 19) occurring following acute removal of volume overload may be the principal cause of low output and death early after Fontan[19,20] and that infants undergoing a *"Hemi-*Fontan" *instead* may better withstand the hemodynamic accompaniments of such geometry changes. Echocardiographic measurements confirm that the wall thickness/cavity ratio markedly increases early after Fontan in those patients who have not undergone previous hemi-Fontan (Figures 20 and 21).

One type of systemic venous baffle is that employed by Puga,[21] deLeval,[22] and Norwood[23] (Figure 22). A "tunnel" is created encompassing the superior and inferior caval orifices (Figure 23). In Norwood's version, the superior caval-right atrial junction is anastomosed side-to-side with the right pulmonary artery. (In many cases now this anastomosis is actually accomplished at an earlier Hemi-Fontan procedure.) The dam preventing superior vena cava flow from reaching the atrium is removed during Fontan completion (Figure 24). The systemic venous baffle is created with a hemi-cylindrical piece of polytetrafluorethylene (Figure 25).

There have only been two sequelae of this kind of baffle: (1) residual peri-baffle leaks (Figure 26), and (2) thrombus formation within (Figure 27), or rarely outside, the systemic venous pathway. The latter is usually easily displayed with subcostal frontal and sagittal views. Peri-baffle leaks have proved difficult to see, even with color flow mapping (Figure 26).

The prevalence of effusions is lower after some fenestration variants[24] and after partial hepatic vein exclusion,[25] although the mechanism is still not clear. Pulmonary artery flow following atriopulmonary anastomosis shows two antegrade peaks, one of which coincides with right atrial systole (Figure 28). Positive pressure retards pulmonary artery flow (Figure 29). Cessation of positive pressure and commencement of spontaneous breathing brings superimposition of normal biphasic pattern on a respiratory-dependent periodicity (Figure 30).

G. Repair of Other Types of Total Anomalous Pulmonary Venous Connection

The goal of this surgery is to create the most patulous connection between the confluence of pulmonary veins and the posterior aspect of the left atrium (Figure 31). The longest dimension is typically horizontal in the case of supracardiac anomalous connection. The anastomosis is usually on the posterosuperior aspect of the left atrium (Figure 32). As with other anastomoses, it is necessary to image in at least two orthogonal views (e.g., frontal and sagittal).

In infracardiac anomalous connection, the longest dimension is typically vertical (Figure 33). The anastomosis is usually on the postero-inferior aspect of the left atrium (Figure 34).

In mixed connection, there is no true confluence. Thus, results of repair depend on the success of reconstructing a confluence before anastomosing it to the left atrium.

The identification of postoperative obstruction[26,27] depends on performing a pullback of the pulsed Doppler sample volume from the confluence to the atrium (Figures 35 and 36). Vander Velde[28] reported an anastomotic area of >0.95 cm^2/m^2 in unobstructed survivors.

Recently, Fogel[29] reported that pulmonary venous obstruction following Fontan operation is often associated with relatively low velocities (Figure 37). The pulmonary venous flow pattern when pulmonary venous obstruction occurs in the patient with single ventricle and a systemic-to-pulmonary artery shunt has not yet been reported.

References

1. Van Praagh R, Harken AH, Delisle G, Ando M, Gross RE. Total anomalous pulmonary venous drainage to the coronary sinus: a revised procedure for its correction. *J Thorac Cardiovasc Surg* 1972; 64:132–135.

2. Williams WH, Zorn-Chelton S, Raviele AA, Michalik RE, Guyton RA, Dooley KJ, Hatcher CR. Extracardiac atrial pedicle conduit repair of partial anomalous pulmonary venous connection to the superior vena cava in children. *Ann Thorac Surg* 1984; 38:345–354.

3. Mustard WT, Keith JD, Trusler GA, Fowler R, Kidd L. The surgical management of transposition of the great vessels. *J Thorac Cardiovasc Surg* 1964; 48:953–958.

4. Williams WG, Trusler GA, Kirklin JW, Blackstone EH, Coles JG, Izukawa T, Freedom RM. Early and late results of a protocol for simple transposition leading to an atrial switch (Mustard) repair. *J Thorac Cardiovasc Surg* 1988; 95:717–726.

5. Ashraf MH, Cotroneo J, DiMarco D, Subramanian S. Fate of long-term survivors of Mustard procedure (inflow repair) for simple and complex transposition of the great arteries. *Ann Thorac Surg* 1986; 42:385–389.

6. Cobanoglu A, Abbruzzese PA, Freimanis I, Garcia CE, Grunkemeier G, Starr A. Pericardial baffle complications following the Mustard operation. *J Thorac Cardiovasc Surg* 1984; 87:371–378.

7. Berman MA, Barash PS, Hellenbrand W, Stansel HC, Talner NS. Late development of severe pulmonary venous obstruction following the Mustard operation. *Circulation* 1977; 56(Suppl II):II91–II94.

8. Smallhorn JF, Gow R, Freedom RM, Trusler GA, Olley P, Pacquet M, Gibbons J, Vlad P. Pulsed Doppler echocardiographic assessment of the pulmonary venous pathway after the Mustard or Senning procedure for transposition of the great arteries. *Circulation* 1986; 73:765–774.

9. Aziz KU, Paul MH, Bharati S, Cole RB, Muster AJ, Lev M, Idriss FS. Two dimensional echocardiographic evaluation of Mustard operation for d-transposition of the great arteries. *Am J Cardiol* 1981; 47:654–664.

10. deLeon VH, Hougen TJ, Norwood WI, Lang P, Marx GR, Castaneda AR. Results of the Senning operation for transposition of the great arteries with intact ventricular septum in neonates. *Circulation* 1984; 70(Suppl I):I-21 through I-25.

11. Matherne GP, Razook JD, Thompson WM, Lane MM, Murray CK, Elkins RC. Senning repair for transposition of the great arteries in the first week of life. *Circulation* 1985; 72:840–845.

12. Senning A. Correction of transposition of the great arteries. *Ann Surg* 1975; 182:287–292.

13. Chin AJ, Sanders SP, Williams RG, Lang P, Norwood WI, Castaneda AR. Two-dimensional echocardiographic assessment of caval and pulmonary venous pathways after the Senning operation. *Am J Cardiol* 1983; 52:118–126.

14. Baudet EM, Hafez A, Choussat A, Roques X. Isolated ventricular inversion with situs solitus: successful surgical repair. *Ann Thorac Surg* 1986; 41:91–94.

15. Guyton RA, Dorsey LM, Silberman MS, Hawkins HK, Williams WH, Hatcher CR. The broadly based pericardial flap. *J Thorac Cardiovasc Surg* 1984; 87:619–625.

16. Turina ML, Siebenmann R, von Segesser L, Schonbeck M, Senning A. Late functional deterioration after atrial correction for transposition of the great arteries. *Circulation* 1989; 80(Suppl I):I-162–I-167.

17. Trowitzsch E, Colan SD, Sanders SP. Global and regional right ventricular function in normal infants and infants with transposition of the great arteries after Senning operation. *Circulation* 1985; 72:1008–1014.

18. Henry WL, Ware J, Gardin JM, Hepner SI, McKay J, Weiner M. Echocardiographic measurements in normal subjects. Growth-related changes that occur between infancy and early adulthood. *Circulation* 1978; 57:278–285.

19. Chin AJ, Franklin WH, Andrews BA, Norwood WI. Changes in ventricular geometry early after Fontan's operation. *Ann Thorac Surg* 1993 (in press).

20. Rychik J, Lieb DR, Jacobs ML, Norwood WI, Chin AJ. Early changes in ventricular geometry following removal of volume overload. *Cardiol in the Young* 1993; 3:12 (abstract).

21. Puga FJ, Chiavarelli M, Hagler DJ. Modification of the Fontan operation applicable to patients with left atrioventricular valve atresia or single atrioventricular valve. *Circulation* 1987; 76(Suppl III):III-53–60.

22. deLeval MR, Kilner P, Gewillig M, Bull C. Total cavopulmonary connection: a logical alternative to atriopulmonary connection for complex Fontan operations. *J Thorac Cardiovasc Surg* 1988; 96:682–695.

23. Norwood WI, Jacobs ML, Murphy JD. Fontan procedure for hypoplastic left heart syndrome. *Ann Thorac Surg* 1992; 54:1025–1029.

24. Bridges ND, Mayer JE, Lock JE, Jonas RA, Hanley FL, Keane JF, Perry SB, et al. Effect of baffle fenestration on outcome of the modified Fontan operation. *Circulation* 1992; 86:1762–1769.

25. Jacobs ML, Norwood WI. Fontan's operation: influence of modifications on morbidity and mortality (submitted).

26. Smallhorn JF, Burrows P, Wilson G, Coles J, Gilday DL, Freedom RM. Two-dimensional and pulsed Doppler echocardiography in the postoperative evaluation of total anomalous pulmonary venous connection. *Circulation* 1987; 76:298–305.

27. Leung MP, Cheung DLC, Lau KC. Echocardiographic diagnosis of anastomotic stricture following surgical correction of supracardiac total anomalous pulmonary venous connection. *Am Heart J* 1987; 114:1518–1520.

28. Van der Velde ME, Parness IA, Colan SD, Spevak PJ, Lock JE, Mayer JE, Sanders SP. Two-dimensional echocardiography in the pre- and postoperative management of total anomalous pulmonary venous connection. *J Am Coll Cardiol* 1991; 18:1746–1751.

29. Fogel MA, Chin AJ. Imaging of pulmonary venous pathway obstruction in patients after the modified Fontan procedure. *J Am Coll Cardiol* 1992; 20:181–190.

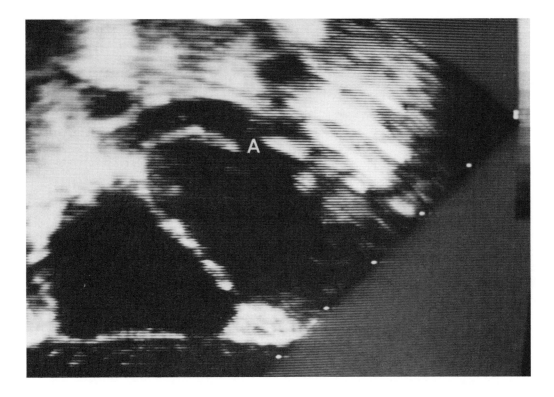

Figure 1: Subcostal frontal view of repair of total anomalous pulmonary venous connection to coronary sinus. The coronary sinus has been unroofed and its ostium completely patch-closed. The narrowest point (A) is thus the junction of the confluence to the proximal coronary sinus.

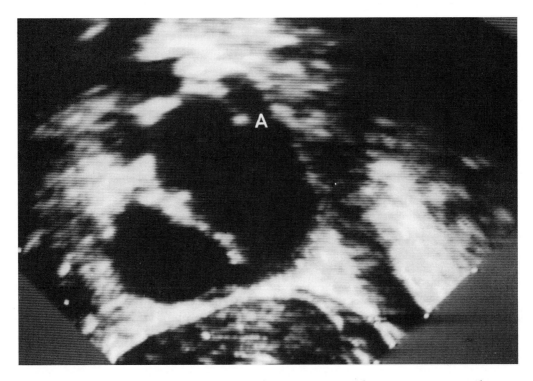

Figure 2: Subcostal sagittal view of patient shown in Figure 1. The coronary sinus roof has been completely excised. The junction (A) between the confluence and the coronary sinus has not been touched.

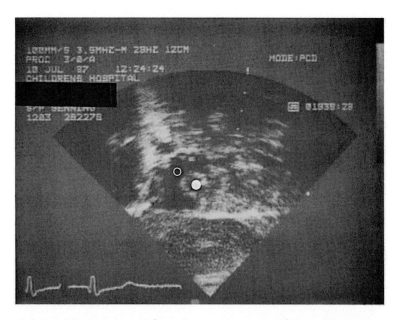

Figure 3: Subcostal frontal view of the pulmonary venous pathway after Senning's operation (open circle). It wraps around the systemic venous pathway (closed circle).

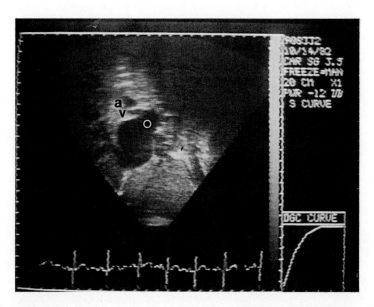

Figure 4: Subcostal sagittal view to the right of the systemic venous pathway. The pulmonary venous pathway's narrowest point is denoted by the open circle. a = right pulmonary artery; v = right upper pulmonary vein.

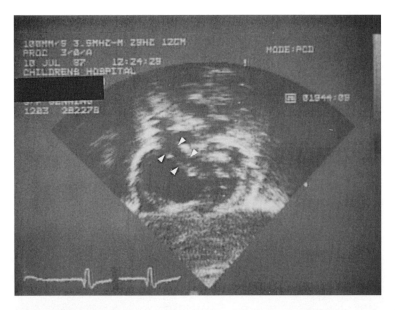

Figure 5: Subcostal left oblique view of the superior vena caval pathway (arrowheads).

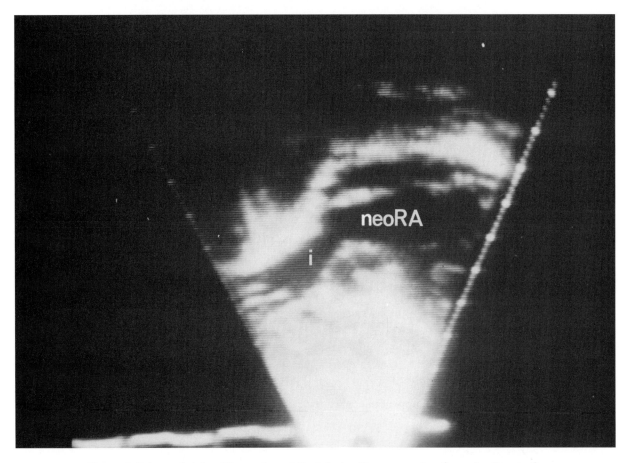

Figure 6: Subcostal right oblique view of the inferior (i) vena caval pathway leading to the neo-right atrium (neo-RA).

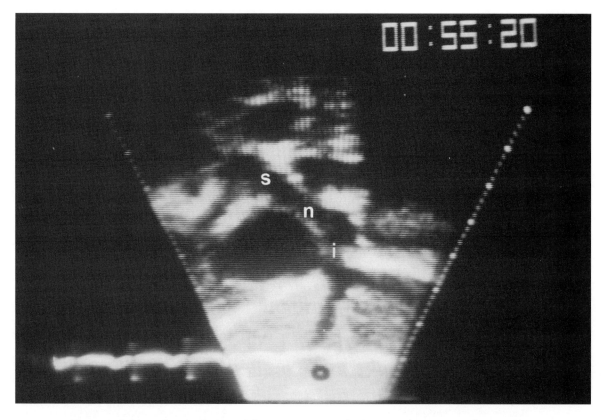

Figure 7: Subcostal sagittal view of the superior (s) and inferior (i) vena cava pathway after Senning's operation. n = neo-right atrium.

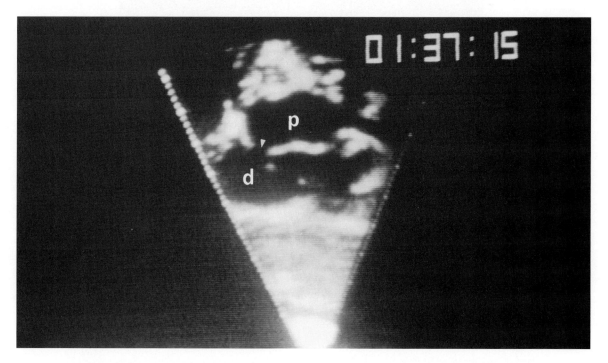

Figure 8: Subcostal frontal view of pulmonary venous pathway obstruction (arrowhead). d = distal portion of pulmonary venous pathway; p = proximal portion of pulmonary venous pathway.

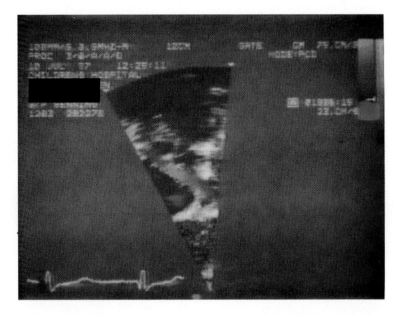

Figure 9: Doppler color flow mapping, sagittal view. At this moment the superior vena caval flow reaches the inferior vena cava.

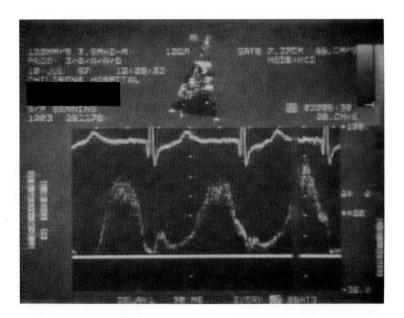

Figure 10: Pulsed Doppler display of pulmonary venous flow, subcostal frontal view. Flow is phasic and laminar.

PULMONARY VENOUS PATHWAY DIMENSION PRODUCT

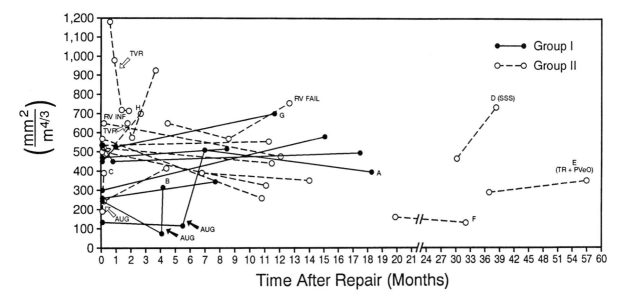

Figure 11: Pulmonary venous pathway dimension product (i.e., frontal dimension normalized to cube root of BSA × sagittal dimension normalized to cube root of BSA) vs. time after Senning repair. Group I = 7 patients repaired as neonates. Group II = 15 patients repaired after the first month of life. AUG = surgical augmentation of pulmonary venous pathway; FAIL = failure; INF = infarction; PVeO = pulmonary venous obstruction; SSS = sick sinus syndrome; TR = tricuspid regurgitation; TVR = tricuspid valve replacement.

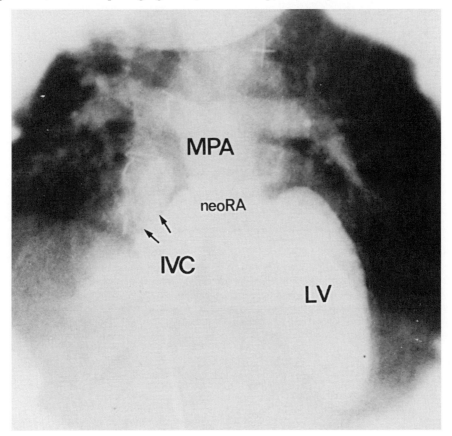

Figure 12: Hepatoclavicular angiogram showing small right-to-left leak in the inferior vena caval (IVC) portion of the systemic venous pathway following Senning's operation. LV = left ventricle; MPA = main pulmonary artery; neoRA = neo-right atrium.

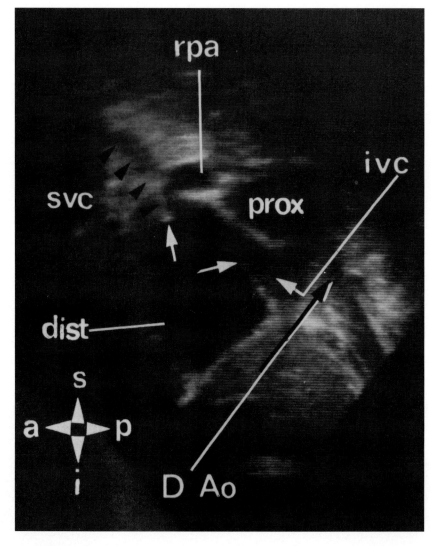

Figure 13: Subcostal sagittal view of the systemic venous pathway following Senning's operation. Much of the suture line involved in the creation of the systemic venous pathway has dehisced, leaving a large atrial level communication (unlabeled arrows). DAo = descending aorta; dist = distal portion of pulmonary venous pathway; ivc = inferior vena cava; prox = proximal portion of pulmonary venous pathway; rpa = right pulmonary artery; svc = superior vena cava. Used with permission of American Journal of Cardiology.

RVED VOLUME

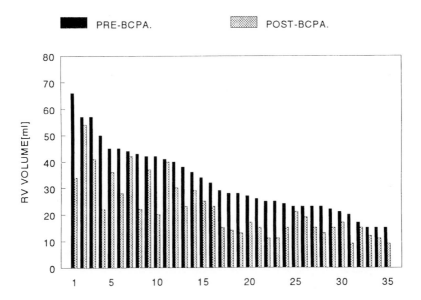

Figure 14: Right ventricular end-diastolic (RVED) volume before and 1 week after Hemi-Fontan (BCPA) for hypoplastic heart syndrome. Used with permission of Elsevier Publishing.

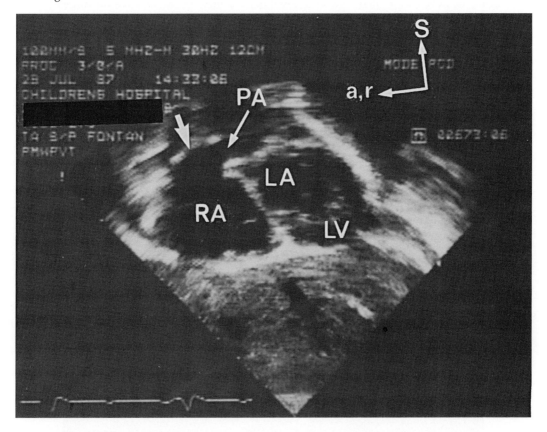

Figure 15: Subcostal left oblique view of atriopulmonary (unlabeled arrow) anastomosis for tricuspid atresia. LA = left atrium; LV = left ventricle; PA = proximal right pulmonary artery; RA = right atrium.

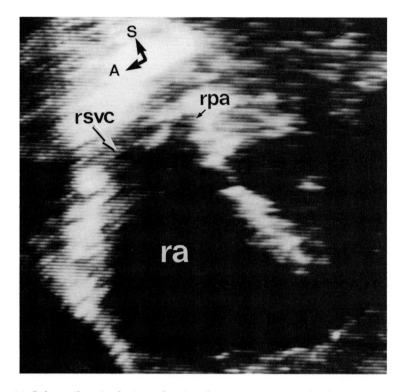

Figure 16: Subcostal sagittal view of atriopulmonary anastomosis. One reason surgeons have abandoned the pulmonary venous baffle is that the right atrium (ra) frequently becomes markedly dilated, as in this patient. Note how the right atrium dwarfs the right pulmonary artery (rpa) and right superior vena cava (rsvc).

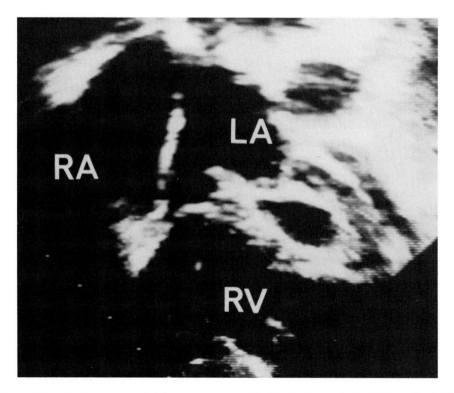

Figure 17: Apical view of a "pulmonary venous" baffle (in hypoplastic left heart) which redirects left atrial blood through the surgically widened atrial septal defect toward the tricuspid valve and right ventricle (RV). RA = right atrium; LA = left atrium.

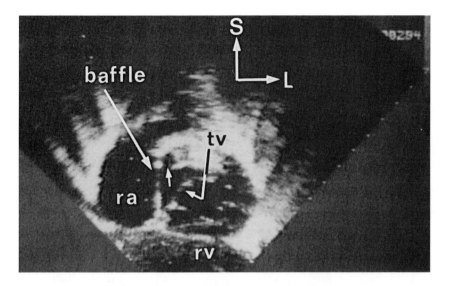

Figure 18: Subcostal frontal view of pulmonary venous baffle in hypoplastic left heart syndrome. Pulmonary venous pathway obstruction (unlabeled arrow) has occurred because the baffle has protruded far to the left. tv = tricuspid valve; ra = right atrium; rv = right ventricle.

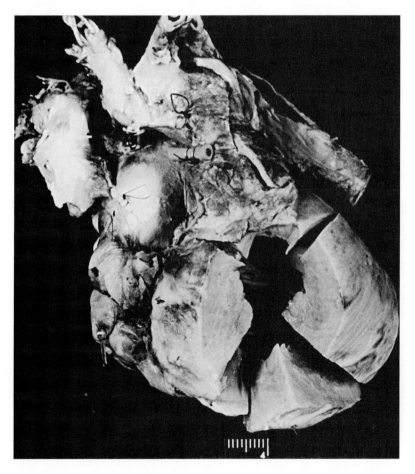

Figure 19: Postmortem view of right ventricle following Fontan operation for hypoplastic left heart syndrome. The total ruler segment is 10 mm. Note the high wall thickness/cavity dimension ratio. This patient had not undergone prior hemi-Fontan. Used with permission of Elsevier Science Publishing.

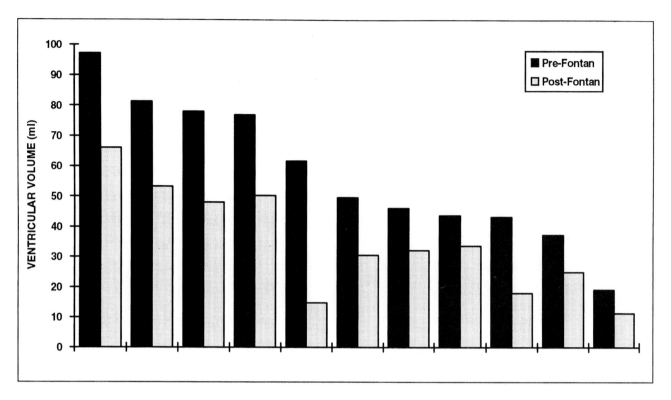

Figure 20: Left ventricular end-diastolic volume before and 1 week after Fontan operation. None of these patients had undergone a prior hemi-Fontan. Used with permission of Elsevier Publishing.

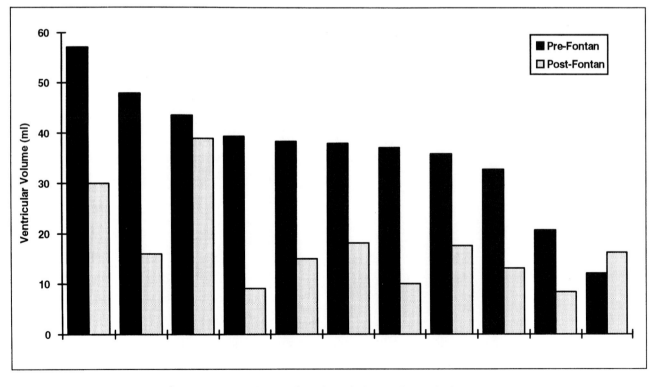

Figure 21: Right ventricular end-diastolic volume before and 1 week after Fontan operation. None of these patients had undergone a prior hemi-Fontan. Used with permission of Elsevier Publishing.

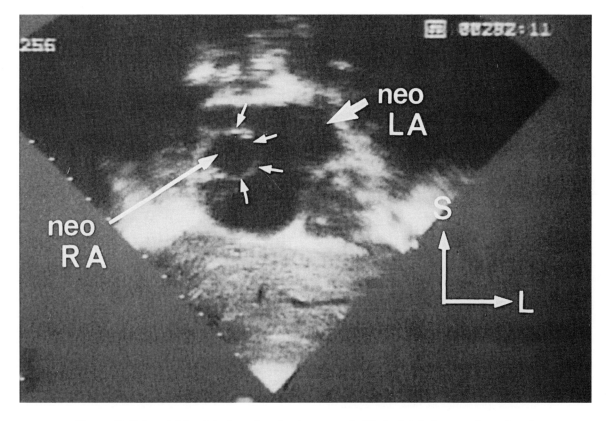

Figure 22: Subcostal frontal view of systemic venous baffle (unlabeled arrows) employed in 1993 modified Fontan operation. neo-LA = neo-left atrium; neo-RA = neo-right atrium. Compare with Figure 3. Note that in the Senning, the neo-RA is to the patient's left. In the Fontan, the neo-RA is to the right.

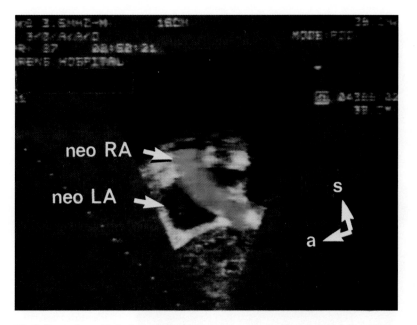

Figure 23: Subcostal sagittal view of the systemic venous pathway following Fontan operation. Note that at this moment inferior vena caval return predominates. (Superior vena cava flow is not seen.)

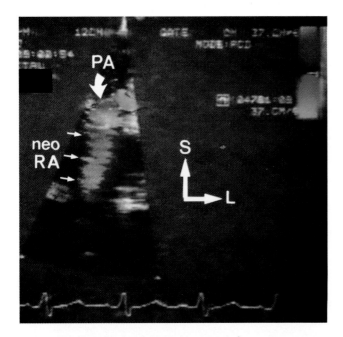

Figure 24: Suprasternal frontal view of the superior vena cava-to-right pulmonary anastomosis-neo RA three-way intersection. The superior caval-right PA anastomosis is formed at the hemi-Fontan stage; to complete the Fontan, the superior vena cava-atrial communication is restored and the inferior vena caval orifice is included by the placement of systemic venous baffle.

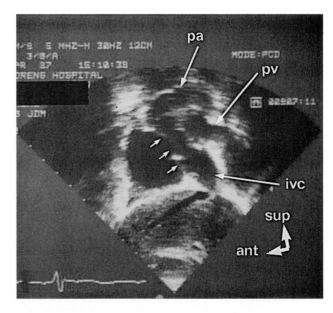

Figure 25: Subcostal sagittal view of the polytetrafluorethylene baffle comprising most of the anterior aspect of the systemic venous pathway (unlabeled arrows). ivc = inferior vena cava; pa = right pulmonary artery; pv = right lower pulmonary vein.

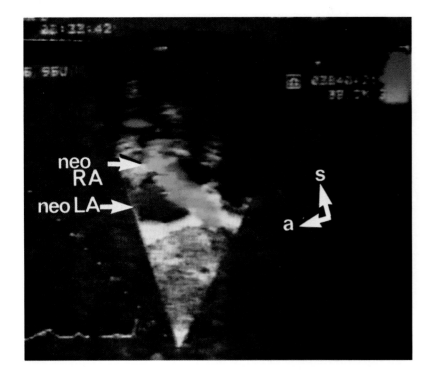

Figure 26: Subcostal sagittal view of Fontan. Doppler color flow mapping facilitates the identification of small residual peri-baffle leaks by providing a sharp color boundary as a background. This patient does not appear to have any atrial-level shunt.

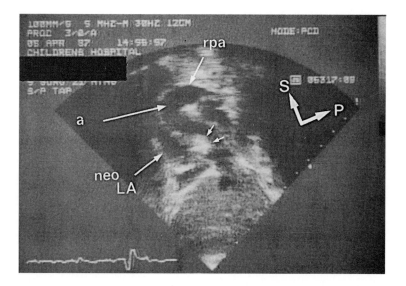

Figure 27: Subcostal sagittal view of a thrombus (unlabeled arrows) within the systemic venous pathway. Compare with Figure 25. a = anastomosis of the superior vena cava-right junction with the right pulmonary artery (rpa).

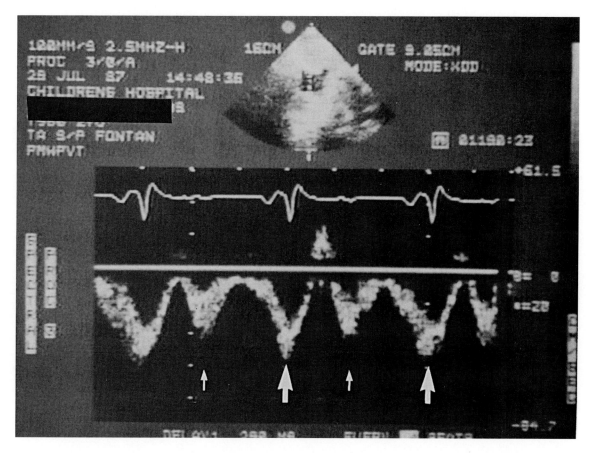

Figure 28: Biphasic antegrade pulmonary artery flow. One peak (large arrow) coincides with right atrial systole.

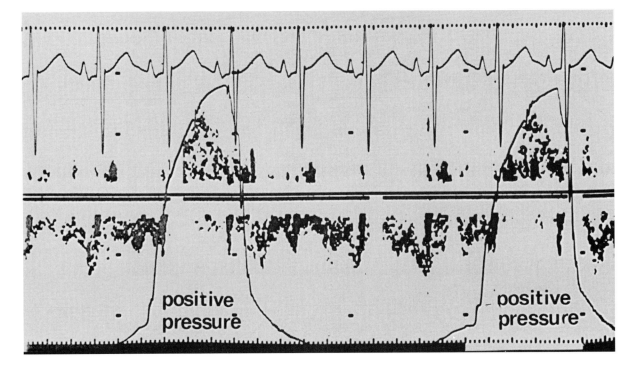

Figure 29: Effect of positive pressure (delivered by ventilator) on pulmonary artery flow. Note that flow becomes retrograde (above baseline) coincident with burst of positive pressure.

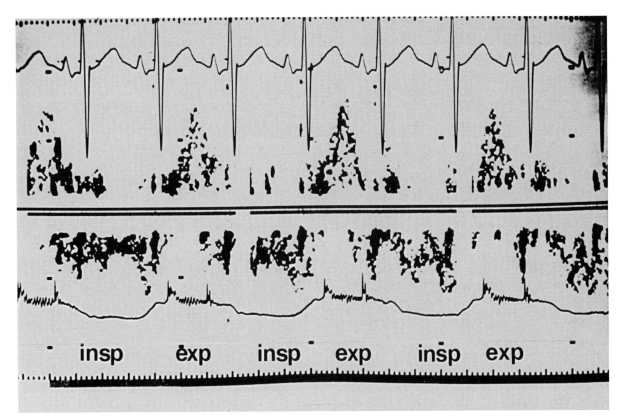

Figure 30: Pulmonary artery flow with spontaneous breathing. Flow is antegrade (below baseline) during inspiration (insp) and retrograde (above baseline) during expiration (exp).

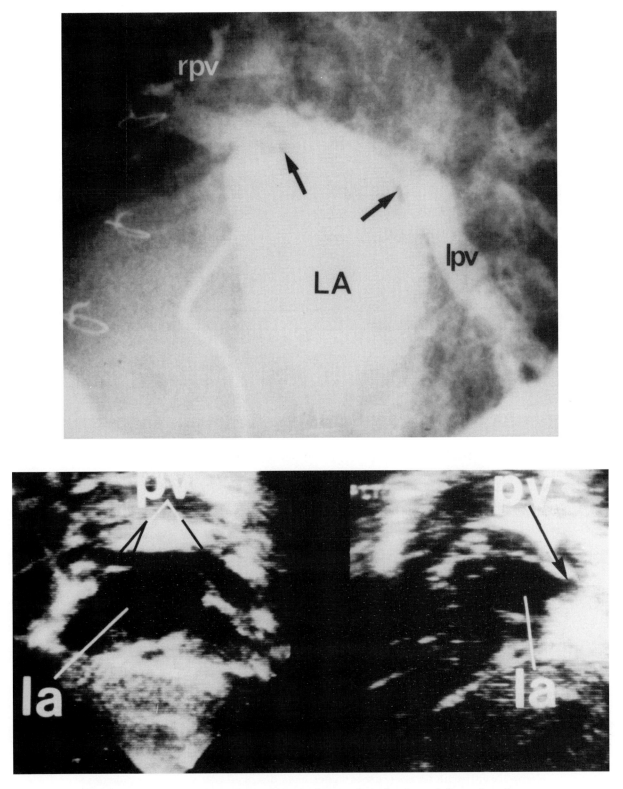

Figure 31: Top: Hepatoclavicular angiogram showing large horizontal dimension of anastomosis (arrows). LA = left atrium; lpv = left pulmonary vein; rpv = right pulmonary vein. **Bottom left:** Subcostal frontal view of patulous anastomosis. **Bottom right:** Subcostal sagittal view of the same anastomosis, illustrating the small vertical dimension.

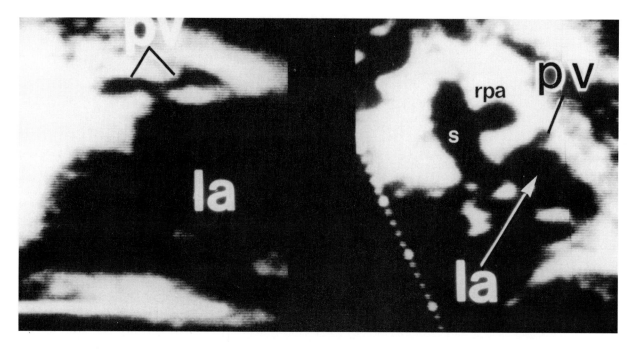

Figure 32: Left: Subcostal frontal view of anastomosis in supracardiac total anomalous pulmonary venous connection. **Right:** Subcostal sagittal view of anastomosis. Note that the anastomosis is situated on the posterosuperior aspect of the left atrium. rpa = right pulmonary artery; s = superior vena cava; pv = pulmonary vein.

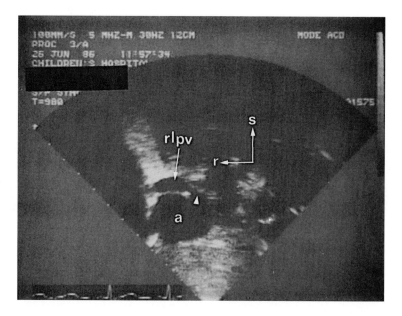

Figure 33: Subcostal frontal view of a patient who had undergone repair of infracardiac total anomalous pulmonary venous connection. This sector is very inferior; the anastomosis (arrowhead) is quite narrow (4 mm in the horizontal direction). rlpv = right lower pulmonary vein.

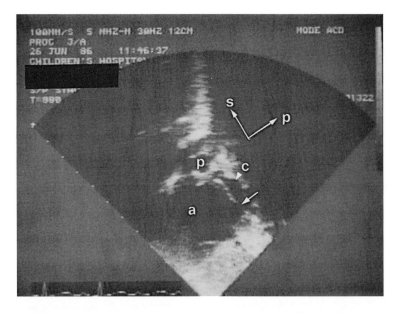

Figure 34: Subcostal sagittal view of patient shown in Figure 33. The confluence (c)-to-atrial (a) anastomosis (unlabeled arrow) is in an extremely inferior location on the back of the left atrium. Its vertical dimension was 5 mm.

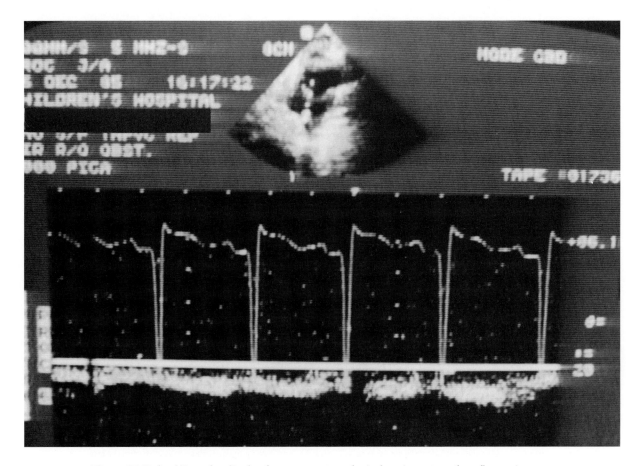

Figure 35: Pulsed Doppler display from suprasternal window (near top of confluence), same patient as shown in Figure 34. Flow is low-velocity, continuous, and laminar.

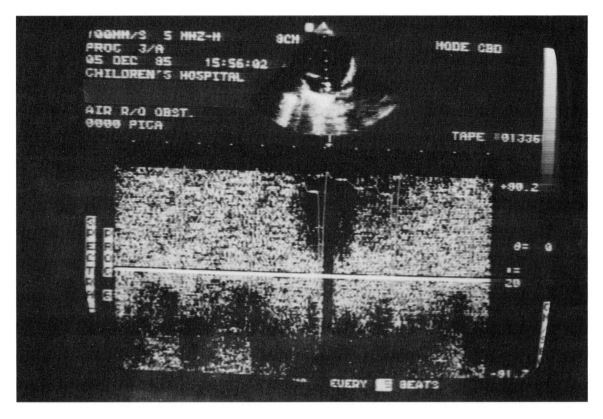

Figure 36: Pulsed Doppler display from subcostal window (adjacent to anastomosis), same patient as in Figure 34. Flow is high-velocity, continuous, and turbulent.

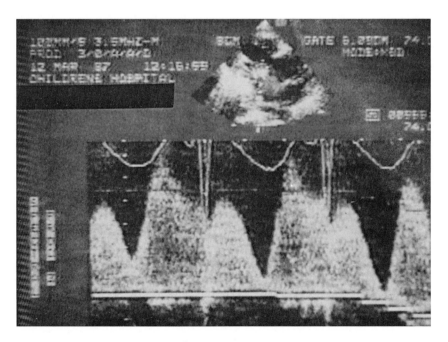

Figure 37: Pulsed Doppler display with sample volume next to anastomosis. Pulmonary venous flow is still phasic and its maximal velocity is <2 m/sec; however, flow is clearly turbulent. This Fontan patient had undergone repair of infracardiac total anomalous pulmonary venous connection as a neonate. The confluence-to-atrial anastomosis was narrow (4 mm diameter) at postmortem examination.

Chapter 32

Surgery of the Atrial Septum

A. Balloon Atrial Septotomy

Rashkind and Miller[1] reported the technique of atrial septal defect (ASD) creation using a balloon-tipped catheter. The success of this technique, still widely used for transposition of the great arteries after a quarter century, depends on the presence of a thin septum primum (flap valve of the foramen ovale). Although the septum primum in the neonate is almost always 1 mm or less in thickness, conspicuous exceptions are some patients with left atrioventricular valve underdevelopment (e.g., hypoplastic left heart syndrome). In the latter, approximately 5% have congenitally closed (or nearly closed) foramen ovale; the thickness of the septum primum is >1 mm in these cases.

The appearance of the fractured septum primum tissue is that of a flail element. There is no doubt that at the extremes of ASD size, two-dimensional echocardiography, with or without color Doppler echocardiography, aids in management. (With a ≤3 mm dimension, the ASD is virtually always severely restrictive; with a ≥8 mm dimension, enlarging the ASD further will not be helpful).

As with the pre-balloon atrial septotomy (BAS) situation, the patient with left atrioventricular valve underdevelopment demands special care. The left oblique view must be utilized because of the unusual topology of the atrial septum in 40% (see Chapter 8, section D). BAS may be more hazardous in this subset than it is in ordinary simple transposition of the great arteries. Whether BAS actually produces a nonrestrictive hole should be assessed with color Doppler imaging in at least two views.

B. Blalock-Hanlon Atrial Septectomy

The position of the Blalock-Hanlon septectomy[2] defect is posterior to the septum primum. It lies in the sinus venosus portion of the septum. Although it could conceivably be mistaken for a natural sinus venosus defect of the superior vena cava type or a sinus venosus defect of the inferior vena cava type, it is typically larger than either of these. The frontal sweep demonstrates the posterior and rightward location of a Blalock-Hanlon defect (Figure 1 and 2).

The sagittal sweep is also useful.

C. Open Atrial Septectomy in Left Atrioventricular Valve Underdevelopment Associated with Leftward Deviation of Superior Attachments of Septum Primum

The widest such excisions frequently leave the appearance of abolishing the distinctive features of the left atrium; in other words, the pulmonary veins appear as though they are draining directly into the right atrium with no intervening chamber. The presumed reason for this appearance is the initial small left atrial cavity size in patients with leftward deviation of superior attachment of septum primum.[3]

Because of this phenomenon, it is difficult to distinguish residual obstruction at the atrial septal level from pulmonary venous ostial stenosis by two-dimensional echocardiography alone. Often the dimension of the pulmonary venous ostium may be similar to the residual ASD. Color Doppler should help in such situations by localizing the site at which there is a change in velocity.

The subcostal frontal view is unreliable (see Chapter 8, section D); the subcostal left oblique view must be used because of the spatial orientation of the septum primum.

D. Closure of the Secundum Atrial Septal Defect

The only residua from this operation that the imaging lab can help diagnose are pericardial effusion, which occurs in roughly one-third of patients,[4] and residual ASD (which is rare except when the method of closure is transcatheter placement[5-7] of a double-disk device). The latter technique is also effectively monitored in the catheterization laboratory by transesophageal imaging.

References

1. Rashkind WJ, Miller WW. Creation of an atrial septal defect without thoracotomy: a palliative approach to complete transposition of the great arteries. *JAMA* 1966; 196:173–174.

2. Blalock A, Hanlon CR. The surgical treatment of complete transposition of the aorta and the pulmonary artery. *Surg Gynecol Obstet* 1950; 90:1–15.

3. Chin AJ, Weinberg PM, Barber G. Subcostal two-dimensional echocardiographic detection of anomalous attachment of septum primum in patients with left atrioventricular valve underdevelopment. *J Am Coll Cardiol* 1990; 15:1645–1653.

4. Chin AJ, Jacobs ML. Etiology of postoperative effusions. *Circulation* 1993; 88:I56 (abstract).

5. Lock JE, Rome JJ, Davis R, Van Praagh S, Perry SB, Van Praagh R, Keane JF. Transcatheter closure of atrial septal defects: experimental studies. *Circulation* 1989; 79:1091–1099.

6. Rome JJ, Keane JF, Perry SB, Spevak PJ, Lock JE. Double umbrella closure of atrial defects: initial clinical applications. *Circulation* 1990; 82:751–758.

7. Hellenbrand WE, Fahey JT, McGowan FX, Weltin GG, Kleinman CS. Transesophageal echocardiographic guidance of transcatheter closure of atrial septal defects. *Am J Cardiol* 1990; 66:207–213.

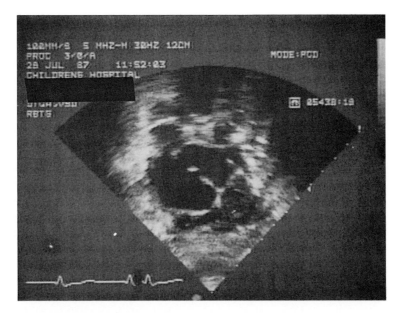

Figure 1: Subcostal frontal sweep at the level of the superior vena cava–right atrial junction. The defect is beginning to be seen.

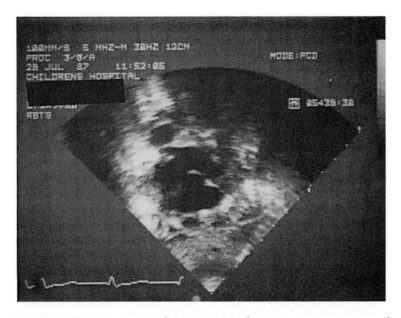

Figure 2: Subcostal frontal sweep slightly inferior to the plane of Figure 1. Note the superior vena cava is no longer visible; however, the defect is even larger than in Figure 1. There is very little distance between the right pulmonary vein and the posterior aspect of the defect.

Chapter 33

The Diaphragm

Two questions involving the diaphragmatic region are: Is there a pleural effusion? and Does the diaphragm move? Pleural supradiaphragmatic effusions in the supine patient usually layer in the posterior thorax. Thus, the transverse abdominal view (Figure 1) will demonstrate a collection posterior to the right lobe of the liver (right hemithorax) or posterior to the stomach (left hemithorax). The effusion can be tracked as the transducer is angled cranially (Figure 2 and 3). As the size of the effusion increases, it becomes easier to visualize collapsed pulmonary parenchyma "floating" within the effusion. The presence of this sign on the left side allows the examiner to distinguish a left pleural effusion from a pericardial effusion.

Another question regarding the diaphragm that can be answered in a straightforward manner is whether there is a phrenic palsy.[1] The most common clinical setting for this question is in the postoperative infant who cannot be successfully liberated from the ventilator. The transverse abdominal view outlines a section of the saddle-shaped hemidiaphragm. In the normal patient, there is a conspicuous change in this outline with inspiration.

Reference

1. Balaji S, Kunovsky P, Sullivan I. Ultrasound in the diagnosis of diaphragmatic paralysis after operation for congenital heart disease. *Br Heart J* 1990; 64:20–22.

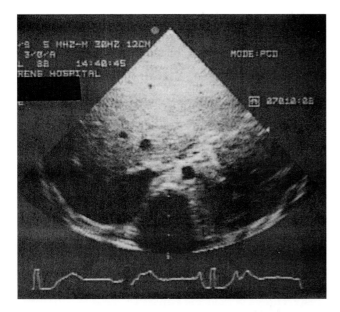

Figure 1: Transverse abdominal view at a level just above the renal poles. The right pleural effusion is seen in the posterior portion of the hemithorax.

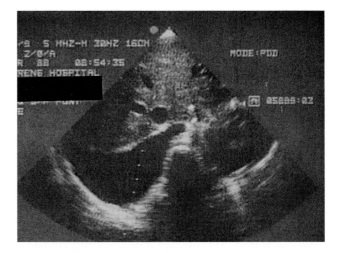

Figure 2: The transducer has begun to be angled cranially from the plane of Figure 1.

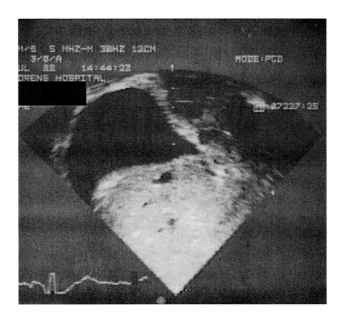

Figure 3: The sector has almost reached the heart. The image orientation has been "flipped" to display the thorax at the top of the screen and the liver at the bottom.

Chapter 34

Postoperative Magnetic Resonance Imaging:
Form and Function

Mark Alan Fogel, MD

A. Three-Dimensional Reconstruction

The technical aspects of three-dimensional reconstruction and its preoperative applications have been discussed in Chapter 20. There are postoperative circumstances where three-dimensional reconstruction may be particularly useful.

1. Extracardiac Conduits and Intracardiac Baffles

There are numerous lesions, such as transposition of the great arteries with a ventricular septal defect and pulmonic stenosis, tetralogy of Fallot with pulmonary atresia and confluent branch pulmonary arteries, as well as certain types of coarctation of the aorta or left ventricular outflow tract obstructions, which are amenable to corrective surgery with external conduits, such as right ventricle-to-pulmonary artery,[1-4] or apical-aortic conduits.[5-7] The course and extent of these conduits may not be appreciated well on either angiocardiography or echocardiography. MRI can obtain better tomographic images of these conduits, but shaded surface displays can give a three-dimensional view of the full course and extent of the conduit (Figure 1), including the presence and location of any stenoses. The image can be rotated about any axis to obtain the best view of the areas in question.

Single ventricles require partitioning of the atria into systemic and pulmonary venous pathways (Fontan reconstruction) so that all systemic venous return is baffled directly into the pulmonary arteries.[8-10] This procedure may cause obstruction in either one of the pathways if the atrial partition is not created correctly[9,10]; therefore, defining the anatomy of the baffle is of practical importance (Figure 2). Transthoracic echocardiography has only been useful in the young patient.

Figure 3 depicts the three-dimensional reconstruction of a patient with supero-inferior ventricles and pseudo criss-cross atrioventricular relationships (see Chapter 14) after a Senning procedure[11-13] (see Chapter 20). With standard tomographic imaging, the spatial relationship of the systemic ("*neo-right*") and pulmonary ("*neo-left*") venous pathways are not well appreciated.

Figure 4 shows a patient with transposition of the great arteries {S,L,L} and tricuspid atresia, with a restrictive bulboventricular foramen causing subaortic stenosis. The patient has had both a Fontan reconstruction and an apical-aortic conduit. Figure 5 shows the three-dimensional reconstruction of the patient shown in Figure 4.

B. Oblique Sectioning

Another type of three-dimensional reconstruction which is performed internally by the computer and displayed in a two-dimensional tomographic format is sectioning the volumetric data set at an *oblique* plane to visualize structures not well seen in the original plane.[14] Similar to conventional three-dimensional reconstruction, the software stacks images (for example, axial) on top of each other noting the thickness of the slice, and, when the oblique plane is prescribed by the user, "cuts" the volumetric data set in that plane by adding up only those pixels defined by that plane and constructing a new image. This image is then interpolated to smooth out the features of the oblique picture. Multiple parallel slices at the oblique angle may be generated to create a new volumetric data set at that angle. The user may also view planes at multiple complex angles by initially prescribing a plane from the original data set and subsequently prescribing planes from the computer-generated images of the oblique planes.

The advantages and uses of this technique are obvious. Oblique sectioning takes considerably less time to accomplish than three-dimensional reconstruction as described above (3 minutes vs. 4–5 hours). Only one volumetric data set needs to be acquired. Any oblique plane through the thorax or oblique volumetric data set may then be created, thus decreasing imaging time on the magnet. The images can be virtually indistinguishable from real-time images. A user may try many planes in a short period of time to obtain the optimal image to display the anatomy. For example, "candy cane views" of coarctation of the aorta may be generated from axial data sets, or in cases of nonconfluent branch pulmonary arteries, sagittal and coronal views can be generated from axial views to "clinch" the diagnosis (nonconfluency in three orthogonal planes).

Figure 6 shows just such a study of nonconfluent branch pulmonary arteries in a patient with hypoplastic left heart syndrome following a bidirectional cavopulmonary anastomosis. The image on the left, an axial image at the level of the pulmonary arteries, clearly shows a separation between branch pulmonary arteries (black and white arrow). However, to be certain that a communication between them does not exist, axial images above and below this one need to be examined. These images may not be clearcut because of a partial volume effect, in which part of the vessel appears in one slice and part in another, making the diagnosis questionable. On the upper and lower right panels are sagittal and coronal computer-generated images, respectively, through the discontinuity on the left image. This clearly shows the nonconfluent nature of the pulmonary arteries. Because this is shown in three orthogonal slices, the diagnosis reaches a high level of certainty.

Oblique sectioning on computer may save scanning time and patient material from trial and error on-line. For example, the short axis of the right ventricular inflow (sinus) needed to be standardized for function analysis (see below) and has yet to be described in the literature. Our definition, based on the left ventricular short axis, is a result of various maneuvers using oblique sectioning and a volumetric data set from a postmortem heart.

The long axis of the right ventricle is defined as a line through the atrioventricular valve plane and intersecting the apex of the sinus portion of the right ventricle; the short axis planes are defined as perpendicular to the long axis. Figure 7 shows the problem encountered. Since the heart can be oriented in multiple directions in the chest, a standard axial view most likely will not show both atrioventricular valve plane and apex in the same picture. As a matter of fact, false-positive identification of the apex may occur [e.g., Figure 7, the right image is in the atrioventricular valve plane and the apex may falsely be identified on this picture. True apex is further caudad (left image)] causing erroneous construction of the short axis. To standardize short axis imaging, a postmortem specimen of a patient with hypoplastic left heart syndrome was scanned, and oblique sectioning was used to determine the optimal algorithm of localizers to isolate the short axis.

Figure 8 shows this algorithm.

C. Spin-Echo Images

There are a number of instances where spin-echo images alone are sometimes sufficient to obtain the postoperative information needed.

1. Pulmonary Artery Size

Especially in older patients, pulmonary artery size may be difficult to visualize. Transverse MRI images are sufficient to determine this accurately. Figure 9 shows a typical case of a patient with hypoplastic left heart syndrome following a Fontan reconstruction. The images clearly show the size of the branch pulmonary arteries and the superior vena cava-to-right pulmonary artery anastomosis.

2. Conduits

Not all conduits need to be reconstructed in three dimensions by MRI to be assessed. The spin-echo images may be sufficient enough for the information needed (see Figure 4).

D. Regional Wall Motion/Strain Analysis

One of the unique features of magnetic resonance imaging is the ability to magnetically tag tissue and observe its motion.[15–17] This has opened the door to a biomechanical analysis of ventricular function. Numerous algorithms have been employed[15–17] in recent years to tag myocardium and blood, and the one described below is named SPAMM (**SPA**tial **M**odulation of **M**agnetization).[16–17]

Tagging is accomplished by "demagnetizing" lines of tissue (a localized presaturation of the tissue) prior to routine cine (gradient echo) imaging. This demagnetization of specific lines of tissue is performed by using a number of gradients and a series of 90° radiofrequency pulses separated in space and time to destroy the spins of the protons along the lines chosen (essentially, a sequence of preparation pulses producing local variations of the z magnetization). After this process is completed, a regular cine sequence is performed, and all of the tissue in the slice becomes magnetized *except for the chosen lines of demagnetization.* If these lines of demagnetization are laid down on the slice as a grid (two sets of parallel lines perpendicular to each other), areas in between "cubes of magnetization" can be tracked throughout the cardiac cycle for motion and deformation (i.e., strain). Therefore, in-plane motion occurring after labeling is visible as distortion and displacement of the initial pattern, and identification and tracking of corresponding landmarks in a temporal sequence of magnetic resonance images permits mapping and accurate quantification of cardiac motion.

Figure 10 displays this technique in pictorial form. In image A, the SPAMM lines are created on a short axis slice through the ventricle for 12 phases through the cardiac cycle 25 msec apart. These images are downloaded onto a Sun workstation, and each intersection point on the grid is uniquely labeled by a "dot" for each imaged phase, as in image B. These "dots" are then connected to create unique triangles through a mathematical process in graph theory called Delaunay triangulation,[18,19] which assures nonoverlapping and uniformity of all the triangles (image C). For wall motion analysis, the centroid of each triangle at each phase is then calculated as depicted in image D and its motion is tracked and displayed in graphical form (image E). In image E, "dots" represent the starting point for each centroid at end-diastole and "tails" represent the direction of subsequent motion. The centroid of the ventricular cavity is found after tracing the endocardial contour at end-diastole, and all quantitative calculations are made (e.g., radial shortening, twist, etc.) relative to this point.

Finite strain analysis relates myocardial deformation during systole relative to end-diastole. In its simplest form, it is the measure of shape change of a given area of myocardium from phase to phase of the cardiac cycle, defined as the final area minus the initial area divided by the final area.

To do this mathematically, from the two-dimensional data sets, even the most complex finite deformation can be decomposed into two length changes and two associated angle changes. These measurements can easily be converted to finite strains of continuum mechanics consisting of two normal strain vectors and two shear strain vectors. Based on the work of Waldman et al.,[20–22] strain calculations use the two-dimensional strain tensor and the method of eigensystem solutions to solve for principle strains (the maximum and minimum strains experienced by each triangle). Principle strain E1 represents the more positive strain value signifying local myocardial compression, while the principle strain in the perpendicular direction E2 represents the less positive (and possibly negative) strain value signifying less local myocardial compression and possibly, elongation. θ1 and θ2 represent the respective angles E1 and E2 make with a global cartesian coordinate system. Underlying assumptions about cardiac muscle are that it is a nonlinear material (i.e., that the force-length curve is nonlinear) and that it is isotropic within each triangle (i.e., the force-length curve is the same in all directions which the force is applied). Figure 11 shows that the data can be displayed in color-coded form superimposed on the anatomical image (image A with the color map directly below), in tabular (image B) or in graphical form (image C).

In summary, this technique allows for the tracking of intramyocardial wall motion and deformation region by region, and has successfully enabled investigators to build wall motion and strain maps[22–26] of the entire ventricle. Furthermore, the blood tagging technique is extremely useful in constructing velocity profiles in vessels and investigating wave propagation in a pulsatile system.

Our laboratory has recently embarked on an extensive investigation of regional myocardial wall motion and strain analysis in patients with functional single ventricles throughout staged Fontan reconstruction. A number of these patients develop poor systolic ventricular function. Our hypothesis is that these patients represent a subgroup that have altered biomechanical properties because of the nature of the surgery performed or the lesion itself. Numerous studies have evaluated wall motion,[23–25] stress, and strain[20–22,26–31] in the *normal* left ventricle, some of the studies basing their work on specific geometric models.[20,21,27–31] There have been no studies to date investigating these parameters in functional single ventricles. The following paragraphs summarize our findings.

To date, we have studied 28 patients (ages 0.4–237 months) at various stages of Fontan reconstruction (23 functional single right ventricles and 5 functional single left ventricles). Of the 23 patients who had a morphological right ventricle as the systemic pumping chamber, 19 had hypoplastic left heart syndrome, 3 had double-outlet right ventricle (with an atrioventricular valve either markedly hypoplastic or atretic) and pulmonic stenosis, and 1 had transposition of the great arteries with mitral hypoplasia, pulmonic stenosis, and multiple ventricular septal defects. Five patients had a morphological left ventricular systemic pumping chamber (used only for twist data, as this group was too small and heterogeneous to make a statistical statement); this group consisted of two patients with pulmonary atresia and intact ventricular septum, two patients with tricuspid atresia, and one patient with double outlet right ventricle, valvar and subvalvar pulmonic stenosis, and a hypoplastic right ventricle.

The 28 patients consisted of 13 studied prior to having bilateral cavopulmonary anastomosis (hemi-Fontan procedure), eight studied following a hemi-Fontan procedure but before Fontan completion, and seven studied after Fontan completion (baffling inferior vena caval blood flow to the pulmonary artery). Basal and apical short axis planes through the ventricular wall were categorized into four distinct regions equally spaced around the slice as well as into regions of interest. Observations of particular interest are:

1. Right ventricular post-Fontan and pre-hemi-Fontan groups had the highest compressive strains (-0.19 ± 0.03, superior wall and -0.18 ± 0.03, inferior wall, respectively) and the post-hemi-Fontan had the least (-0.14 ± 0.03, inferior wall) (Figure 12). Pre-hemi-Fontan patients, *regardless of ventricular morphology,* reached maximum compressive strain 25 msec earlier than other surgical subgroups.

2. Regional heterogeneity of strain, assessed by the coefficient of variation, was *least* in the post-Fontan group in two of four regions in the basal slice and in one of four at the apex.

3. Post-Fontan patients had endocardial-to-epicardial strain ratios that were different from the other surgical subgroups as well as from normals, while the pre- and post-hemi-Fontan patients had basal-to-apical short axis strain ratios different from post-Fontan and normal patients.

4. Functional single left ventricles had a different strain distribution across region and surgical subgroup from functional single right ventricles (Figure 13).

5. Contrary to the normal human adult left ventricle which twists *counterclockwise* (Figure 14, image C and D), 26 of 28 functional single ventricles *regardless of ventricular morphology,* twisted *clockwise* in one region, counterclockwise in another, and had a transitional zone of no twist (Figures 15 and 16). This transitional zone had the highest strains of all the regions.

6. Radial contraction was greatest in the superior wall of the single right ventricle pre-hemi-Fontan and post-Fontan groups while all three surgical subgroups in functional single left ventricles had their superior and anterior walls performing the most radial motion. *Inferior* walls of all surgical subgroups, *regardless of ventricular morphology,* performed the *least* radial contraction and in some instances, moved paradoxically (Figures 14–16).

7. The hypoplastic left ventricle in patients with hypoplastic left heart syndrome appears to do no contraction and gets "pulled along for the ride" by the posterior wall (septal wall) of the right ventricle (Figure 14, image A).

Markedly different strain characteristics were noted at each stage of Fontan reconstruction, across various wall regions and between ventricular morphological groups. Marked differences were also noted in regional wall motion throughout Fontan reconstruction regardless of ventricular morphology, and differences in strains and radial wall motion were noted across various wall regions and surgical subgroups. Whether baffle placement, deep hypothermic circulatory arrest, or time-dependent adaptation is responsible, the findings of abnormal twisting, increased strain in the transition zone, and marked differences in regional wall radial contraction may play an important role in the energetics of the heart and the long-term viability of the single ventricle.

References

1. Rastelli GC, Wallace RB, Ongley PA. Complete repair of transposition of the great arteries with pulmonic stenosis: a review and report of a case corrected by using a new surgical technique. *Circulation* 1969; 39:83–95.

2. Olin CL, Ritter DG, McGoon DC, Wallace RB, Danielson GK. Pulmonary atresia: Surgical consideration and results in 103 patients undergoing definitive repair. *Circulation* 1976; 54 (Suppl III):III-35–III-40.

3. Alfieri O, Locatelli G, Bianchi T, Vanini V, Parenzan L. Repair of tetralogy of Fallot after Waterston anastomosis. *J Thorac Cardiovasc Surg* 1979; 77:826–831.

4. Rastelli GC, Ongley PA, Davis GD, Kirklin JW. Surgical repair for pulmonary valve atresia with coronary-pulmonary artery fistula: report of case. *Mayo Clin Proc* 1965; 40:521.

5. Norwood WI, Lang P, Castaneda AR, Murphy JD. Management of infants with left ventricular outflow obstruction by conduit interposition between the ventricular apex and thoracic aorta. *J Thorac Cardiovasc Surg* 1983; 85:771–776.

6. DiDonato RM, Danielson GK, McGoon DC, Driscoll DJ, Julsrud PR, Edwards WD. Left ventricle-aortic conduits in pediatric patients. *J Thorac Cardiovasc Surg* 1984; 88:82–91.

7. Shuford WH, Sybers RG, Hogan GB. *The Aortic Arch and Its Malformations*. Charles C Thomas, Springfield, 1974, pp 215–244.

8. Fontan F, Baudet E. Surgical repair of tricuspid atresia. *Thorax* 1971; 26:240–8.

9. Di Carlo D, Marcelletti C, Nijveld A, Lubber LJ, Becker AE. The Fontan procedure in the absence of the interatrial septum: failure of its principle? *J Thorac Cardiovasc Surg* 1983; 85:923–927.

10. Puga FJ, Chiavarelli M, Hagler DJ. Modification of the Fontan operation applicable to patients with left atrioventricular valve atresia or single atrioventricular valve. *Circulation* 1987; 76(Suppl III):III-53–III-60.

11. Senning A. Surgical correction of transposition of the great vessels. *Surgery* 1959; 45:966.

12. Quaegebeur JM, Rohmer J, Brom AJ, Tinkelenberg J. Revival of the Senning operation in the treatment of transposition of the great arteries. *Thorax* 1977; 32:517–524.

13. Parenzan L, Locatelli G, Alfieri O, Villani M, Invernizzi G. The Senning procedure for transposition of the great arteries. *J Thorac Cardiovasc Surg* 1978; 76:305–11.

14. Hoffman EA, Gnanaprakasam D, Gupta KB, Hoford JD, Kugelmass SD, Kulaweic RS. VIDA: an environment for multidimensional image display and analysis. *Proc SPIE* 1992; 1660:694–711.

15. Zerhouni EA, Parish DM, Rogers WJ, Yang A, Shapiro EP. Human heart tagging with MR imaging: A method for non-invasive assessment of myocardial motion. *Radiology* 1988; 169:59–63.

16. Axel L, Dougherty L. MR imaging of motion with spatial modulation of magnetization. *Radiology* 1989; 171:841–845.

17. Axel L, Dougherty L. Heart wall motion: improved method of spatial modulation of magnetization for MR imaging. *Radiology* 1989; 172:349–350.

18. De Floriani L. Surface representations based on triangular grids. *Visual Computer* 1987; 3:27–50.

19. Lee DT, Schachter BJ. Two algorithms for constructing a Delaunay triangulation. *Intl J Computer Info Sci* 1980; 9:219–242.

20. Waldman LK, Fung YC, Covell JW. Transmural myocardial deformation in the canine left ventricle. *Circ Res* 1985; 57:152–163.

21. Hunter PJ, Smaill BH. The analysis of the heart: a continuum approach. *Prog Biophys Molec Biol* 1988; 52:101–164.

22. Gupta KB, Bogdan AA, Fellows KE, Hoffman EA. Finite strains using SPAMM in normal human left ventricles. *Circulation* 1991; 84 (Suppl II): II-159 (abstract).

23. Buchhalter MB, Weiss JL, Rogers WJ, Zerhouni EA, Weisfeldt ML, Beyar R, Shapiro EP. Noninvasive quantification of left ventricular rotational deformation in normal humans using magnetic resonance imaging myocardial tagging. *Circulation* 1990; 81:1236–1244.

24. Clark NR, Reichek N, Bergey P, Hoffman EA, Brownson D, Palmon L, Axel L. Circumferential myocardial shortening in the normal human left ventricle: assessment by magnetic resonance imaging using spatial modulation of magnetization. *Circulation* 1991; 84:67–74.

25. Rogers WJ, Shapiro EP, Weiss JL, Buchhalter MB, Rademakers FE, Weisfeldt ML, Zerhouni EA. Quantification of and correction for left ventricular long-axis shortening by magnetic resonance tissue tagging and slice isolation. *Circulation* 1991; 84:721–731.

26. Moore C, O'Dell W, McVeigh E, Zerhouni E. Three dimensional myocardial strains in humans using bi-planar tagged MRI in Book of Abstracts, Tenth Annual Meeting, San Francisco. Berkeley, Society of Magnetic Resonance in Medicine, 1991, vol. 1.

27. Young AA, Hunter PJ, Samill BH. Epicardial surface estimation from coronary cineangiograms. *Computer Vision, Graphics and Image Processing* 1989; 47:111–127.

28. Burns JW, Covell JW, Myers R, Ross J. Comparison of directly measured left ventricular wall stress and stress calculated from geometric reference figures. *Circ Res* 1971; 28:611–621.

29. McHale PA, Greenfield JC. Evaluation of several geometric models for estimation of left ventricular circumferential wall stress. *Circ Res* 1973; 33:303–312.

30. Fiegl EO, Fry DL. Intramural myocardial shear during the cardiac cycle. *Circ Res* 1964; 14:536–540.

31. Donders JJ, Beneken JE. Computer model of cardiac muscle mechanics. *Cardiovasc Res* 1971; Suppl I:34–50.

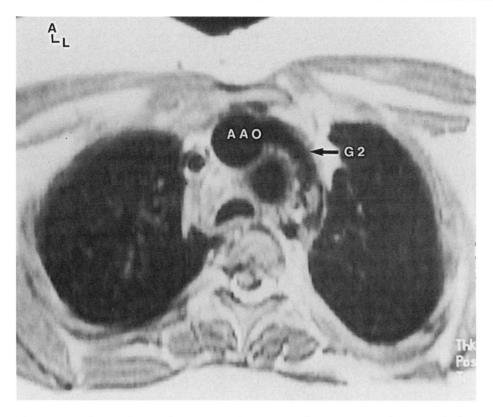

Figure 1: Axial (A) and sagittal (B) images of a patient with coarctation of the aorta who has had two bypass grafts of his coarctation. Each data set displays different aspects of the anatomy, but no one image displays all the needed information. Anterior (C) and lateral (D) views of a shaded surface display for the external conduits shown in Figure 1, depicting the origins and insertions of both grafts, in one data set. A = anterior; AAo = ascending aorta; DAo = ascending aorta; G1 = graft 1; G2 = graft 2; L = lateral; P = posterior; S = superior. (Pictures courtesy of Paul M. Weinberg, MD.)

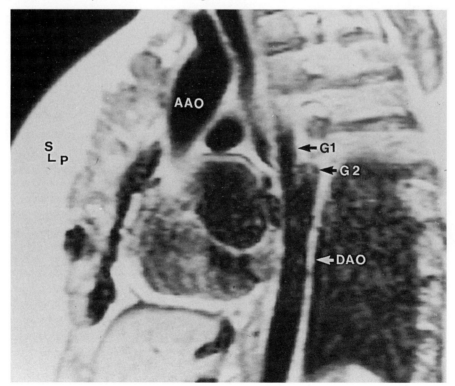

Figure 1B.

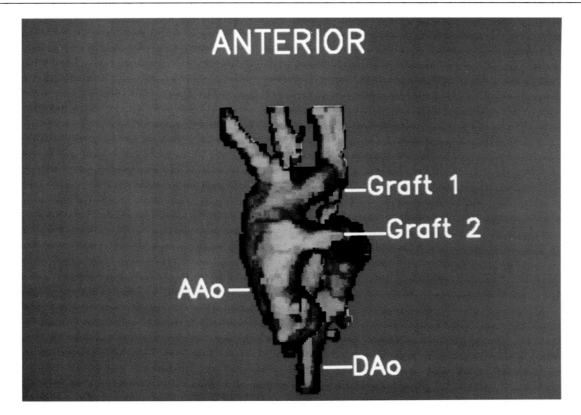

Figure 1C.

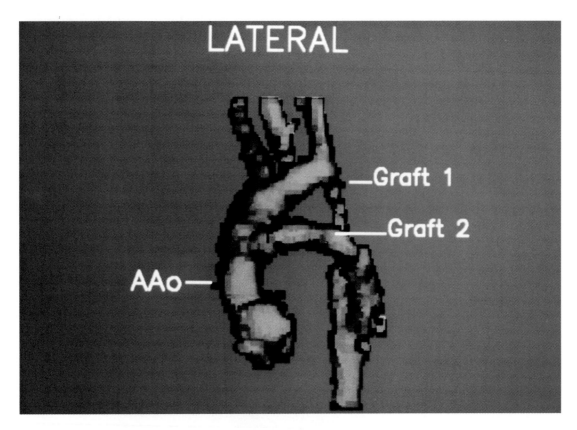

Figure 1D.

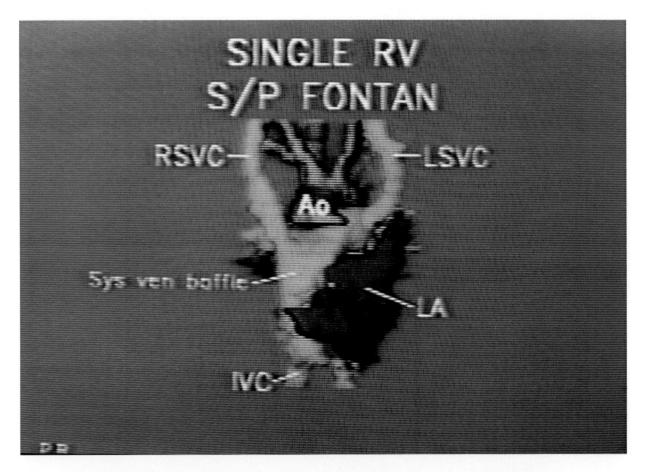

Figure 2: Anterior (A and B) and transverse (C) views of a patient with single right ventricle and left superior vena cava after a Fontan procedure and LSVC-to-LPA anastomosis. The anterior view (A) shows both systemic and pulmonary venous pathways and their relationships to each other. The anterior view of only the systemic venous pathway (B) shows the entire length of the cavopulmonary connection to the branch pulmonary arteries. The transverse view (C) also gives a superior view of both systemic and pulmonary venous pathways from above. Posterior is at the top; anterior is at the bottom. Ao = aorta; IVC = inferior vena cava; LA = left atrium (pulmonary venous pathway); LAA = left atrial appendage; LPA = left pulmonary artery; LPV = left pulmonary vein; LSVC = left superior vena cava; RPA = right pulmonary artery; RPV = right pulmonary vein; LSVC = left superior vena cava; RPA = right pulmonary artery; RPV = right pulmonary vein; RSVC = right superior vena cava; RV = right ventricle; S/P = status post; Sys ven baffle = systemic venous pathway. (Pictures courtesy of Paul M. Weinberg, MD.)

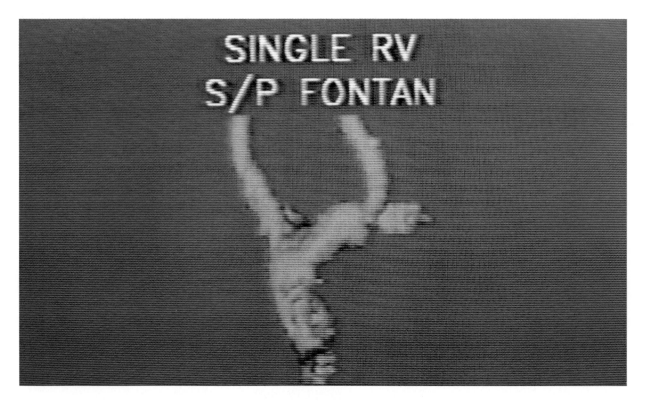

Figure 2B.

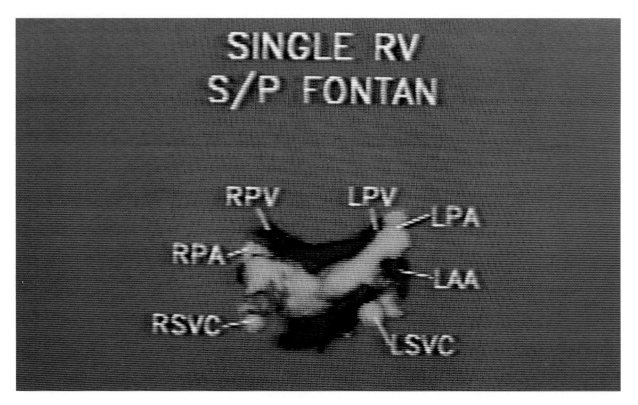

Figure 2C.

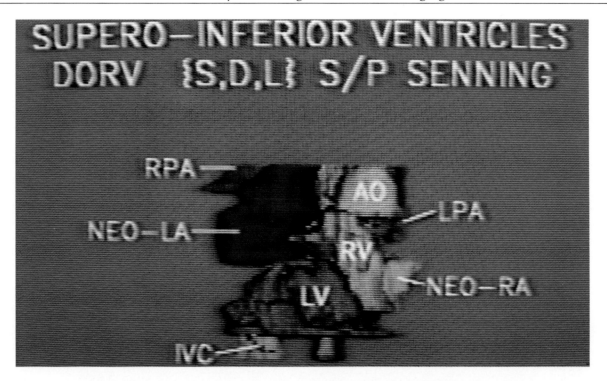

Figure 3: Three-dimensional reconstruction of a patient with superoinferior ventricles and pseudo criss-cross atrioventricular relationships after a Senning procedure. (A) Anterior view shows the superoinferior relationship of the ventricles, and (B) the transverse view shows the relationships of the "*neo-right*" and "*neo-left*" atrium. If various structures are removed in the transverse views (Figures C and D), the viewer can appreciate what is meant by the criss-cross relationship of the atrioventricular valves. AAo = ascending aorta; Ao = aorta; DORV = double outlet right ventricle; IVC = inferior vena cava; LPA = left pulmonary artery; LPV'S = left pulmonary veins; LV = left ventricle; MV = mitral valve; neo-LA = pulmonary venous pathway; neo-RA = systemic venous pathway; RPA = right pulmonary artery; RPV'S = right pulmonary veins; RV = right ventricle; S/P = status post; SVC = superior vena cava; TV = tricuspid valve. (Pictures courtesy of Paul M. Weinberg, MD.)

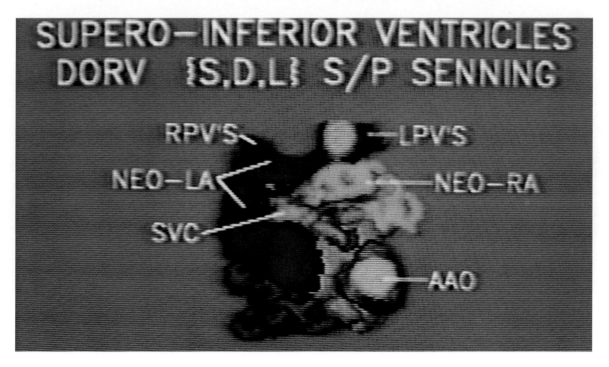

Figure 3B.

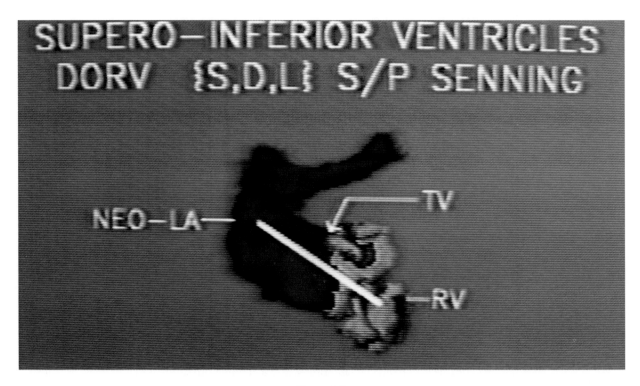

Figure 3C.

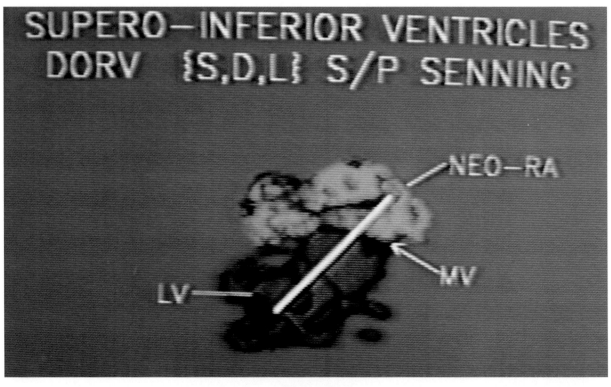

Figure 3D.

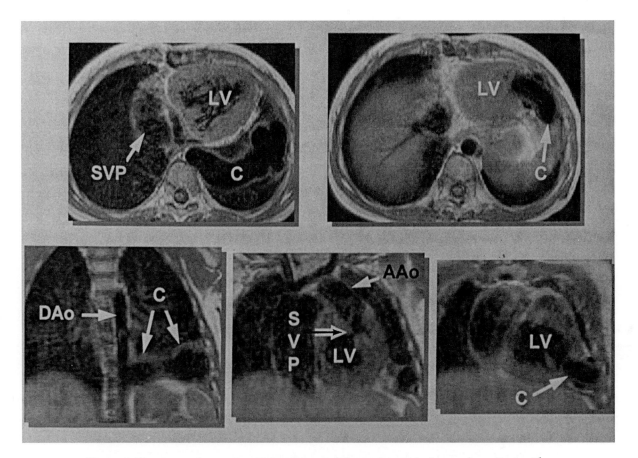

Figure 4: Transverse (upper images) and coronal (lower images) planes of a patient with transposition of the great arteries {S,L,L}, and tricuspid atresia, with a restrictive bulboventricular foramen causing subaortic stenosis. The patient has both a Fontan reconstruction and an apical-to-descending aortic conduit. The narrowed bulboventricular foramen is also clearly seen (black and white arrow). Upper images from left to right go from superior to inferior. Lower images from left to right go from posterior to anterior. AAo = ascending aorta; C = apical to aortic conduit; DAo = descending aorta; LV = left ventricle; SVP = systemic venous pathway.

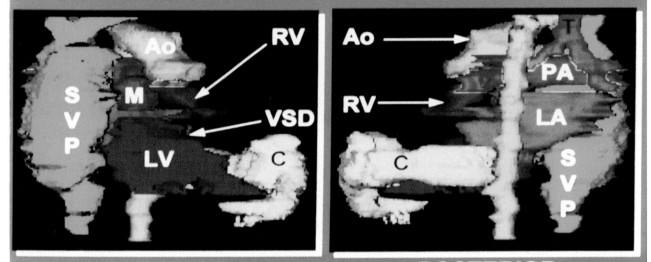

Figure 5: Three-dimensional reconstruction of the patient is shown in Figure 4. Anterior and posterior views (A) as well as transverse and lateral images (B) display the perspective necessary to fully appreciate the relationships both conduits have to each other and the important cardiac structures. With various structures removed (Figures C and D), this is even more clearly seen: (1) the relationship of the apical-to-aortic conduit to the left ventricular apex and to the descending aorta and (2) the Fontan baffle with the pulmonary arteries. Also note that the three-dimensional images clearly show the pulmonary artery coming from the right-sided left ventricle and the aorta coming from a diminutive left-sided right ventricle. Ao = aortic; Ap → Ao = apical to aortic; C = apical-aortic conduit; D = division of main pulmonary artery from central pulmonary arteries; LA = left atrium; LPA = left pulmonary artery; LV = left ventricle; MPA, M = main pulmonary artery; PA = central pulmonary arteries; RPA = right pulmonary artery; RV = right ventricle; S/P = status post; SVP = systemic venous pathway; T = trachea; TGA{S,L,L} = transposition of the great arteries with situs solitus of the atria, L-looped ventricles, L-malposition of the great vessels; VSD = ventricular septal defect.

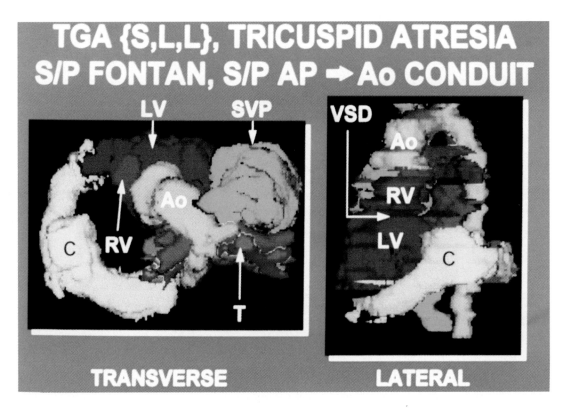

Figure 5B.

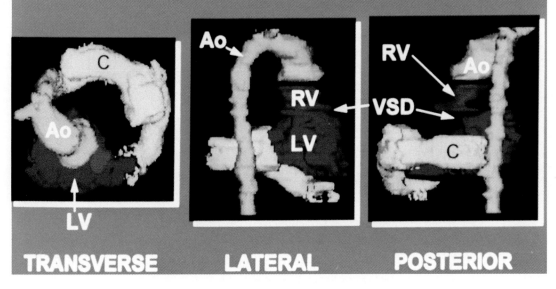

Figure 5C.

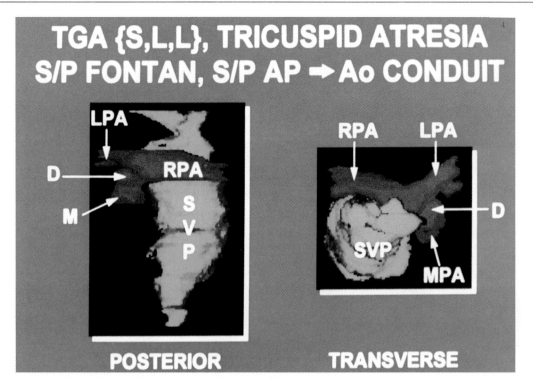

Figure 5D.

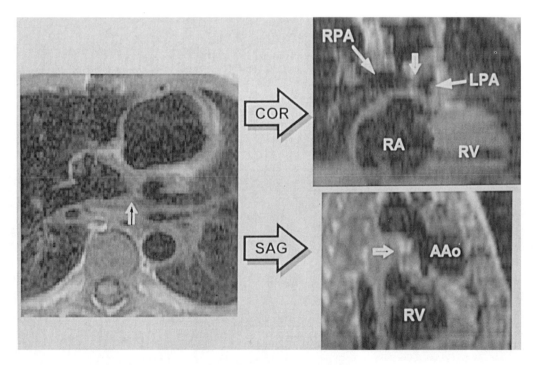

Figure 6: MRI of nonconfluent branch pulmonary arteries in a patient with hypoplastic left heart syndrome after a bidirectional cavopulmonary anastomosis. The image on the left, an axial image at the level of the pulmonary arteries, clearly shows a separation between branch pulmonary arteries (clear arrow). Images on the upper right and lower right are sagittal and coronal computer-generated images respectively, through the discontinuity on the left image. The nonconfluent nature of the pulmonary arteries (black and white arrows) is seen. AAo = ascending aorta; COR = coronal reconstruction; LPA = left pulmonary artery; RA = right atrium; RPA = right pulmonary artery; RV = right ventricle; SAG = sagittal reconstruction.

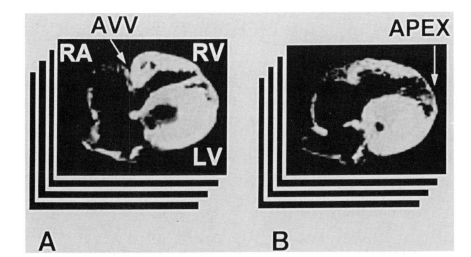

Figure 7: A and B: MRI of a postmortem specimen of a patient with hypoplastic left heart syndrome. Since the heart can be oriented in multiple directions in the chest, a standard axial view most likely will not obtain both atrioventricular valve plane and apex in the same picture. The right image is in the atrioventricular valve plane and the apex may falsely be identified on this picture. The true apex is further caudad 5 mm (left image), possibly causing erroneous isolation of the short axis. AVV = atrioventricular valve; LV = left ventricle; RA = right atrium; RV = right ventricle.

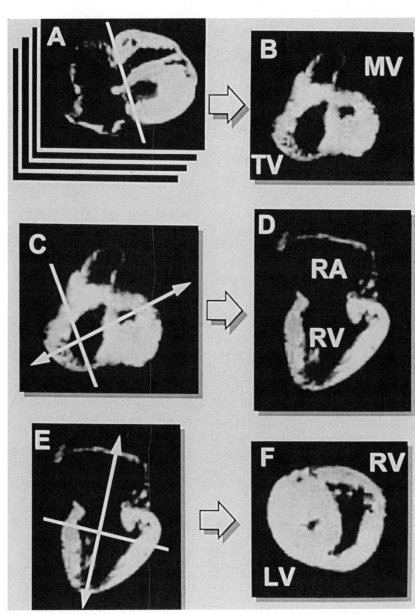

Figure 8: Algorithm displaying the steps to isolate the short axis of the right ventricle. An axial image is identified with both atrioventricular valves (or their remnants) (A) and an oblique plane (white line) is cut through them at this level which is computer-generated (B), showing both mitral and tricuspid valves in cross-section. If an imaginary line is drawn through the center of both valves (image C, double arrow line) and a volumetric data set of images are obtained perpendicular to this, one picture will by necessity contain the atrioventricular valve and the apex (the long axis, image D). If an imaginary line is again drawn through the middle of the atrioventricular valve and the apex (image E, double arrow line) and a volumetric data set of images are obtained perpendicular to this, the short axis will be obtained (image F). LV = left ventricle; MV = mitral valve; RA = right atrium; RV = right ventricle; TV = tricuspid valve.

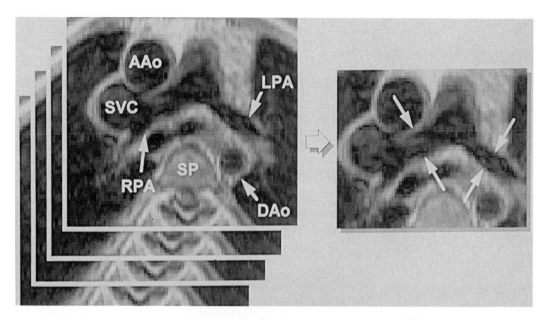

Figure 9: A patient with hypoplastic left heart syndrome after Fontan reconstruction. The images clearly show the size of the branch pulmonary arteries and the superior vena cava-to-right pulmonary artery anastomosis. The image on the right is a magnification of the region of interest on the left. AAo = ascending aorta; DAo = descending aorta; LPA = left pulmonary artery; RPA = right pulmonary artery; SP = spine; SVC = superior vena cava.

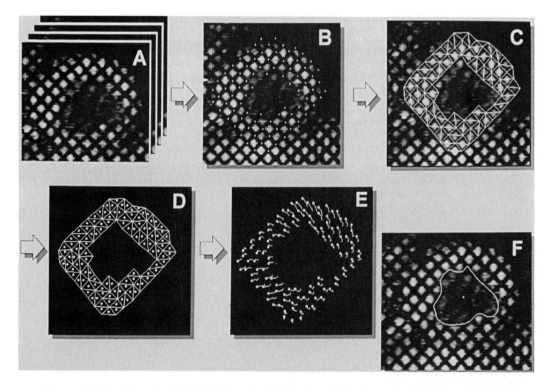

Figure 10: Creation of a SPAMM image and technique to track regional wall motion. (A) SPAMM lines are created on a short axis slice through the ventricle. (B) Each intersection point on the grid is uniquely labeled by a "dot" for each imaged phase. (C) These "dots" are then connected to create unique triangles. (D) For wall motion analysis, the centroid of each triangle at each phase is then calculated. (E) Motion is tracked and displayed in graphical form (see text). (F) The centroid of the ventricular cavity is found after tracing the endocardial contour at end-diastole.

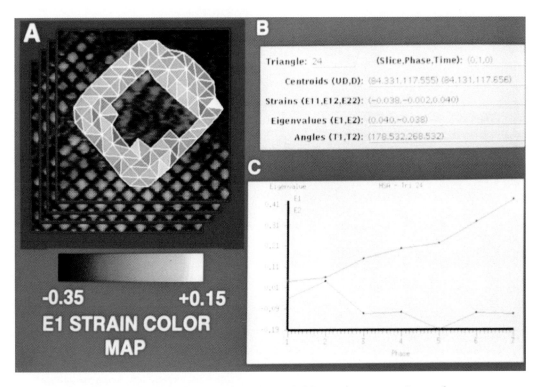

Figure 11: Strain data can be displayed in color-coded form superimposed upon the anatomical image (image A with the color map directly below), in tabular (image B) or in graphical form (image C).

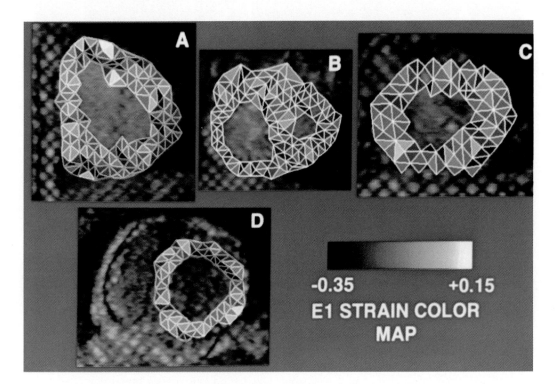

Figure 12: Color-coded strain data in patients with functional single right ventricles after a stage I reconstruction (A), post-hemi-Fontan (B), post Fontan (C), and normal left ventricle (D). E1 strain color map is in the lower left corner.

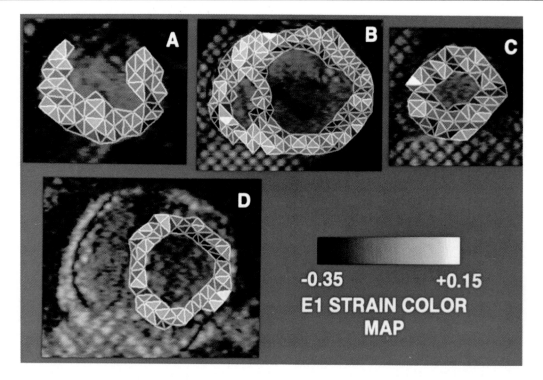

Figure 13: Color-coded strain data in patients with functional single left ventricles after a stage I reconstruction (A), post-hemi-Fontan (B), post-Fontan (C), and normal left ventricle (D). E1 strain color map is in the lower right corner.

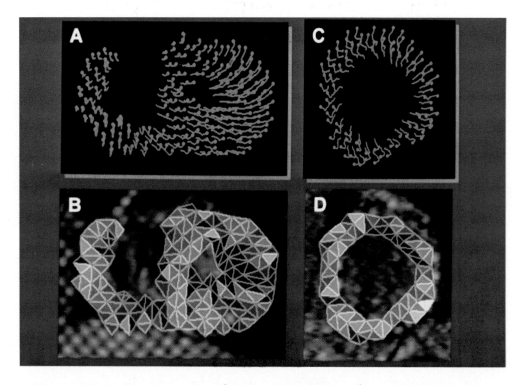

Figure 14: Twist data displayed graphically (upper images) with corresponding anatomical and strain data (lower images) of a patient with hypoplastic left heart syndrome (A and B) and the normal left ventricle (C and D). Note how the normal systemic pumping chamber twists counterclockwise initially across the entire short axis (C) while the single right ventricle twists clockwise in one region, counterclockwise in another, and there is a transitional zone of no twist (A). Also note how the hypoplastic left ventricle just gets "pulled along for the ride" by the septal wall anteriorly (to the left of the picture).

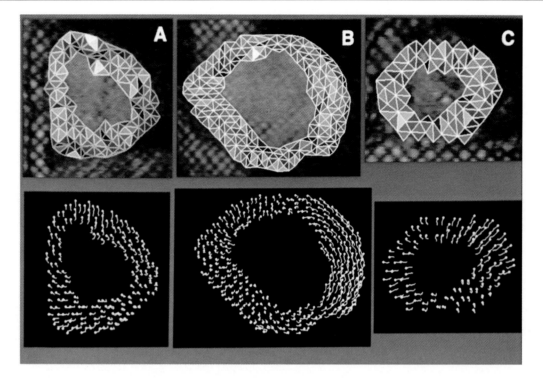

Figure 15: Strain data (upper images) with their corresponding regional wall motion data below of patients with functional single right ventricles following a stage I reconstruction (A), post-hemi-Fontan (B), and post-Fontan completion (C). Note how the single right ventricle twists clockwise in one region, counterclockwise in another, and there is a transitional zone of no twist.

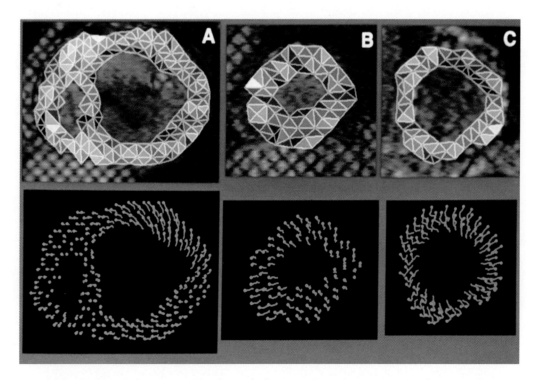

Figure 16: Strain data (upper images) with their corresponding regional wall motion data below of patients with functional single left ventricles following a stage I reconstruction (A), post-hemi-Fontan (B), and post-Fontan completion (C). Note how the single left ventricle twists clockwise in one region, counterclockwise in another, and there is a transitional zone of no twist.

Index

385